Biliary Atresia: Aetiology, Diagnosis and Treatment

Biliary Atresia: Aetiology, Diagnosis and Treatment

Editor

Claus Petersen

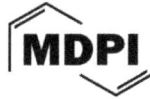 Basel • Beijing • Wuhan • Barcelona • Belgrade • Novi Sad • Cluj • Manchester

Editor
Claus Petersen
Department of Pediatric
Surgery, Hannover Medical
School
Hannover
Germany

Editorial Office
MDPI
St. Alban-Anlage 66
4052 Basel, Switzerland

This is a reprint of articles from the Special Issue published online in the open access journal *Journal of Clinical Medicine* (ISSN 2077-0383) (available at: https://www.mdpi.com/journal/jcm/special_issues/Biliary-Atresia).

For citation purposes, cite each article independently as indicated on the article page online and as indicated below:

Lastname, A.A.; Lastname, B.B. Article Title. *Journal Name* **Year**, *Volume Number*, Page Range.

ISBN 978-3-7258-1217-2 (Hbk)
ISBN 978-3-7258-1218-9 (PDF)
doi.org/10.3390/books978-3-7258-1218-9

© 2024 by the authors. Articles in this book are Open Access and distributed under the Creative Commons Attribution (CC BY) license. The book as a whole is distributed by MDPI under the terms and conditions of the Creative Commons Attribution-NonCommercial-NoDerivs (CC BY-NC-ND) license.

Contents

About the Editor vii

Preface ix

Nimish Godbole, Iiris Nyholm, Maria Hukkinen, Joseph R. Davidson, Athanasios Tyraskis, Katja Eloranta, et al.
Prognostic and Pathophysiologic Significance of IL-8 (CXCL8) in Biliary Atresia
Reprinted from: *Journal of Clinical Medicine* **2021**, *10*, 2705, doi:10.3390/jcm10122705 1

Nobuhiro Takahashi, Daigo Ochiai, Yohei Yamada, Masumi Tamagawa, Hiroki Kanamori, Mototoshi Kato, et al.
Prepregnancy Assessment of Liver Function to Predict Perinatal and Postpregnancy Outcomes in Biliary Atresia Patients with Native Liver
Reprinted from: *Journal of Clinical Medicine* **2021**, *10*, 3956, doi:10.3390/jcm10173956 14

Mark Davenport, Ancuta Muntean and Nedim Hadzic
Biliary Atresia: Clinical Phenotypes and Aetiological Heterogeneity
Reprinted from: *Journal of Clinical Medicine* **2021**, *10*, 5675, doi:10.3390/jcm10235675 22

Joachim F. Kuebler, Omid Madadi-Sanjani, Eva D. Pfister, Ulrich Baumann, David Fortmann, Johannes Leonhardt, et al.
Adjuvant Therapy with Budesonide Post-Kasai Reduces the Need for Liver Transplantation in Biliary Atresia
Reprinted from: *Journal of Clinical Medicine* **2021**, *10*, 5758, doi:10.3390/jcm10245758 33

Ana M. Calinescu, Omid Madadi-Sanjani, Cara Mack, Richard A. Schreiber, Riccardo Superina, Deirdre Kelly, et al.
Cholangitis Definition and Treatment after Kasai Hepatoportoenterostomy for Biliary Atresia: A Delphi Process and International Expert Panel
Reprinted from: *Journal of Clinical Medicine* **2022**, *11*, 494, doi:10.3390/jcm11030494 42

Björn Fischler, Piotr Czubkowski, Antal Dezsofi, Ulrika Liliemark, Piotr Socha, Ronald J. Sokol, et al.
Incidence, Impact and Treatment of Ongoing CMV Infection in Patients with Biliary Atresia in Four European Centres
Reprinted from: *Journal of Clinical Medicine* **2022**, *11*, 945, doi:10.3390/jcm11040945 59

Richard A. Schreiber, Sanjiv Harpavat, Jan B. F. Hulscher and Barbara E. Wildhaber
Biliary Atresia in 2021: Epidemiology, Screening and Public Policy
Reprinted from: *Journal of Clinical Medicine* **2022**, *11*, 999, doi:10.3390/jcm11040999 65

Ana M. Calinescu, Anne-Laure Rougemont, Mehrak Anooshiravani, Nathalie M. Rock, Valerie A. McLin and Barbara E. Wildhaber
Features of Nodules in Explants of Children Undergoing Liver Transplantation for Biliary Atresia
Reprinted from: *Journal of Clinical Medicine* **2022**, *11*, 1578, doi:10.3390/jcm11061578 80

Jean de Ville de Goyet, Toni Illhardt, Christophe Chardot, Peace N. Dike, Ulrich Baumann, Katherine Brandt, et al.
Variability of Care and Access to Transplantation for Children with Biliary Atresia Who Need a Liver Replacement
Reprinted from: *Journal of Clinical Medicine* **2022**, *11*, 2142, doi:10.3390/jcm11082142 92

Caroline P. Lemoine, John P. LeShock, Katherine A. Brandt and Riccardo Superina
Primary Liver Transplantation vs. Transplant after Kasai Portoenterostomy for Infants with Biliary Atresia
Reprinted from: *Journal of Clinical Medicine* 2022, 11, 3012, doi:10.3390/jcm11113012 . . . . **114**

Sarah Mohamedaly, Claire S. Levy, Cathrine Korsholm, Anas Alkhani, Katherine Rosenberg, Judith F. Ashouri, et al.
Hepatic Ly6C^{Lo} Non-Classical Monocytes Have Increased Nr4a1 (Nur77) in Murine Biliary Atresia
Reprinted from: *Journal of Clinical Medicine* 2022, 11, 5290, doi:10.3390/jcm11185290 . . . . **127**

Caroline P. Lemoine, Hector Melin-Aldana, Katherine A. Brandt and Riccardo Superina
Identification of Early Clinical and Histological Factors Predictive of Kasai Portoenterostomy Failure
Reprinted from: *Journal of Clinical Medicine* 2022, 11, 6523, doi:10.3390/jcm11216523 . . . . **139**

Mark Davenport, Omid Madadi-Sanjani, Christophe Chardot, Henkjan J. Verkade, Saul J. Karpen and Claus Petersen
Surgical and Medical Aspects of the Initial Treatment of Biliary Atresia: Position Paper
Reprinted from: *Journal of Clinical Medicine* 2022, 11, 6601, doi:10.3390/jcm11216601 . . . . **149**

Maria Janowska, Joanna B. Bierła, Magdalena Kaleta, Aldona Wierzbicka-Rucińska, Piotr Czubkowski, Ewelina Kanarek, et al.
The Impact of a CMV Infection on the Expression of Selected Immunological Parameters in Liver Tissue in Children with Biliary Atresia
Reprinted from: *Journal of Clinical Medicine* 2022, 11, 7269, doi:10.3390/jcm11247269 . . . . **158**

Anas Alkhani, Cathrine Korsholm, Claire S. Levy, Sarah Mohamedaly, Caroline C. Duwaerts, Eric M. Pietras, et al.
Neonatal Hepatic Myeloid Progenitors Expand and Propagate Liver Injury in Mice
Reprinted from: *Journal of Clinical Medicine* 2023, 12, 337, doi:10.3390/jcm12010337 . . . . **168**

Deirdre Kelly, Marianne Samyn and Kathleen B. Schwarz
Biliary Atresia in Adolescence and Adult Life: Medical, Surgical and Psychological Aspects
Reprinted from: *Journal of Clinical Medicine* 2023, 12, 1594, doi:10.3390/jcm12041594 . . . . **183**

Caroline P. Lemoine, Omid Madadi-Sanjani, Claus Petersen, Christophe Chardot, Jean de Ville de Goyet and Riccardo Superina
Pediatric Liver and Transplant Surgery: Results of an International Survey and Expert Consensus Recommendations
Reprinted from: *Journal of Clinical Medicine* 2023, 12, 3229, doi:10.3390/jcm12093229 . . . . **197**

About the Editor

Claus Petersen

Claus Petersen was board-certified for general and paediatric surgery before being appointed to the Hannover Medical School (MHH). There, he established an interdisciplinary working group for biliary atresia and related diseases (BARD). Clinical and basic research led to more than 60 peer-reviewed publications and 20 national and international awards. Between 1999 and 2022, he also organized four international and interdisciplinary congresses and founded the BARD Society. He was also co-founder of ERN-rare-liver, a Europe-wide initiative for reference centre networks for rare diseases. The paediatric surgery department at the MHH became a reference centre for biliary atresia and remains so to this day. Towards the end of his clinical work, C. Petersen also became a member of the EASL–Lancet Liver Commission, whose report "Protecting the next generation of Europeans against liver disease complications and premature mortality" was published in 2021.

Preface

Biliary atresia and related diseases (BARD) are continuously gaining more interest, particularly because biliary atresia is the most frequent indication for paediatric liver transplantation. Interdisciplinary clinical studies as well as basic research are still mandatory to elucidate the enigmatic aetiology of most of these rare diseases. The present Special Issue includes investigations and studies originating from several interdisciplinary working groups. We hope that the articles meet the readers´ expectations and provide an impetus for further and consecutive projects. International initiatives like BARD and ERN-rare-liver, whose websites can easily be found, are going to join scientific forces and clinical cooperation in order to improve the mid- and long-term survival of patients with a native liver. The editor and the authors appreciate the support of MDPI in providing open source publishing.

Claus Petersen
Editor

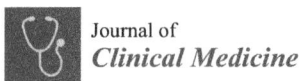

Article

Prognostic and Pathophysiologic Significance of IL-8 (CXCL8) in Biliary Atresia

Nimish Godbole [1,2], Iiris Nyholm [1,2], Maria Hukkinen [1,2], Joseph R. Davidson [3,4], Athanasios Tyraskis [4], Katja Eloranta [1], Noora Andersson [1], Jouko Lohi [5], Päivi Heikkilä [5], Antti Kyrönlahti [1], Marjut Pihlajoki [1], Mark Davenport [4], Markku Heikinheimo [1,6] and Mikko P. Pakarinen [1,2,*]

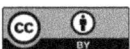

Citation: Godbole, N.; Nyholm, I.; Hukkinen, M.; Davidson, J.R.; Tyraskis, A.; Eloranta, K.; Andersson, N.; Lohi, J.; Heikkilä, P.; Kyrönlahti, A.; et al. Prognostic and Pathophysiologic Significance of IL-8 (CXCL8) in Biliary Atresia. *J. Clin. Med.* **2021**, *10*, 2705. https://doi.org/10.3390/jcm10122705

Academic Editor: Claus Petersen

Received: 20 May 2021
Accepted: 16 June 2021
Published: 18 June 2021

Publisher's Note: MDPI stays neutral with regard to jurisdictional claims in published maps and institutional affiliations.

Copyright: © 2021 by the authors. Licensee MDPI, Basel, Switzerland. This article is an open access article distributed under the terms and conditions of the Creative Commons Attribution (CC BY) license (https://creativecommons.org/licenses/by/4.0/).

[1] Pediatric Research Center, Children's Hospital, University of Helsinki and Helsinki University Hospital, 00029 Helsinki, Finland; nimish.godbole@helsinki.fi (N.G.); iiris.nyholm@helsinki.fi (I.N.); maria.hukkinen@hus.fi (M.H.); katja.eloranta@helsinki.fi (K.E.); noora.andersson@helsinki.fi (N.A.); antti.kyronlahti@helsinki.fi (A.K.); marjut.pihlajoki@helsinki.fi (M.P.); markku.heikinheimo@helsinki.fi (M.H.)
[2] Section of Pediatric Surgery, Pediatric Liver and Gut Research Group and Pediatric Research Center, Children's Hospital, University of Helsinki and Helsinki University Hospital, 00029 Helsinki, Finland
[3] Department of Pediatric Surgery, GOS-UCL Institute of Child Health, London WC1N 1EH, UK; joseph.davidson@doctors.org.uk
[4] Department of Pediatric Surgery, King's College Hospital, London SE5 9RS, UK; thanost88@gmail.com (A.T.); markdav2@ntlworld.com (M.D.)
[5] Department of Pathology, University of Helsinki and Helsinki University Hospital, 00029 Helsinki, Finland; jouko.lohi@hus.fi (J.L.); paivi.heikkila@hus.fi (P.H.)
[6] Department of Pediatrics, Washington University in St. Louis, St. Louis, MO 63130, USA
* Correspondence: mikko.pakarinen@hus.fi

Abstract: Interleukin (IL)-8 (CXCL8), a chemokine involved in neutrophil recruitment, has been implicated in ductular reaction and liver fibrogenesis. We studied liver and serum IL-8 expression in a large biliary atresia (BA) cohort and explored its prognostic and pathophysiological potential. IL-8 expression was assessed in liver utilizing quantitative polymerase chain reaction (qPCR), immunohistochemistry and in situ hybridization and in serum using an enzyme-linked immunosorbent assay, among 115 BA patients, 10 disease controls and 68 normal controls. Results were correlated to portoenterostomy (PE) outcomes, biochemical and histological liver injury, transcriptional markers of fibrosis and cholangiocytes, and expression of other related cytokines. IL-8 was markedly overexpressed in liver and serum of BA patients at PE ($n = 88$) and in serum samples obtained during postoperative follow-up ($n = 40$). IL-8 expression in the liver was predominantly in cholangiocytes within areas of ductular reaction. Liver *IL-8* mRNA expression correlated positively with its serum concentration, bile ductular proliferation, Metavir fibrosis stage, and transcriptional markers of activated myofibroblasts (*ACTA2*) and cholangiocytes (*KRT19*). Taken together, IL-8 may mediate liver injury in BA by promoting ductular reaction and associated liver fibrogenesis. Prognostic value of serum IL-8 to predict native liver survival was limited and confined to the postoperative period after PE.

Keywords: biomarker; cholangiocyte; ductular reaction; liver fibrosis; pediatric liver disease

1. Introduction

Biliary atresia (BA), presenting in the neonatal period, is characterized by fibroinflammatory obliteration of the extra- and intrahepatic bile ducts. Although its exact etiology remains elusive, previous studies have at times suggested a developmental, dysfunctional immune response or environmental toxin hypotheses either individually or in some combination [1,2]. Untreated, the resulting bile duct disruption and cholestasis rapidly progresses to fatal biliary cirrhosis and end-stage liver disease within 2 years from birth [2,3]. The current management of BA involves an early attempt at restoration of bile flow with excision of the obliterated extrahepatic bile ducts and biliary reconstruction using a Roux jejunal loop (portoenterostomy (PE)) [2]. Consequent normalization of serum bilirubin levels is then regarded as a successful outcome. Although PE is successful in over half of the patients, progressive fibrosis continues in their native livers necessitating liver transplantation (LT) in the majority of patients before the age of 20 years [3]. Consequently, BA is the leading cause of LT in children [4].

The highly variable surgical prognosis of BA necessitates intensive postoperative monitoring [5]. Reliable tools for prediction of the outcome of PE and progression of liver injury are limited [5,6], but urgently needed for individualized patient follow-up, family counselling and early prediction of the need for LT as well as interventional studies [7]. A chemokine, interleukin (IL)-8 or CXCL8, mediates innate immune activation and regulates neutrophil recruitment and degranulation [8]. Increased IL-8 expression has been linked with reactive cholangiocytes in ductular reaction (DR) and progression of liver fibrosis in other chronic liver diseases in accordance with the ability of IL-8 to induce alpha-smooth muscle actin (α-SMA), a marker of myofibroblast activation [9,10]. Numerous studies have shown that *IL-8* expression is increased in patients with BA and experimental data suggest that IL-8 might contribute to disease progression [8,11–13]. However, a recent study has reported that tissue and serum levels of IL-8 of BA patients at the time of PE were not related to the outcome [14]. Thus the pathophysiological significance and the role of IL-8 as a biomarker for liver injury and thereby its predictive ability for PE outcomes has not been yet fully established [3].

The aim of this study was to explore the prognostic and pathophysiological potential of IL-8 in BA by assessing its serum and liver expression in a controlled manner. We hypothesized that by correlating with liver fibrogenesis, *IL-8* expression could serve as a valuable prognostic biomarker for the success of PE and native liver survival thereafter. To this end, we assessed liver expression and serum levels of IL-8 and other connected cytokines including IL-18, IL-33, tumor necrosis factor-alpha (TNFα) and interferon gamma (IFN-γ) at PE. We extend previous knowledge by addressing *IL-8* expression also during postoperative follow-up and by relating IL-8 in a large patient cohort to histological liver fibrosis, bile ductular proliferation and transcriptional markers indicative of active liver fibrogenesis and cholangiocytes as well as surgical outcomes.

2. Materials and Methods
2.1. Patients and Controls

This was a retrospective observational study. We included all BA patients with stored serum or liver samples, who had undergone PE at King's College Hospital, London, UK, during 2005–2013 or the Children's Hospital, University of Helsinki, Finland during 2012–2018. Of the 115 included patients representing 33% and 90% of all patients operated on in London and Helsinki during the same eras, 75 had available samples obtained at PE, 27 during post-PE follow-up and 13 at both time points (Table 1). Follow-up samples were collected from stable patients in Helsinki during 2012–2018, where serum samples were obtained at least yearly and liver biopsies at 1 year post-PE and once in 5 years thereafter as a part of routine clinical follow-up [15]. Wedge liver biopsies were taken at PE, and ultrasound guided core needle biopsies under general anesthesia for endoscopic variceal surveillance as described previously [15]. Liver biopsy is not part of the clinical management of patients post-operatively at King's College Hospital. All PE surgeries were open and postoperative steroids, ursodeoxycholic acid and antibiotics were routinely used in both centers [15]. The diagnosis of BA was confirmed by histopathological assessment of bile duct remnants in both centers.

Table 1. Baseline patient characteristics and included study samples for all patients (*n* = 115), this included patients with samples only at portoenterostomy (PE) (*n* = 75) and patients with samples only at follow-up (*n* = 27) as well as 13 patients with samples both at PE and follow-up. Data are median (interquartile range) or frequencies (%).

	All Patients (*n* = 115)	Patients at PE (*n* = 88)	Patients at Follow Up (*n* = 40)
Age at PE, days	56 (41–76)	55 (41–75)	56 (35–76)
Follow up after PE, years	3.6 (1.1–9.7)	2.1 (0.7–6.6)	9 (3.6–11.7)
Type of BA, *n* (%) 1 or 2 3	 5 (4%) 110 (96%)	 1 (1%) 87 (99%)	 5 (13%) 35 (87%)
Splenic malformation, *n* (%)	17 (15%)	11 (13%)	8 (20%)
Cystic disease, *n* (%)	15 (13%)	12 (14%)	5 (13%)
Clearance of Jaundice, *n* (%)	74 (64%)	47 (53%)	38 (95%)
Liver transplantation, *n* (%)	56 (49%)	49 (56%)	10 (25%)
Age at liver transplantation, year	1.5 (0.8–3.0)	1.2 (0.7–2.3)	6.9 (2.5–9.4)
Died without transplantation, *n*	3	3	0
Liver biochemistry			
Bilirubin total, µmol/L	132 (18–167)	145 (124–177)	10 (5–17)
GGT (U/L)	329 (107–673)	572 (235–873)	62 (25–162)
AST (U/L)	165 (94–232)	196 (143–260)	74 (52–122)
ALT (U/L)	84 (44–123)	112 (64–163)	48 (24–98)
APRi	0.84 (0.49–1.43)	0.83 (0.5–1.23)	1.2 (0.48–1.92)
Included serum and liver samples			
Number of patients with Serum IL-8 samples	*n* = 109	*n* = 77	*n* = 40
Number of Serum IL-8 samples/patient	1	1	3 (2–4)
Number of patients with liver biopsies	*n* = 82	*n* = 66	*n* = 22
Number of liver biopsies/patient	1	1	2 (1–2)

BA: biliary atresia; PE: portoenterostomy; GGT: gamma-glutamyl transferase; AST: aspartate transaminase; ALT: alanine aminotransferase; APRi: AST-to-platelet ratio index; IL-8: Interleukin-8.

Serum samples from 68 generally healthy pediatric day surgery patients and 10 pediatric donor liver biopsies were used as normal controls, and 10 liver biopsies from children with other cholestatic disorders as disease controls. Clinical details of disease controls are displayed in Supplementary Table S1.

2.2. Liver Biochemistry and Histology

Serum levels of bilirubin, alanine aminotransferase (ALT), aspartate transaminase (AST), AST-to-platelet ratio index (APRi) and gamma-glutamyl transferase (GGT) were measured by the local hospital laboratories. Liver biopsies were graded for fibrosis using the Metavir staging and scored for cholangiocyte marker cytokeratin (CK)-7 positive bile ductular proliferation (0–2) and portal inflammatory cell infiltration (0–3) by an experienced pediatric liver pathologist blinded to the clinical data as described previously [15,16].

2.3. Serum Cytokine Levels

Serum concentrations of IL-8, IL-18 and TNF-α were determined using commercially available Q-Plex multiplex ELISA (enzyme-linked immune sorbent assay) array kits (Quansys Bioscience, Logan, UT, USA) following the manufacturer's instructions.

2.4. Liver mRNA Expression

RNA from liver biopsies was extracted using the RNeasy Mini Kit (QIAGEN, Frederick, MD, USA). RNA concentration was assessed spectrophotometrically. mRNA expression of IL-8, IL-18, IL-33, TNF-α, IFNG, COL1A2, ACTA2, KRT7 and KRT19 were analyzed in triplicate by quantitative real-time polymerase chain reaction (qPCR) using Custom RT Profiler PCR Array (CAPH12366A) (QIAGEN SABiosciences, Frederick, MD, USA) on BIO-RAD CFX384 Real-Time System (Bio-Rad, Hercules, CA, USA) according to the manufacturer's instructions. ACTA2 (marker of myofibroblast activation) and COL1A2 (marker of collagen production) were studied as surrogates for active liver fibrogenesis, and KRT7 and KRT19 as cholangiocyte markers, while HPRT1, GAPDH, ACTB and B2M were used as housekeeping genes. Quantification of target gene mRNA expression was performed using the $\Delta\Delta Ct$ method and expressed after normalization to housekeeping genes and relative to normal control subjects.

2.5. Immunohistochemistry

Formalin fixed, paraffin embedded (FFPE) sections were deparaffinized, hydrated, and treated with target retrieval solution pH 9 (Dako - Agilent Technologies, Glostrup, Denmark). Commercially available antibody for IL-8 (rabbit polyclonal, AHC0881, ThermoFisher Scientific, Waltham, MA, USA) was used at a dilution of 1:3000 along with the Novolink TM polymer detection system (Leica biosystems Newcastle Ltd, Newcastle Upon Tyne, UK). Primary antibody was incubated overnight at 40 °C. Images were generated using 3DHISTECH Panoramic 250 FLASH II digital slide scanner at Genome biology unit supported by HiLIFE and the Faculty of Medicine, University of Helsinki, and Biocenter Finland.

2.6. RNA In Situ Hybridization

RNA in situ hybridization was performed on fresh 4.5 μm FFPE tissue sections using RNAscope Multiplex Fluorescent Reagent Kit Version 2 (#323100, Advanced Cell Diagnostics, Newark, CA, USA) for target detection according to the manual. Tissue sections were baked for 1 h at 60 °C, then deparaffinized and treated with hydrogen peroxide for 10 min at room temperature (RT). Target retrieval was performed for 15 min at 98 °C, followed by protease plus treatment for 15 min at 40 °C. All probes (Hs-ONECUT1 (HNF6) #490081, Hs-IL-8 #310381, 3-Plex negative control probe dapB #320871 and 3-plex positive control probe, POLR2A, PPIB, UBC #320861, Advanced Cell Diagnostics, Newark, CA, USA) were hybridized for 2 h at 40 °C followed by signal amplification and developing of HRP channels undertaken according to the manual. TSA Plus fluorophores fluorescein (1:1000 dilution), Cyanine 3 (1:1500 dilution) and Cyanine 5 (1:3000 dilution) (NEL744001KT, PerkinElmer, Waltham, MA, USA) were used for signal detection. The sections were counterstained with DAPI (4′, 6-diamidino-2-phenylindole) and mounted with ProLong Gold Antifade Mountant (P36930, Invitrogen ThermoFisher Scientific, Waltham, MA, USA). Tissue sections were scanned using 3DHISTECH Panoramic 250 FLASH II digital slide scanner at Genome Biology Unit (Research Programs Unit, Faculty of Medicine, University of Helsinki, Biocenter, Finland) using 1×20 magnification with extended focus and 7 focus levels.

2.7. Statistical Methods

Unless otherwise stated, continuous variables were expressed as medians with interquartile ranges and compared using the Mann–Whitney U test. Multiple group comparisons were undertaken using the Kruskal–Wallis test. Correlations were tested with Spearman's rank correlation between different variables analyzed from the same liver biopsy or from simultaneously obtained liver and serum samples. To address effects of different expression levels on native liver survival, Kaplan–Meier analysis with log-rank test was used to predict native liver survival between tertiles for serum IL-8 concentration and relative liver mRNA expression. $p < 0.05$ was considered as statistically significant and all analyses were done on RStudio version 1.2.5033 (RStudio, Boston, MA, USA). Numbers throughout the analysis may be discrepant, owing to differing samples available from relevant time points (Table 1). These are given in each section of the Results.

2.8. Ethics

The study protocol was approved by the local hospital ethical committees. All procedures followed were in accordance with the ethical standards of the responsibility committee on human experimentation (institutional/national) and with the Helsinki Declaration of 1975, as revised in 2008. The study was approved by the hospital ethical committee (protocol number 345/03/1372008) and the institutional review board on 21 July 2017 (§68 HUS/149/2017) and also by the National Research Ethics Committee of the UK (12/WA/0282 and 18/SC/0058). An informed consent for use of samples in research was obtained from all patients.

3. Results

3.1. Patient Characteristics

Patient characteristics are listed in Table 1. The median patient age at the time of surgery was 56 days (41–76), and 96% of the children presented with type 3 BA. Following PE, 74 (64%) of the patients normalized their serum bilirubin (<20 µmol/L), and 56 (49%) underwent LT at median age of 1.5 years (interquartile range (IQR) 0.8–3.0). Native liver survival was 77% (95% confidence interval (CI) 70–85), 69% (95% CI 61–78) and 56% (95% CI 47–66) at 1, 2 and 5 years respectively.

3.2. Liver Expression and Serum Levels of Interleukin-8 (IL-8) Were Increased and Intercorrelated

Liver *IL-8* mRNA expression was markedly increased at PE ($n = 66$), when compared to both disease (by 16-fold) and normal (by 9-fold) control groups ($p < 0.001$) (Figure 1a). Similar to the upregulated liver expression, we found a significant, over 15-fold increase ($p < 0.001$) in IL-8 serum levels at PE ($n = 77$) compared to normal controls (Figure 1b). Both liver mRNA expression and serum levels of IL-8 peaked at and within one year after PE and declined thereafter, although serum IL-8 levels remained significantly above normal control values. A positive intercorrelation ($r = 0.53$, $p < 0.01$, $n = 70$) was observed between liver mRNA expression and serum concentrations of IL-8 (Supplementary Figure S1).

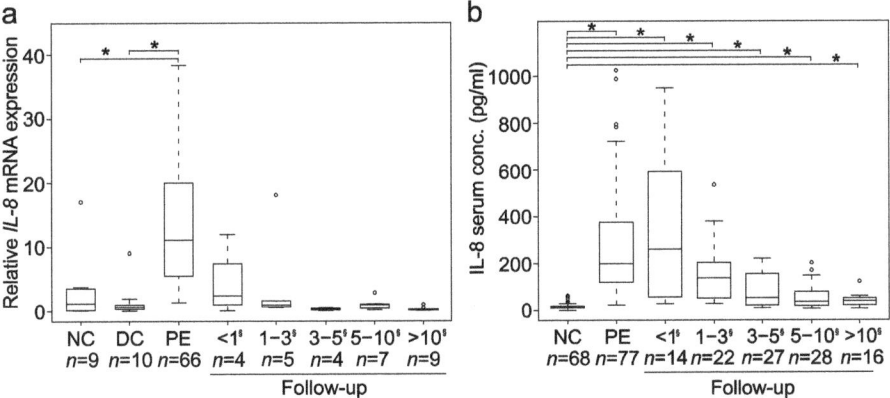

Figure 1. Liver and serum expression of interleukin-8 (IL-8). Box plots (median, interquartile range and 90th percentile) of (**a**) liver IL-8 mRNA expression (fold-change) and (**b**) serum IL-8 concentration (pg/mL) in normal controls (NC), disease controls (DC), biliary atresia patients at portoenterostomy (PE) and during follow-up following PE * $p < 0.05$ § = Years after PE. circles = outliers.

The patient age at PE positively correlated with liver *IL-8* mRNA expression ($r = 0.32$, $p < 0.01$, $n = 66$) and IL-8 serum levels ($r = 0.31$, $p < 0.01$, $n = 77$). At PE, the patients with splenic malformation showed lower liver IL-8 mRNA expression (5.51 (3.95–7.22) fold, n = 10) than those without (13.31 (6.37–21.07) fold, n = 54, p = 0.02), but median serum IL-8 concentrations were similar in patients with (164 (116–225) pg/mL, n = 9) and without (208 (121–381) pg/mL, n = 68, p = 0.44) splenic malformation. *IL-8* liver mRNA expression (14.9 ± 10.7 vs. 11.6 ± 9.92) fold, p = 0.288) and serum levels (394 ± 613 vs. 372 ± 204 pg/mL, p = 0.823) were comparable in the London and Helsinki samples.

3.3. Liver IL-8 Expression Predominantly Localized to Cholangiocytes

As studied with immunohistochemistry *IL-8* expression localized to cholangiocytes in the bile ducts within the normal liver (Figure 2a). In BA livers, enhanced *IL-8* expression was mainly observed in cholangiocytes within areas of DR and also in the cytoplasm of surrounding cells, most likely representing inflammatory cells. *IL-8* expression was more prominent at PE (Figure 2b) than during the follow up (Figure 2c). The findings were confirmed using in situ hybridization for IL8 and a hepatocyte marker HNF6, showing *IL-8* expression in bile duct cholangiocytes in the normal liver, and a predominant *IL-8* expression in the DR areas and cholangiocytes instead of hepatocytes in biliary atresia patients.

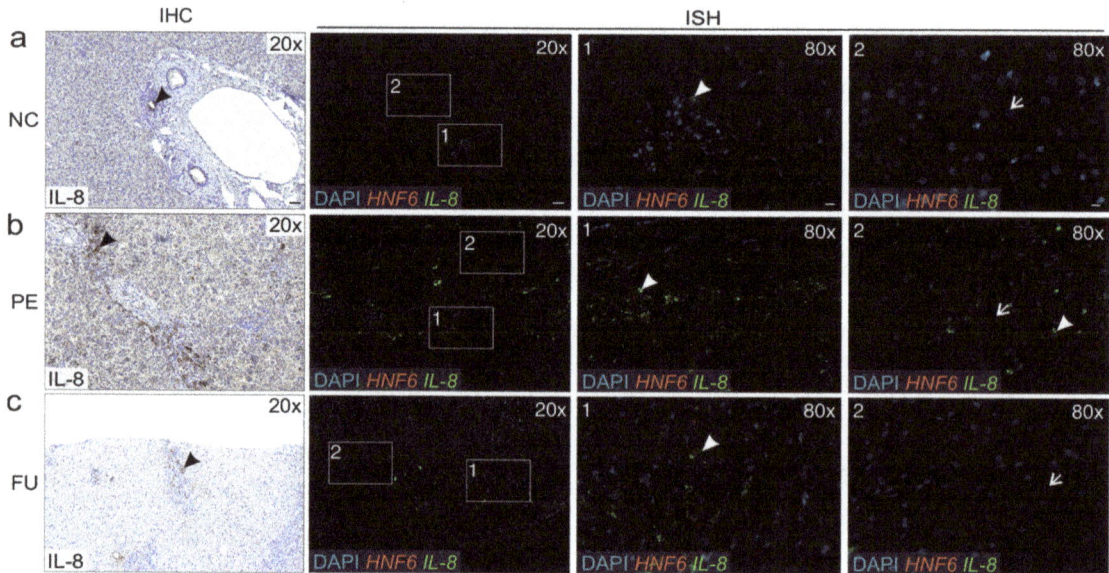

Figure 2. Representative liver expression of *IL-8* on immunohistochemistry (IHC) and in situ hybridization (ISH) in (**a**) normal control (NC), (**b**) biliary atresia patient at portoenterostomy (PE) and (**c**) during follow-up (FU) after PE. ISH includes two magnified images (80×) from each of the original (20×) image focused on (1) the area of ductular reaction (DR) and (2) hepatocyte rich parenchymal area. Arrow heads (black and white filled) point to IL-8 expressing cells (brown in IHC and green in ISH) while arrows (white filled) point to a hepatocyte marker HNF6 expressing cells in ISH. Note the expression of *IL-8* in bile duct cholangiocytes in the normal liver, while IL-8 is strongly expressed in the DR area and cholangiocytes instead of hepatocytes in biliary atresia patients. Scale bar = 50 µm (20×)/10 µm (80×).

3.4. IL-8 Associated with Liver Fibrosis, Ductular Reaction and Liver Injury

Liver *IL-8* mRNA expression correlated positively with the Metavir fibrosis stage at PE (r = 0.28, p = 0.04, n = 51) and in follow-up biopsies (r = 0.44, p = 0.05; n = 19), and with fibrosis markers *ACTA2* encoding for α-SMA and *COL1A2* encoding for collagen type 1 (Figure 3). Liver *IL-8* expression correlated positively with bile ductular proliferation (r = 0.45, p < 00.1, n = 70) and cholangiocyte markers *KRT19* encoding for CK-19 and *KRT7* encoding for CK-7 (Figure 3). No correlation with portal inflammation score was observed (r = 0.14, p = 0.26, n = 67). *IL-8* mRNA expression correlated positively with bilirubin (r = 0.51, p < 0.01), AST (r = 0.48, p < 0.01), ALT (r = 0.53, p < 0.01) and GGT (r = 0.51, p < 0.0, n = 70 for all) and with APRi during follow-up (r = 0.54, p = 0.04, n = 15).

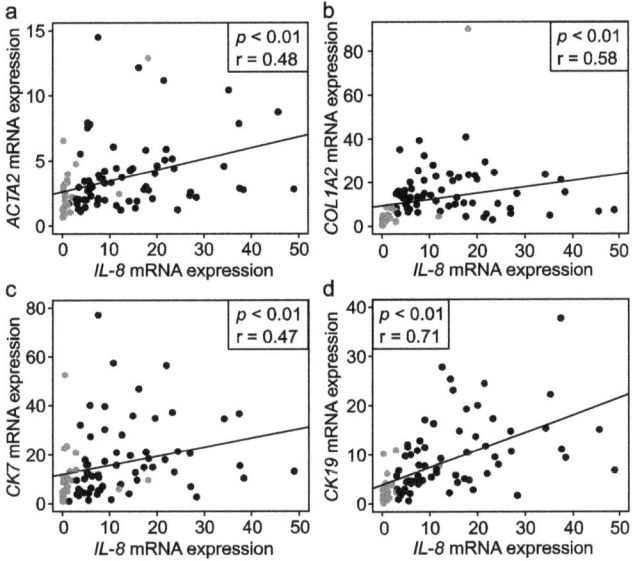

Figure 3. Correlations between liver *IL-8* expression and transcriptional markers of fibrogenesis and cholangiocytes. Scatterplot for correlation between relative liver *IL-8* mRNA expression and (**a**) *ACTA2* (**b**) *COL1A2* (**c**) *KRT7* and (**d**) *KRT19*. Black dots represent samples obtained at portoenterostomy (PE) and grey dots represent follow up samples.

At PE, serum IL-8 levels correlated with GGT (r = 0.27, p = 0.02, n = 77), whereas in the follow up serum samples, IL-8 not only correlated positively with GGT (r = 0.75, p < 0.01), but also with bilirubin (r = 0.58, p < 0.01), AST (r = 0.71, p < 0.01), and ALT (r = 0.69, p < 0.01; n = 36 for all). Although serum IL-8 levels correlated positively with bile ductular proliferation (r = 0.51, p < 0.01, n = 101), *COL1A2* (r = 0.29, p = 0.01, n = 69) and *KRT19* (r = 0.31, p < 0.01, n = 68), no significant correlations with the Metavir fibrosis stage, portal inflammation score, *ACTA2* or *KRT7* expression were observed.

3.5. IL-8 Had Limited Ability to Predict Portoenterostomy (PE) Outcomes

At PE, median serum levels of IL-8 were similar in patients (n = 41) who normalized serum bilirubin after PE (191 (128–327) pg/mL) when compared to those (n = 36) who remained jaundiced [208 (112–409) pg/mL, p = 0.54]. Liver IL-8 mRNA expression was also not significantly different between patients who cleared their jaundice and who did not (Supplementary Figure S2). However, when divided into tertiles based on their liver IL-8 expression level, the patients with the lowest IL-8 expression at PE showed significantly higher 1-year native liver survival (p = 0.03) compared to those with the highest expression, while no difference was seen in their 2- and 5-year native liver survival (Figure 4a). There was no difference in native liver survival rates at 1, 2 or 5 years between serum IL-8 tertiles measured at PE (Figure 4b).

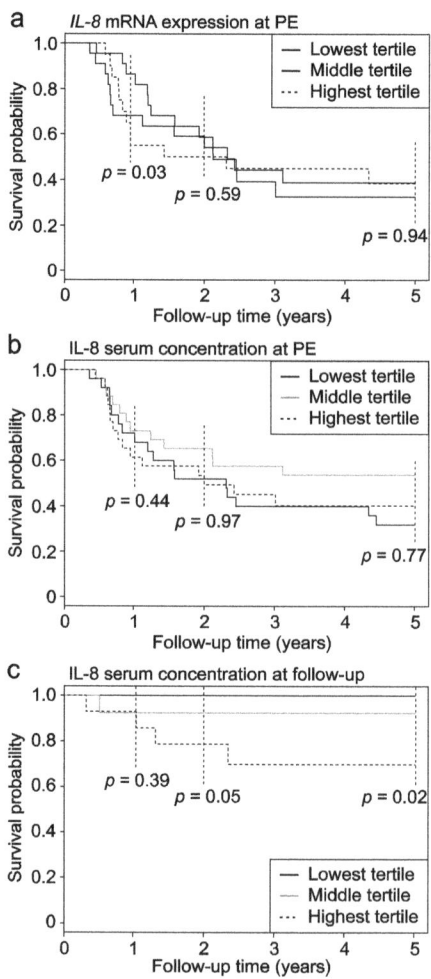

Figure 4. Native liver survival according to tertiles for IL-8 expression. Kaplan–Meier survival curves for native liver survival according to tertiles of (**a**) liver *IL-8* mRNA expression at portoenterostomy (PE) (*n* = 64), (**b**) serum IL-8 concentration at PE (*n* = 77), and (**c**) serum IL-8 concentration measured at the first follow-up sample (*n* = 40).

3.6. Serum IL-8 Associated with Native Liver Survival during Post-PE Follow-Up

Forty patients underwent median two (range, 1–6) follow-up serum IL-8 measurements after PE. The first follow-up measurement was performed 2.9 (1.1–4.2) years postoperatively, and the median period between the first and last measurement was 3.4 (0.18–5.4) years. Ten of these 40 patients underwent LT 3.8 (1.1–6.2) years after PE, while 30 patients had survived with their native livers for 6.7 (2.9–9.2) years. The first (154 (130–310) vs. 48.0 (32–197) pg/mL, p = 0.03), the last (117 (65–269) vs. 35.4 (20–86) pg/mL, p = 0.01) and the average (147 (108–289) vs. 44.0 (28–164) pg/mL, p = 0.02) postoperative serum IL-8 level was significantly higher among the patients who were later transplanted when compared to those who continued to survive with their native liver. In addition, the patients in the lowest serum IL-8 tertile of the first postoperative measurement showed significantly higher native liver survival than the patients in the highest tertile (Figure 4c).

3.7. Expression of Cytokines Connected to IL-8

As shown in Figure 5, expression of other cytokines connected to IL-8 changed less consistently, although *IL-18* (n = 66) mRNA expression was also significantly increased both at PE ($p < 0.01$) and <1 year after PE ($p < 0.01$). Despite IL-8 correlating positively with IL-18 at transcriptional level (r = 0.56, $p < 0.01$; n = 95) and in serum (r = 0.28, $p < 0.01$; n = 107), the postoperative *IL-18* expression remained unchanged. While TNF-α showed slightly increased postoperative serum concentration among patients, it along with *IFN-γ* and *IL-33* did not show any significant overexpression at transcriptional level. However, also *TNF-α* (r = 0.40, $p < 0.01$, n = 90), *IFN-γ* (r = 0.26, $p = 0.01$, n = 84) and *IL-33* (r = 0.46, $p < 0.01$, n = 90) positively correlated with *IL-8* mRNA expression in the liver while *TNF-α* also correlated with IL-8 in serum (r = 0.14, $p = 0.04$, n = 107).

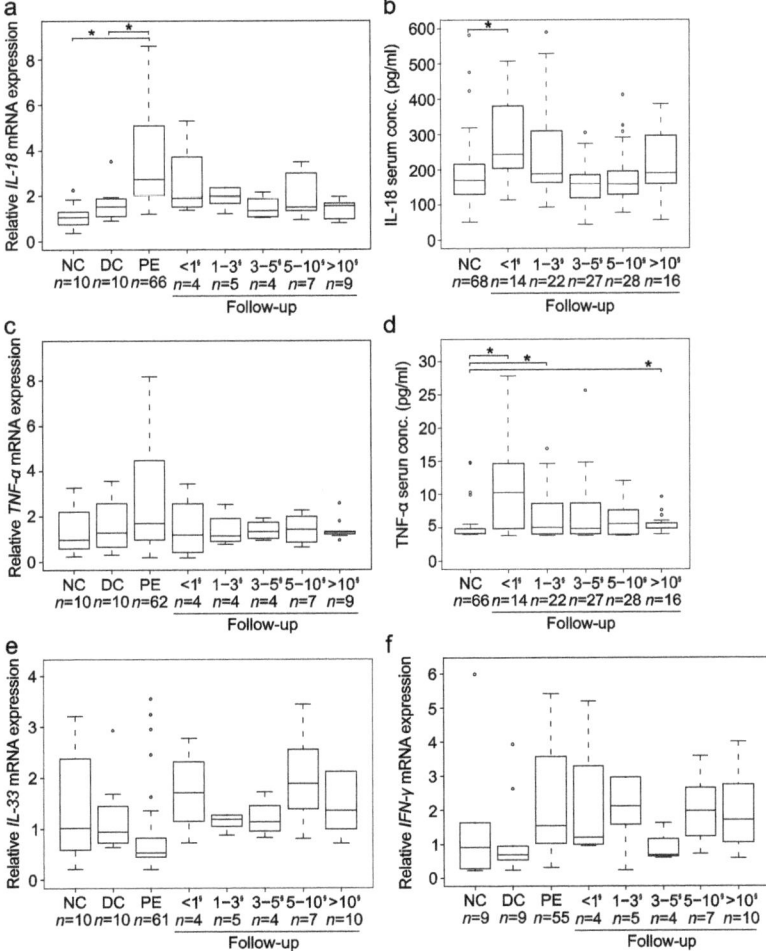

Figure 5. Expression of several cytokines related to IL-8. Box plots (median, interquartile range and 90th percentile) of (**a**) liver *IL-18* mRNA expression (fold-change) and (**b**) serum IL-18 concentration (pg/mL), (**c**) liver *TNF* mRNA expression, (**d**) serum tumor necrosis factor-alpha (TNF-α) concentration (pg/mL), (**e**) liver *IL-33* mRNA expression, and (**f**) liver *IFN* mRNA expression in normal controls (NC), disease controls (DC), biliary atresia patients at portoenterostomy (PE) and during follow-up following PE * $p < 0.05$. § = Years after PE circles = outliers.

4. Discussion

In this study we have comprehensively addressed the prognostic value of liver and serum expression of IL-8 for PE outcomes in a large number of BA patients in relation to histological liver fibrosis, (transcriptional) markers of liver fibrogenesis and cholangiocytes as well as biochemical markers of liver injury. We demonstrated marked parallel increases in liver and serum expression of IL-8, which were specific for IL-8 among several other cytokines studied. Although liver *IL-8* expression was associated with histological liver fibrosis, and surrogate markers of liver fibrogenesis as well as bile ductular proliferation and cholangiocytes at the mRNA level, serum IL-8 levels were associated with further survival with native liver only in samples obtained during postoperative follow-up after PE. Our findings suggest that although IL-8 may have a distinctive pathophysiological role in BA by promoting DR and liver fibrogenesis, prognostic value of serum IL-8 in predicting PE outcomes is limited to the postoperative follow-up period after PE.

Prolonged immune activation with the release of several proinflammatory cytokines in the affected liver is considered vital for the developing fibrosis and liver damage in BA [17]. At the time of PE, an inflammatory infiltrate associated with DR and fibrosis along the portal tracts occurs [16,18]. Liver fibrosis progresses, also following successful PE surgery, for largely unknown reasons [15], but has been attributed to activation of hepatic stellate cells and portal myofibroblasts by cytokines derived from Kupffer cells and reactive cholangiocytes of DR [3,5,19,20], leading to the deposition of an extra cellular matrix and collagen. In accordance with previous experimental observations [11], our findings suggest that IL-8 is involved with the above outlined liver injury cascade in BA, and that the involvement was specific to IL-8 as several other cytokines studied failed to show enhanced expression to a comparable degree. Not only was *IL-8* distinctively overexpressed in BA livers, but also correlated with histological fibrosis, bile ductular proliferation and transcriptional markers of fibrogenesis and cholangiocytes. In addition, liver *IL-8* expression was localized to cholangiocytes in the areas of DR in accordance with previous findings in adult cholestatic liver diseases [21]. We can only speculate as to the underlying reasons for the lower correlation of liver *IL-8* mRNA expression with the Metavir stage than with ACTA2 or COL1A2. One possible reason could be that the Metavir stage is a class variable as opposed to mRNA expression being a continuous variable, which may skew the correlation between them. There is also a notable overlap between histological scoring of adjoining Metavir stages, especially between stages 2 and 3. Histological portal inflammation score gives a crude estimation of all inflammatory cells present in portal areas, and the missing correlation between portal inflammation and *IL-8* expression might be related to similar limitations as outlined above for histological fibrosis score.

Overexpression of IL-8 peaked at and within one year after PE and gradually decreased thereafter. The early expression peak may be attributable to the combined effects of overt cholestasis, vigorous bile ductular proliferation and inflammation before surgical re-establishment of bile flow as well as plausibly causative viral infection directly inflicting the initial bile duct damage [1,3,17]. The fact that liver *IL-8* expression showed only limited prognostic value for PE outcomes suggest a non-decisive but complementary role of IL-8 as an indicator for the success of PE or as a mediator for the progression of postoperative liver injury in BA. Contrary to liver *IL-8* expression, serum IL-8 showed no association with histological liver fibrosis and only weak correlations with surrogate markers of liver injury measured by qPCR, explaining the poor predictive value of serum IL-8 at PE. Our findings are in accordance with a recent study among 57 BA patients, where serum and liver IL-8 concentration measured at PE was unrelated to 2-year native liver survival following PE [14].

Interestingly, the increased post-PE expression profile of serum IL-8 followed that of cholangitis episodes, frequency of which is reported to predominate the first postoperative year with a prompt subsequent decline [22–24]. It has been previously shown that expression of *IL-8* in human biliary epithelial cells is stimulated by proinflammatory cytokines

IL-1β and TNF-α, and lipopolysaccharide produced by gram negative bacteria, which are commonly causative microbes underlying BA associated cholangitis [21,23,25,26]. In the early disease phase, enhanced secretion by an augmented peripheral immature B-cell population seems to be an important source of elevated serum IL-8 [27]. Serum TNF-α and IL-18 levels have been shown to be significantly increased within 6 months of PE surgery [28]. Here, liver and serum expression patterns of TNF-α followed those of IL-8 and their liver mRNA expression correlated with each other. Based on these data, we hypothesize that besides persisting DR, bacterial cholangitis may have contributed to the increased postoperative serum IL-8 levels, and may help to explain their association with native liver survival as recurrent postoperative cholangitis episodes are known to relate with the need of liver transplantation following PE [29].

In accordance with previous reports, serum IL-8 levels positively correlated with biochemical liver injury markers such as bilirubin, GGT and transaminases during postoperative follow-up, reflecting progression of cholestasis and liver injury [30]. The significant correlation of IL-8 with bile ductular proliferation and GGT both at PE and during follow-up reinforces the connection between IL-8 and bile duct injury at both time points. We hypothesize that the increased serum IL-8 levels mainly reflected active DR, while postoperative serum levels may have been contributed by bacterial cholangitis. However, the shift from a predominantly inflammatory liver injury phenotype at PE to the one predominated by DR and fibrosis may have also allowed their more specific detection and accurate prediction by serum IL-8 during follow-up [15,31].

The main limitations of this study include the retrospective design, which is unavoidably associated with inaccuracies in data collection and missing data points. Although we were not able to prospectively include consecutive patients, PE age, occurrence of associated malformations, anatomic type of BA, clearance of jaundice rate and native liver survival among the included patients were well represented in previously described BA cohorts from Europe [32,33]. While we were able to include a relatively large number of BA patients at PE and during follow-up, the number of patients with simultaneous postoperative liver and serum specimens remained limited. Moreover, serum samples were not collected during cholangitis episodes, precluding our ability to address the actual relationship between serum IL-8 concentration and cholangitis, which should be addressed in future studies. Most of the follow-up serum IL-8 measurements were performed after 2 years of PE, which introduces a selection bias and precludes any conclusions regarding the early postoperative period. Finally, our findings concerning follow-up studies may not be generalizable to patient cohorts with different postoperative treatment regimens.

5. Conclusions

Our data showed significant and distinctive overexpression of IL-8 by cholangiocytes within DR in BA patients both at PE and during postoperative follow-up. Despite the IL-8 overexpression in the liver, increased serum IL-8 levels associated weakly with decreased native liver survival only during the postoperative period following PE.

Supplementary Materials: The following are available online at https://www.mdpi.com/article/10.3390/jcm10122705/s1, Figure S1: Correlation between liver and serum expression of IL-8, Figure S2: Liver and serum expression of IL-8 in relation to clearance of jaundice after portoenterostomy, Table S1: Baseline characteristics of disease control patients.

Author Contributions: Conceptualization, M.P.P. and M.H. (Markku Heikinheimo); methodology, M.P.P., M.H. (Markku Heikinheimo), A.K., M.P., M.H. (Maria Hukkinen), K.E., N.G. and I.N.; validation, N.G.; formal analysis, N.G., M.P.P., M.H. (Markku Heikinheimo) and A.K.; investigation, N.G., N.A., J.L. and P.H.; resources, M.P.P., M.H. (Markku Heikinheimo), J.R.D., A.T. and M.D.; visualization, N.G. and M.P.; writing—original draft, N.G., M.P.P., M.H. (Markku Heikinheimo) and A.K.; writing—review and editing, all authors; supervision, M.P.P., M.H. (Markku Heikinheimo) and A.K.; project administration and funding acquisition, M.P.P. and M.H. (Markku Heikinheimo). All authors have read and agreed to the published version of the manuscript.

Funding: This research was funded by Sigrid Juselius Foundation (M.P.P., M.H. (Markku Heikinheimo)), Finnish Pediatric Research Foundation (M.P.P.), Helsinki University Hospital Fund (M.P.P., M.H. (Markku Heikinheimo)) and Finska Läkaresällskapet M.H. (Markku Heikinheimo). Open access funding provided by University of Helsinki.

Institutional Review Board Statement: The study was conducted according to the guidelines of the Declaration of Helsinki, and was approved by the Helsinki Hospital ethical committee (protocol number 345/03/1372008) and the institutional review board on 21 July 2017 (§68 HUS/149/2017) and also by the National Research Ethics Committee of the UK (12/WA/0282 and 18/SC/0058).

Informed Consent Statement: Informed consent was obtained from all subjects involved in the study.

Acknowledgments: The authors would like to acknowledge the excellent technical assistance by Tuike Helmiö.

Conflicts of Interest: The authors declare no conflict of interest. The funders had no role in the design of the study; in the collection, analyses, or interpretation of data; in the writing of the manuscript; or in the decision to publish the results.

References

1. Lakshminarayanan, B.; Davenport, M. Biliary atresia: A comprehensive review. *J. Autoimmun.* **2016**, *73*, 1–9. [CrossRef]
2. Hartley, J.L.; Davenport, M.; Kelly, D.A. Biliary atresia. *Lancet* **2009**, *14*, 1704–1713. [CrossRef]
3. Bezerra, J.A.; Wells, R.G.; Mack, C.L.; Karpen, S.J.; Hoofnagle, J.; Doo, E.; Sokol, R.J. BILIARY ATRESIA: Clinical and Research Challenges for the 21st Century. *Hepatology* **2018**, *68*, 1163–1173. [CrossRef] [PubMed]
4. Sundaram, S.S.; Mack, C.L.; Feldman, A.G.; Sokol, R.J. Biliary Atresia: Indications and Timing of Liver Transplantation and Optimization of Pre-Transplant Care. *Liver Transpl.* **2017**, *23*, 96–109. [CrossRef] [PubMed]
5. Hukkinen, M.; Pihlajoki, M.; Pakarinen, M.P. Predicting native liver injury and survival in biliary atresia. *Semin. Pediatr. Surg.* **2020**, *29*, 150943. [CrossRef] [PubMed]
6. Grieve, A.; Makin, E.; Davenport, M. Aspartate Aminotransferase-to-Platelet Ratio index (APRi) in infants with biliary atresia: Prognostic value at presentation. *J. Pediatr. Surg.* **2013**, *48*, 789–795. [CrossRef] [PubMed]
7. Karpen, S.J.; Kelly, D.; Mack, C.; Stein, P. Ileal bile acid transporter inhibition as an anticholestatic therapeutic target in biliary atresia and other cholestatic disorders. *Hepatol. Int.* **2020**, *14*, 677–689. [CrossRef] [PubMed]
8. Dong, R.; Zheng, S. Interleukin-8: A critical chemokine in biliary atresia. *J. Gastroenterol. Hepatol.* **2015**, *30*, 970–976. [CrossRef]
9. Clément, S.; Pascarella, S.; Conzelmann, S.; Gonelle-Gispert, C.; Guilloux, K.; Negro, F. The hepatitis C virus core protein indirectly induces alpha-smooth muscle actin expression in hepatic stellate cells via interleukin-8. *J. Hepatol.* **2010**, *52*, 635–643. [CrossRef]
10. Langhans, B.; Krämer, B.; Louis, M.; Nischalke, H.D.; Hüneburg, R.; Staratschek-Jox, A.; Odenthal, M.; Manekeller, S.; Schepke, M.; Kalff, J.; et al. Intrahepatic IL-8 producing Foxp3+CD4+ regulatory T cells and fibrogenesis in chronic hepatitis C. *J. Hepatol.* **2013**, *59*, 229–235. [CrossRef] [PubMed]
11. Arafa, R.S.; Haie, O.M.A.; El-Azab, D.S.; Abdel-Rahman, A.M.; Sira, M.M. Significant hepatic expression of IL-2 and IL-8 in biliary atresia compared with other neonatal cholestatic disorders. *Cytokine* **2016**, *79*, 59–65. [CrossRef]
12. Bessho, K.; Mourya, R.; Shivakumar, P.; Walters, S.; Magee, J.C.; Rao, M.; Jegga, A.G.; Bezerra, J.A. Gene expression signature for biliary atresia and a role for interleukin-8 in pathogenesis of experimental disease. *Hepatology* **2014**, *60*, 211–223. [CrossRef]
13. El-Faramawy, A.A.M.; E El-Shazly, L.B.; A Abbass, A.; Ismail, H.A.B. Serum IL-6 and IL-8 in infants with biliary atresia in comparison to intrahepatic cholestasis. *Trop. Gastroenterol.* **2011**, *32*, 50–55.
14. Madadi-Sanjani, O.; Kuebler, J.F.; Dippel, S.; Gigina, A.; Falk, C.S.; Vieten, G.; Petersen, C.; Klemann, C. Long-term outcome and necessity of liver transplantation in infants with biliary atresia are independent of cytokine milieu in native liver and serum. *Cytokine* **2018**, *111*, 382–388. [CrossRef]
15. Hukkinen, M.; Kerola, A.; Lohi, J.; Heikkilä, P.; Merras-Salmio, L.; Jahnukainen, T.; Koivusalo, A.; Jalanko, H.; Pakarinen, M.P. Treatment Policy and Liver Histopathology Predict Biliary Atresia Outcomes: Results after National Centralization and Protocol Biopsies. *J. Am. Coll. Surg.* **2018**, *226*, 46–57.e1. [CrossRef]
16. Lampela, H.; Kosola, S.; Heikkilä, P.; Lohi, J.; Jalanko, H.; Pakarinen, M.P. Native liver histology after successful portoenterostomy in biliary atresia. *J. Clin. Gastroenterol.* **2014**, *48*, 721–728. [CrossRef]
17. Bessho, K.; Bezerra, J.A. Biliary Atresia: Will Blocking Inflammation Tame the Disease? *Annu. Rev. Med.* **2011**, *62*, 171–185. [CrossRef] [PubMed]
18. Mack, C.L.; Tucker, R.M.; Sokol, R.J.; Karrer, F.M.; Kotzin, B.L.; Whitington, P.F.; Miller, S.D. Biliary Atresia Is Associated with CD4+ Th1 Cell–Mediated Portal Tract Inflammation. *Pediatr. Res.* **2004**, *56*, 79–87. [CrossRef] [PubMed]
19. Ramm, G.A.; Nair-Shalliker, V.; Bridle, K.R.; Shepherd, R.W.; Crawford, D.H.G. Contribution of Hepatic Parenchymal and Nonparenchymal Cells to Hepatic Fibrogenesis in Biliary Atresia. *Am. J. Pathol.* **1998**, *153*, 527–535. [CrossRef]
20. Deng, Y.-H.; Pu, C.-L.; Li, Y.-C.; Zhu, J.; Xiang, C.; Zhang, M.-M.; Guo, C.-B. Analysis of Biliary Epithelial-Mesenchymal Transition in Portal Tract Fibrogenesis in Biliary Atresia. *Dig. Dis. Sci.* **2010**, *56*, 731–740. [CrossRef] [PubMed]

21. Isse, K.; Harada, K.; Nakanuma, Y. IL-8 expression by biliary epithelial cells is associated with neutrophilic infiltration and reactive bile ductules. *Liver Int.* **2007**, *27*, 672–680. [CrossRef]
22. Cheng, K.; Molleston, J.P.; Bennett, W.E. Cholangitis in Patients With Biliary Atresia Receiving Hepatoportoenterostomy: A National Database Study. *J. Pediatr. Gastroenterol. Nutr.* **2020**, *71*, 452–458. [CrossRef] [PubMed]
23. Ecoffey, C.; Rothman, E.; Bernard, O.; Hadchouel, M.; Valayer, J.; Alagille, D. Bacterial cholangitis after surgery for biliary atresia. *J. Pediatr.* **1987**, *111*, 824–829. [CrossRef]
24. Baek, S.H.; Kang, J.-M.; Ihn, K.; Han, S.J.; Koh, H.; Ahn, J.G. The Epidemiology and Etiology of Cholangitis After Kasai Portoenterostomy in Patients With Biliary Atresia. *J. Pediatr. Gastroenterol. Nutr.* **2020**, *70*, 171–177. [CrossRef] [PubMed]
25. Chung, P.H.Y.; Tam, P.K.H.; Wong, K.K.Y. Does the identity of the bacteria matter in post-Kasai cholangitis? A comparison between simple and intractable cholangitis. *J. Pediatr. Surg.* **2018**, *53*, 2409–2411. [CrossRef] [PubMed]
26. Ni, Y.-H.; Hsu, H.-Y.; Wu, E.-T.; Chen, H.-L.; Lee, P.-I.; Chang, M.H.; Lai, H.-S. Bacterial cholangitis in patients with biliary atresia: Impact on short-term outcome. *Pediatr. Surg. Int.* **2001**, *17*, 390–395. [CrossRef]
27. Zhang, Y.; Zhou, L.; Gu, G.; Feng, M.; Ding, X.; Xia, Q.; Lu, L. CXCL8 high inflammatory B cells in the peripheral blood of patients with biliary atresia are involved in disease progression. *Immunol. Cell Biol.* **2020**, *98*, 682–692. [CrossRef] [PubMed]
28. Narayanaswamy, B.; Gonde, C.; Tredger, J.M.; Hussain, M.; Vergani, D.; Davenport, M. Serial circulating markers of inflammation in biliary atresia—Evolution of the post-operative inflammatory process. *Hepatology* **2007**, *46*, 180–187. [CrossRef]
29. Koga, H.; Wada, M.; Nakamura, H.; Miyano, G.; Okawada, M.; Lane, G.J.; Okazaki, T.; Yamataka, A. Factors influencing jaundice-free survival with the native liver in post-portoenterostomy biliary atresia patients: Results from a single institution. *J. Pediatr. Surg.* **2013**, *48*, 2368–2372. [CrossRef]
30. Honsawek, S.; Chongsrisawat, V.; Vejchapipat, P.; Thawornsuk, N.; Tangkijvanich, P.; Poovorawan, Y. Serum interleukin-8 in children with biliary atresia: Relationship with disease stage and biochemical parameters. *Pediatr. Surg. Int.* **2004**, *21*, 73–77. [CrossRef]
31. Kerola, A.; Lampela, H.; Lohi, J.; Heikkilä, P.; Mutanen, A.; Jalanko, H.; Pakarinen, M.P. Molecular signature of active fibrogenesis prevails in biliary atresia after successful portoenterostomy. *Surgery* **2017**, *162*, 548–556. [CrossRef] [PubMed]
32. Pakarinen, M.P.; Johansen, L.S.; Svensson, J.F.; Bjørnland, K.; Gatzinsky, V.; Stenström, P.; Koivusalo, A.; Kvist, N.; Almström, M.; Emblem, R.; et al. Outcomes of biliary atresia in the Nordic countries-a multicenter study of 158 patients during 2005–2016. *J. Pediatr. Surg.* **2018**, *53*, 1509–1515. [CrossRef] [PubMed]
33. Davenport, M.; Ong, E.; Sharif, K.; Alizai, N.; McClean, P.; Hadzic, N.; Kelly, D.A. Biliary atresia in England and Wales: Results of centralization and new benchmark. *J. Pediatr. Surg.* **2011**, *46*, 1689–1694. [CrossRef] [PubMed]

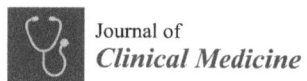
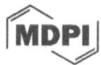

Brief Report

Prepregnancy Assessment of Liver Function to Predict Perinatal and Postpregnancy Outcomes in Biliary Atresia Patients with Native Liver

Nobuhiro Takahashi [1,†], Daigo Ochiai [2,†], Yohei Yamada [1,*], Masumi Tamagawa [2], Hiroki Kanamori [1], Mototoshi Kato [1], Satoru Ikenoue [2], Yoshifumi Kasuga [2], Tatsuo Kuroda [1] and Mamoru Tanaka [2]

1. Department of Pediatric Surgery, Keio University School of Medicine, Tokyo 160-8582, Japan; tkhsnbhr430@keio.jp (N.T.); kanamori06@keio.jp (H.K.); mototoshi77@keio.jp (M.K.); kuroda-t@z8.keio.jp (T.K.)
2. Department of Obstetrics and Gynecology, Keio University School of Medicine, Tokyo 160-8582, Japan; ochiaidaigo@keio.jp (D.O.); akiyama_3_tohoku@yahoo.co.jp (M.T.); ikenouesatoru@me.com (S.I.); 17yoshi23.k@gmail.com (Y.K.); mtanaka@keio.jp (M.T.)
* Correspondence: yohei.z7@keio.jp; Tel.: +81-3-3353-1211
† These authors contributed equally to this work.

Abstract: Considering that some biliary atresia (BA) survivors with native liver have reached reproductive age and face long-lasting complications, specific attention needs to be paid to pregnant cases. This study aimed to investigate the relationship between liver function, perinatal outcomes, and prognosis. A database review was conducted to identify pregnant BA cases with native liver and perinatal data, and clinical information on BA-related complications was analyzed. Perinatal serum cholinesterase (ChE) levels, model for end-stage liver-disease (MELD) score, and platelet trends were analyzed, and the association between these indicators and perinatal outcomes was investigated. Patients were categorized into three groups according to the perinatal clinical outcomes: favorable (term babies with or without several episodes of cholangitis; $n = 3$), borderline (term baby and following liver dysfunction; $n = 1$), and unfavorable (premature delivery with subsequent liver failure; $n = 1$). Lower serum ChE levels, lower platelet counts, and higher MELD scores were observed in the unfavorable category. Borderline and unfavorable patients displayed a continuous increase in MELD score, with one eventually needing a liver transplantation. Pregnancy in patients with BA requires special attention. Serum ChE levels, platelet counts, and MELD scores are all important markers for predicting perinatal prognosis.

Keywords: pregnancy; biliary atresia; chorine esterase; MELD score; liver transplantation

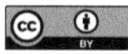

1. Introduction

Kasai portoenterostomy has been widely accepted as the primary method of surgical treatment for biliary atresia (BA), and early diagnosis and timely surgery are known to have a significant impact on long-term prognosis [1–3]. Owing to an improvement in clinical outcomes, an increasing number of BA patients can survive with native liver until adulthood. However, some long-term survivors of the Kasai procedure face and suffer from life-long complications, such as portal hypertension and recurrent cholangitis [4,5]. In pregnant women with native liver after BA surgery, such complications can be exacerbated by pregnancy-associated physiology [6]. Therefore, endoscopic surveillance for esophageal varices is recommended, along with the prompt initiation of antibiotic treatment for cholangitis [7].

Among pregnant patients with BA and native liver, both favorable and unfavorable perinatal courses are reported mainly because of complications, and some develop liver failure after pregnancy [6,8–11]. Sasaki et al. [9] revealed that a history of cholangitis and variceal breeding prior to pregnancy led to recurrent complications during pregnancy.

Kuroda et al. [8,12] reported that the level of serum cholinesterase (ChE), which is synthesized mainly in hepatocytes and reduced in liver dysfunction, at puberty may predict pregnancy safety. To date, 58 live births in 40 pregnant BA patients have been published; however, little is known about the precise pre-pregnancy status of liver function and long-term clinical course after pregnancy [13].

In 2011, Westbrook et al. [14] demonstrated the efficacy of the model for end-stage liver disease (MELD) score in predicting outcomes in cirrhotic patients during pregnancy. In BA patients, given that the MELD score often fails to reflect the severity of BA-specific clinical symptoms, risk evaluation for pregnancy in BA patients remains unclear. Therefore, in the current study, sequential changes in the MELD score, platelet count, and serum ChE in five patients with BA were investigated during pregnancy, and their predictive efficacy for perinatal outcome and maternal prognosis are discussed.

2. Materials and Methods

2.1. Study Design

A database review was conducted to identify pregnant women who conceived after BA surgery and delivered at Keio University Hospital, between 1 April 2010 and 31 March 2020. Owing to the retrospective design of this study, opt-out consent was obtained. The study was approved by the research ethics review board of Keio University (20150103).

2.2. Data Collection

Antenatal data, such as maternal demographic information (age, race, parity, pre-existing chronic diseases, exposure to alcohol, tobacco, and other teratogens), mode of conception, ultrasound findings, and obstetrical complications were collected retrospectively. Delivery information, including birth weight, gestational age at delivery, Apgar scores, and neonatal complications were reviewed. Additionally, we collected information on BA-related complications, including the clinical symptoms of portal hypertension (gastroesophageal varices and thrombocytopenia), coagulopathy, liver dysfunction, and cholangitis. Furthermore, biochemical data on liver function, including serum ChE level, MELD score, and platelet count during the perinatal period and after pregnancy, were collected at various periods during pregnancy. The MELD score was calculated using the following formula [15]:

$$\text{MELD} = 3.78 \times \log_e\{serum\ bilirubin\ (\text{mg}/\text{dL})\} + 11.2 \times \log_e(PT - INR) \\ + 9.6 \times \log_e\{serum\ creatinine(\text{mg}/\text{dL})\} + 6.43 \quad (1)$$

3. Results

3.1. Patients

During the study period, a total of 5880 pregnant patients delivered at Keio University Hospital. Among them, five were identified as pregnant after BA surgery with native liver (Table 1).

3.2. Maternal Characteristics and Obstetrical Outcomes

Table 1 shows the maternal characteristics and obstetric outcomes. Perinatal outcomes after BA surgery were divided into three groups on the basis thereof: favorable (stable maternal condition with minimal complication and term baby [$n = 3$]; Patients 1–3), borderline (complication during pregnancy with subsequent worsening maternal liver function but term baby [$n = 1$]; Patient 4), and unfavorable (complication during pregnancy with subsequent deterioration of liver function and premature delivery [$n = 1$]; Patient 5).

Table 1. Maternal characteristics and perinatal outcomes. LTx, liver transplantation; GA, gestational age; BA, biliary atresia; VD, vaginal delivery; CS, cesarean section; GE varices, gastroesophageal varices.

Patient	Maternal Age	Nulli-Parity	Mode of Delivery	GA at Delivery (Weeks/Days)	BW	Changes in BA Complication during the Perinatal Period		
						Prepregnancy	during Pregnancy	Postpartum
1	30	Yes	VD	39 w 4 d	2980 g	None	None	None
2	32	Yes	VD	36 w 6 d	2578 g	Cholangitis	Recurrence of cholangitis	Recurrence of cholangitis
3	39	No	VD	36 w 5 d	2690 g	Cholangitis	Recurrence of cholangitis	Recurrence of cholangitis
4	40	No	CS	37 w 3 d	2590 g	Cholangitis GE varices Thrombocytopenia	Recurrence of cholangitis Exacerbation of GE varices Thrombocytopenia	Recurrence of cholangitis Exacerbation of GE varices Thrombocytopenia Liver dysfunction
5	34	Yes	CS	30 w 0 d	842 g	GE varices Thrombocytopenia Ascites	Rupture of GE varices Hepatic encephalopathy Thrombocytopenia Ascites Liver dysfunction	Exacerbation of GE varices Hepatic encephalopathy Thrombocytopenia Ascites Liver dysfunction

The median gestational age at delivery was 37 weeks (range: 30–40 weeks), and the median birth weight was 2590 g (range: 842–2980 g). All patients delivered after 36 weeks of gestation, except for unfavorable patient. Three patients (Patients 2–4) developed cholangitis around the second trimester and were treated with antimicrobial agents. Two patients experienced deterioration of esophageal varices: one underwent endoscopic variceal ligation (EVL) treatment in endoscopic survey (Patient 4), and the other experienced a rupture of varices and underwent EVL (Patient 5).

3.3. Maternal Liver Function during the Perinatal Period

The MELD score, platelet count, and ChE were plotted during the perinatal period (Figure 1A–C). In the favorable group (Patients 1–3), maternal serum ChE levels, which are known as indicators of hepatic functional reserve, decreased during pregnancy but recovered to prepregnancy levels after each delivery. In Patient 5 (unfavorable), their low ChE level (below 200 U/L) prior to conception decreased further and did not recover to the baseline after delivery. In Patient 4 (borderline), a relatively high ChE (above 200 U/L) was seen prior to conception; however, the ChE level in this patient decreased earlier than that in the favorable group and did not return to the baseline. In the favorable group, a transient rise in the MELD score was observed, and this reflected complications such as cholangitis. The MELD score returned to the prepregnancy level after the deliveries. By contrast, a continuous uptrend in the MELD score was observed in Patients 4 and 5 after the deliveries. During the perinatal period, the platelet counts were above $10 \times 10^4/\mu L$ in the favorable group and below $10 \times 10^4/\mu L$ in Patients 4 and 5.

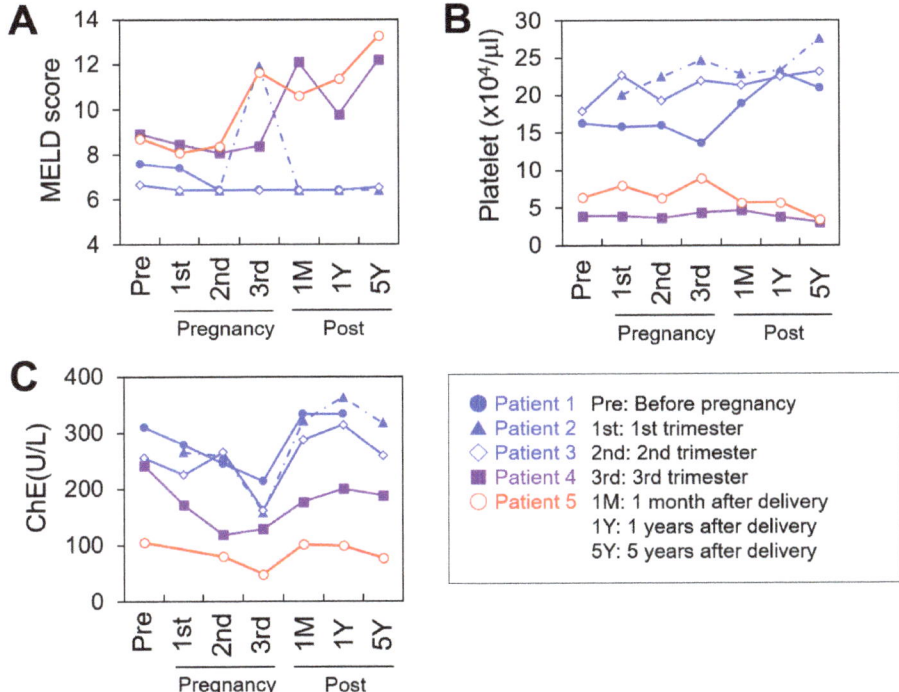

Figure 1. The model for end-stage liver disease (MELD) score (**A**), platelet count (**B**), and cholinesterase (ChE) plot (**C**) during the perinatal period. Pre: Before pregnancy, 1st: 1st trimester, 2nd: 2nd trimester, 3rd: 3rd trimester, 1M: 1 month after delivery, 1Y: 1 year after delivery, 5Y: 5 years after delivery.

3.4. Maternal Prognosis after Delivery

In the favorable group, Patients 2 and 3 experienced a few episodes of cholangitis after pregnancy, which were successfully treated with antibiotics. Patients 1, 2, and 3 (favorable group) were in stable condition two, six, and seven years after delivery, respectively. In Patient 4 (borderline) and Patient 5 (unfavorable), liver function deteriorated gradually after delivery (Figure 1A–C). Patient 5 was listed for deceased donor liver transplantation eight years after delivery and underwent liver transplantation two years later. Unfortunately, Patient 5 died after surgery because of surgical complications. Patient 4 retained her native liver for 6.4 years after delivery with slowly deteriorating liver function.

3.5. Individual Clinical Courses in Pregnancy

3.5.1. Patient 1: Favorable Case

A 30-year-old gravida 2, para 0 pregnant woman with no past episodes of cholangitis was referred to our hospital because of a history of BA. Fortunately, she did not experience BA-related complications, such as portal hypertension, liver dysfunction, and recurrent cholangitis. She regularly attended the preconception checkup with a pediatric surgeon and conceived spontaneously in a planned manner. At 22 weeks of gestation, gastrointestinal endoscopy did not reveal any signs of esophageal or gastric varices. Her pregnancy was uneventful until the day of delivery, and she vaginally delivered a healthy female infant weighing 2980 g at 39 weeks of gestation. Her postpartum course was uneventful, and she was in a stable condition for 1.8 year after delivery without any complications.

3.5.2. Patient 2: Favorable Case

A 32-year-old gravida 1, para 0 pregnant woman was referred to our hospital because of her history of BA. She experienced an episode of cholangitis after Kasai procedure and then interrupted a routine checkup with a pediatric surgeon because her postoperative course was uneventful. She conceived spontaneously in an unplanned manner. She was diagnosed with hilar bile lake and splenomegaly but did not exhibit liver dysfunction, thrombocytopenia, or esophageal varices. Her pregnancy was uneventful, but she experienced recurrent cholangitis. Thus, she was treated with antimicrobial agents at 24 and 29 weeks of gestation. To prevent liver damage caused by repeated cholangitis, labor induction was performed at 36 weeks of gestation. She vaginally delivered a healthy female infant weighing 2578 g. Her postpartum course was uneventful. Although she experienced a few episodes of cholangitis after delivery, she maintained stable liver function for 5.8 years after the delivery.

3.5.3. Patient 3: Favorable Case

A 39-year-old gravida 2, para 1 pregnant woman was referred to our hospital. She had at least seven episodes of cholangitis developed after 18 years old. When she was 37 years old, she delivered vaginally at 39 weeks of gestation and developed cholangitis postpartum. Although she experienced recurrent cholangitis, she did not follow the regularly attended checkup with a pediatric surgeon and conceived spontaneously in a planned manner. Her pregnancy was uneventful, but she experienced cholangitis and was treated with antimicrobial agents at 21 weeks of gestation. During pregnancy, cholangitis recurred four times, and she was treated with antimicrobial agents each time. To prevent liver damage caused by repeated cholangitis, labor induction was performed at 36 weeks of gestation, and she vaginally delivered a healthy male infant weighing 2690 g. Her postpartum course was uneventful. Cholangitis recurred at one and five years after delivery. However, her liver function remained at a good level, and she was alive for 6.8 years after her delivery.

3.5.4. Patient 4: Borderline Case

A 40-year-old gravida 2, para 1 woman with a history of vaginal delivery at 39 weeks of gestation when she was 31 years old was referred to our hospital. She had experienced esophageal varices treated with EVL and some episodes of cholangitis. She started fertility treatment at her discretion and conceived spontaneously during the fertility treatment. At 25 weeks of gestation, cholangitis developed, and she required antimicrobial therapy. At 26 weeks of gestation, gastrointestinal endoscopy revealed worsening of esophageal and gastric varices, and EVL was performed. Fortunately, her pregnancy was uneventful until the day of delivery. At 37 weeks of gestation, a 2590 g healthy male infant was delivered by an elective cesarean section under general anesthesia because of low platelet count ($5.3 \times 10^4/\mu L$). During the postpartum period, pancytopenia and cholangitis were exacerbated. She is alive 6.4 years after delivery, but her liver function has gradually worsened. Liver transplantation was considered.

3.5.5. Patient 5: Unfavorable Case

A 34-year-old gravida 1, para 0 pregnant woman was referred to our hospital at 28 weeks of gestation. Although she experienced several times of cholangitis, she interrupted a routine checkup with a pediatric surgeon at 29 years of age. She was diagnosed with esophageal varices at another hospital, and her condition was treated with EVL. She spontaneously conceived and underwent prenatal checkup at our hospital. At 25 weeks of pregnancy, she was transferred to our emergency room owing to rupture of esophageal varices and received EVL treatment and blood transfusion. She developed hepatic encephalopathy. At 29 weeks and 5 days of gestation, she was diagnosed with fetal growth restriction associated with oligohydramnios, and the estimated fetal weight was 900 g (−2.9 SD) with a 19 mm amniotic fluid pocket. At 30 weeks and 0 days, the patient underwent an emergency cesarean section because of non-reassuring fetal status. An 842 g male infant was delivered, with Apgar scores of four and eight at 1 and 5 min, respectively. Considering that abnormal bleeding due to coagulopathy occurred during the operation, massive blood transfusion and uterine artery embolization were required to stop the bleeding. The total volume of blood loss during delivery was 8700 mL. Her MELD score increased to 11, 13, and 21 at 1, 5, and 10 years after delivery, respectively. Eventually, she underwent liver transplantation 10 years after delivery, but she died in the perioperative period, owing to massive bleeding.

4. Discussion

We demonstrated the details of five perinatal courses in patients after BA surgery (Table 1), which can be summarized as follows: three term babies were successfully born with stable postpartum maternal condition (favorable), one term baby was born with worsening maternal liver function (borderline), and one premature delivery at approximately 30 weeks of gestation with subsequent maternal liver failure 8 years after delivery (unfavorable) [6,11].

Perinatal outcomes after BA surgery with native liver depend on prepregnancy maternal conditions, including frequent episodes of cholangitis and severity of portal hypertension manifesting gastrointestinal bleeding (Table 1) [10,11]. Cholestasis and variceal bleeding commonly occur during the second and third trimesters presumably because of high abdominal pressure, characteristic profiles of steroid hormones, expansion of maternal blood volume, and compression of the inferior vena cava [13,14]. In the current study, some patients (even in the favorable category) developed cholangitis, and their esophageal varices deteriorated; thus, BA patients with a known history of such complications before pregnancy should be followed strictly during the perinatal period.

We analyzed the potential predictors of perinatal outcomes, including the MELD score, platelet count, and serum ChE. The MELD score is an established predictor of survival in patients with liver cirrhosis. Previously, Westbrook et al. [14] demonstrated that a MELD score ≥ 10 was a useful predictor of significant liver-related complications in patients with liver cirrhosis during pregnancy. By contrast, a MELD score ≤ 6 was indicated as an assuring cutoff value. In addition, a platelet count of $<11.0 \times 10^4/\mu L$ was a reliable indicator of the presence of esophageal varices in patients with cirrhosis.

The mean prepregnancy MELD scores in the favorable, unfavorable, and borderline groups were 6.9, 8.7, and 8.9, respectively. These results suggest that MELD scores between 6 and 10 may lead to unfavorable outcomes; however, further studies are warranted to obtain more accurate cutoff values. To obtain a more precise prediction, we advocate the incorporation of platelet count and ChE into our risk stratification. The presence of esophageal varices in Patients 4 and 5, which was consistent with their low platelet counts before pregnancy, corroborated the previous findings, thus leading us to suggest that low platelet count should raise awareness of the presence of esophageal varices in patients with BA. Finally, serum ChE levels <200, which indicate a significantly impaired hepatic functional reserve [16,17], were observed in Patient 5 and resulted in unfavorable perinatal outcomes. In Patient 4, a prenatal ChE >200 led to a borderline outcome as her liver function gradually worsened after pregnancy. Long-term postpartum outcome of liver function in BA patients is still unclear, and, given that the difference in MELD scores and platelet counts between Patients 4 and 5 was minimal, serum ChE may add additional information to delineate a safer pregnancy plan.

The limitations of this study include its retrospective nature, small number of patients, and absence of histological findings to corroborate liver cirrhosis. Additionally, the postpartum deterioration of liver function in Patients 4 and 5 may not be relevant to pregnancy but may reflect the natural course of BA.

Nevertheless, these findings showed the possibility that the combination of the MELD score, platelet count, and serum ChE level is useful for predicting perinatal outcomes even though the absolute cutoff values have not yet been determined, and longitudinal workup enables the delineation of the potential risks of hepatic insufficiency. If an unfavorable course is predicted beforehand, women should be informed of every possibility, including serious complications for both the mother and fetus. Early liver transplantation may be indicated in such cases. In addition, even if preconceptual prediction is favorable, strict follow-up in the perinatal period is mandatory in the pregnancy of patients with BA.

5. Conclusions

In conclusion, pregnancy in patients with BA sometimes experience several types of complications and requires special attention. Serum ChE levels, platelet counts, and MELD scores have a potential to be important markers for predicting perinatal prognosis.

Author Contributions: Conceptualization, N.T., D.O., Y.Y.; methodology, N.T., Y.Y., D.O. and M.T. (Masumi Tamagawa); data curation, N.T., D.O., Y.Y., M.T. (Masumi Tamagawa), H.K., M.K., S.I., Y.K.; Project administration, N.T., D.O., Y.Y.; writing—original draft preparation, N.T., D.O.; writing—review and editing, Y.Y., T.K. and M.T. (Mamoru Tanaka); Supervision, D.O., Y.Y., T.K. and M.T. (Mamoru Tanaka); funding acquisition, M.T. (Mamoru Tanaka). All authors have read and agreed to the published version of the manuscript.

Funding: This research was funded by Japan Society for the Promotion of Science (JSPS) KAKENHI, Grant No. 19K22602.

Institutional Review Board Statement: The study was conducted according to the guidelines of the Declaration of Helsinki, and approved by the Institutional Review Board of Keio University Hospital (20150103).

Informed Consent Statement: This study is retrospective study and Informed consent was obtained in the form of opt-out.

Data Availability Statement: The data presented in this study are available on request from the corresponding author. The data are not publicly available due to patients' privacy.

Acknowledgments: We would like to acknowledge the members of the perinatal team of Keio University Hospital for their help with the data collection for this study.

Conflicts of Interest: The authors declare no conflict of interest. The funders had no role in the design of the study; in the collection, analyses, or interpretation of data; in the writing of the manuscript, or in the decision to publish the results.

References

1. Kasai, M.; Kimura, S.; Asakura, Y.; Suzuki, H.; Taira, Y.; Ohashi, E. Surgical treatment of biliary atresia. *J. Pediatr. Surg.* **1968**, *3*, 665–675.
2. Serinet, M.O.; Wildhaber, B.E.; Broué, P.; Lachaux, A.; Sarles, J.; Jacquemin, E.; Gauthier, F.; Chardot, C. Impact of age at Kasai operation on its results in late childhood and adolescence: A rational basis for biliary atresia screening. *Pediatrics* **2009**, *123*, 1280–1286. [CrossRef] [PubMed]
3. Nio, M.; Sasaki, H.; Wada, M.; Kazama, T.; Nishi, K.; Tanaka, H. Impact of age at Kasai operation on short- and long-term outcomes of type III biliary atresia at a single institution. *J. Pediatr. Surg.* **2010**, *45*, 2361–2363. [CrossRef] [PubMed]
4. Ng, V.L.; Haber, B.H.; Magee, J.C.; Miethke, A.; Murray, K.F.; Michail, S.; Karpen, S.J.; Kerkar, N.; Molleston, J.P.; Romero, R.; et al. Childhood Liver Disease Research and Education Network (CHiLDREN). Medical status of 219 children with biliary atresia surviving long-term with their native livers: Results from a North American multicenter consortium. *J. Pediatr.* **2014**, *165*, 539–546.e2. [CrossRef] [PubMed]
5. Hadzić, N.; Davenport, M.; Tizzard, S.; Singer, J.; Howard, E.R.; Mieli-Vergani, G. Long-term survival following Kasai portoenterostomy: Is chronic liver disease inevitable? *J. Pediatr. Gastroenterol. Nutr.* **2003**, *37*, 430–433. [CrossRef] [PubMed]
6. Shimaoka, S.; Ohi, R.; Saeki, M.; Miyano, T.; Tanaka, K.; Shiraki, K.; Nio, M. Japanese Biliary Atresia Society. Problems during and after pregnancy of former biliary atresia patients treated successfully by the Kasai procedure. *J. Pediatr. Surg.* **2001**, *36*, 349–351. [CrossRef] [PubMed]
7. Ando, H.; Inomata, Y.; Iwanaka, T.; Kuroda, T.; Nio, M.; Matsui, A.; Yoshida, M. Japanese Biliary Atresia Society. Clinical practice guidelines for biliary atresia in Japan: A secondary publication of the abbreviated version translated into English. *J. Hepatobiliary Pancreat Sci.* **2021**, *28*, 55–61. [CrossRef] [PubMed]
8. Kuroda, T.; Saeki, M.; Morikawa, N.; Fuchimoto, Y. Biliary atresia and pregnancy: Puberty may be an important point for predicting the outcome. *J. Pediatr. Surg.* **2005**, *40*, 1852–1855. [CrossRef] [PubMed]
9. Sasaki, H.; Nio, M.; Hayashi, Y.; Ishii, T.; Sano, N.; Ohi, R. Problems during and after pregnancy in female patients with biliary atresia. *J. Pediatr. Surg.* **2007**, *42*, 1329–1332. [CrossRef] [PubMed]
10. O'Sullivan, O.E.; Crosby, D.; Byrne, B.; Regan, C. Pregnancy complicated by portal hypertension secondary to biliary atresia. *Case Rep. Obstet. Gynecol.* **2013**, *2013*, 421386. [CrossRef] [PubMed]
11. Samyn, M.; Davenport, M.; Jain, V.; Hadzic, N.; Joshi, D.; Heneghan, M.; Dhawan, A.; Heaton, N. Young People with Biliary Atresia Requiring Liver Transplantation: A Distinct Population Requiring Specialist Care. *Transplantation* **2019**, *103*, e99–e107. [CrossRef] [PubMed]
12. Kuroda, T.; Saeki, M.; Morikawa, N.; Watanabe, K. Management of adult biliary atresia patients: Should hard work and pregnancy be discouraged? *J. Pediatr. Surg.* **2007**, *42*, 2106–2109. [CrossRef] [PubMed]
13. Samyn, M. Transitional care of biliary atresia. *Semin. Pediatr. Surg.* **2020**, *29*, 150948. [CrossRef] [PubMed]
14. Westbrook, R.H.; Yeoman, A.D.; O'Grady, J.G.; Harrison, P.M.; Devlin, J.; Heneghan, M.A. Model for end-stage liver disease score predicts outcome in cirrhotic patients during pregnancy. *Clin. Gastroenterol. Hepatol.* **2011**, *9*, 694–699. [CrossRef] [PubMed]
15. Kim, W.R.; Biggins, S.W.; Kremers, W.K.; Wiesner, R.H.; Kamath, P.S.; Benson, J.T.; Edwards, E.; Therneau, T.M. Hyponatremia and mortality among patients on the liver-transplant waiting list. *N. Engl. J. Med.* **2008**, *359*, 1018–1026. [CrossRef] [PubMed]
16. Pathak, B.; Sheibani, L.; Lee, R.H. Cholestasis of pregnancy. *Obstet Gynecol. Clin. N. Am.* **2010**, *37*, 269–282. [CrossRef] [PubMed]
17. Tan, J.; Surti, B.; Saab, S. Pregnancy and cirrhosis. *Liver Transpl.* **2008**, *14*, 1081–1091. [CrossRef] [PubMed]

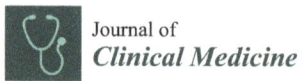

Review

Biliary Atresia: Clinical Phenotypes and Aetiological Heterogeneity

Mark Davenport [1,*], Ancuta Muntean [1] and Nedim Hadzic [2]

[1] Department of Pediatric Surgery, Kings College Hospital, London SE5 9RS, UK; ancuta.muntean@nhs.net
[2] Department of Paediatric Hepatology, Kings College Hospital, London SE5 9RS, UK; nedim.hadzic@kcl.ac.uk
* Correspondence: markdav2@ntlworld.com; Tel.: +44-203-299-3350; Fax: +44-203-299-4021

Abstract: Biliary atresia (BA) is an obliterative condition of the biliary tract that presents with persistent jaundice and pale stools typically in the first few weeks of life. While this phenotypic signature may be broadly similar by the time of presentation, it is likely that this is only the final common pathway with a number of possible preceding causative factors and disparate pathogenic mechanisms—i.e., aetiological heterogeneity. Certainly, there are distinguishable variants which suggest a higher degree of aetiological homogeneity such as the syndromic variants of biliary atresia splenic malformation or cat-eye syndrome, which implicate an early developmental mechanism. In others, the presence of synchronous viral infection also make this plausible as an aetiological agent though it is likely that disease onset is from the perinatal period. In the majority of cases, currently termed isolated BA, there are still too few clues as to aetiology or indeed pathogenesis.

Keywords: biliary atresia; Kasai operation; liver transplant; etiology; adjuvant therapy

1. Introduction

Biliary atresia (BA) is an obliterative condition of the biliary tract that presents with persistent jaundice, pale stools and dark urine in the first weeks of life and, if left untreated, ultimately leads to cirrhosis and end-stage liver failure (Figure 1). Beyond this unchallenged statement, much of the rest are observational facts and hypothetical speculation. This is certainly the case for its aetiology if not its post-natal pathogenesis [1]. The aim of this chapter is to review the spectrum of BA as it presents to the clinician reinforcing this concept of aetiological heterogeneity as a principle feature of the disease itself.

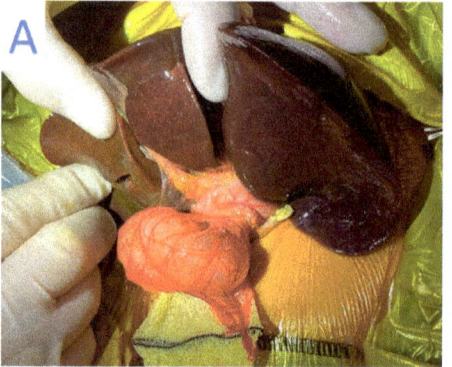
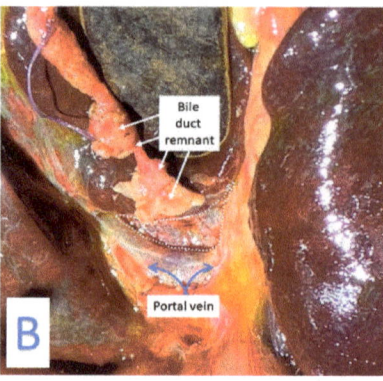

Figure 1. (**A**) Biliary atresia: Liver is mobilized and exteriorized to expose the porta hepatis. (**B**): Dissection of the Porta Hepatis. The bile duct remnant has been transected and is lying on segment 4 of the retracted liver. The white dotted area outlines the extent of the porta hepatis which will then be anastomosed to the Roux jejunal loop.

Geographical Variation and Incidence

The incidence of BA is markedly variable across the world, ranging from about 1:5–10,000 live births in Taiwan [2] and Japan [3] and presumably in China to about 1:15,000–19,000 in Europe [4,5]. The incidence in North America tends to parallel the latter estimates, with the most recent data based on US billing returns at 1:22,000 [6] and 1:19,000 based on Canadian Registry data [7]. Interestingly, both these later studies have suggested that its incidence has increased over the past 20 years, although the explanation is far from clear and has certainly not been suggested elsewhere. The incidence in other parts of the world such as the Indian sub-continent, South America and Africa is less clear in the absence of national studies. Aetiological heterogeneity is one obvious explanation of such variation with the proportion of different variants changing with the local environment or some genetic predisposition.

Some national studies have looked at racial composition for evidence of variation. Evans et al. reported the national New Zealand series quoting an incidence of 1 in 5285 in those of Māori ancestry compared to about 1 in 16,000 live-births for those of European ancestry [8]. Our own experience in England and Wales supports a significant ethnic variation so there is a significant variation by health region from 1 in 14,000 in London the region with the highest non-white ethnicity (40.4%) to 1 in 22,700 for North-West England with one of the lowest non-white ethnicity proportions (14.6%) (Figure 2).

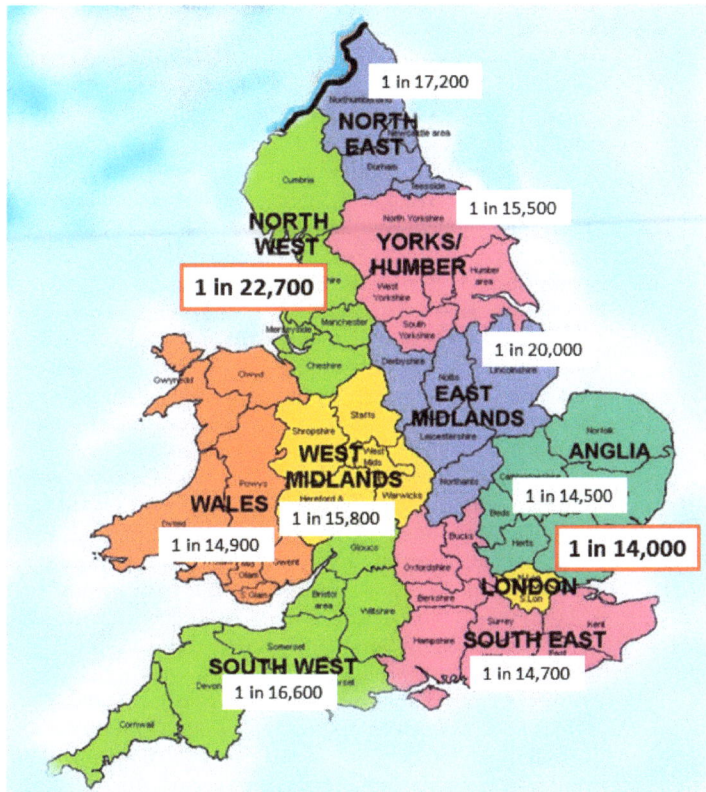

Figure 2. Variation in prevalence of Biliary Atresia in England and Wales (*n* = 713, 1999–2015).

Whether there is some kind of genetic predisposition is not known. Most of the work on this subject has emerged from varying parts of the world, but notably China with initial identification of *ADD3* and *XPNPEP1* mutations in a Han Chinese population [9] and more recently a spectrum of biallelic deleterious variants in liver-expressed "ciliary genes" [10]. However, the degree of risk seems small, as the latter study implies only a two-fold increase in risk compared to normal.

2. Aetiological Heterogeneity

From a clinical perspective, we can separate BA into distinct categories featuring common characteristics (Table 1).

Table 1. Etiological heterogeneity—clinical categories of Biliary Atresia.

Category		Associated Clinical Features
Isolated BA (70–80%)		
Syndromic BA (10–15%)	BASM	Polysplenia, asplenia, situs inversus, pre-duodenal portal vein, absence of IVC, CHD, malrotation.
	Cat-eye syndrome	Coloboma, ano-rectal atresia, CHD et al.
	"Non-syndromic"	e.g., Esophageal atresia, jejunal atresia, cleft palate et al.
Cystic BA (5–10%)		Antenatal or postnatal detected cyst at porta hepatis.
CMV IgM + ve BA (~10%)		Defined by CMV IgM + ve antibodies. ↑age at KPE, ↑AST ↑spleen size. Th1 predominant mononuclear infiltrate in liver

CHD—congenital heart disease, IVC—inferior vena cava, AST—aspartate aminotransferase, CMV—cytomegalovirus, KPE—portoenterostomy.

2.1. Syndromic Biliary Atresia

We recognise two syndromes where BA is a key feature (Table 1). The commonest of these is the Biliary Atresia Splenic Malformation (BASM) syndrome, which accounts for about 10–15% of European and American series [11,12], but is distinctly rare in Chinese and Japanese series (<2%) [13,14]. For instance, Zhan et al. reviewed 851 cases from five centres in mainland China [13]. There were only two (i.e., 0.23%) with situs inversus and four (i.e., 0.5%) with polysplenia—both hallmarks of BASM. In Japan, there is a reported incidence of about 4% from the Sendai series [14]. By comparison, we have an incidence of 14% in our national registry of infants from England and Wales (1999–2000) (unpublished observation).

The phenotype of BASM is unmistakable and can be characterised by a host of visceral anomalies. The splenic malformation is typically polysplenia, but sometimes can be asplenia or double spleen [11,15]. The other obvious and evident visceral anomalies are: situs inversus, present in about 30–40% of patients with and without malrotation; preduodenal portal vein and a complete absence of the intrahepatic vena cava. Cardiac anomalies are apparent in about half the cases overall, but there is lack of a consistent cardiac phenotype. Indeed, when we reviewed our experience of biliary atresia-associated cardiac anomalies ($n = 37$), features indicative of BASM were present in 48% [16].

Therefore, how might we explain BASM? The biliary system develops in two distinct phases. Firstly, the extrahepatic bile duct arises as an outpouching of the foregut at Carnegie embryo stage 11 (4th week) and is essentially complete at about Carnegie embryo stage 17 (6th week) with a patent common duct and gallbladder, all in intimate contact with the developing, predominantly haematopoietic, liver. The other constituents within the liver at this stage are the hepatoblasts, which then differentiate into hepatocytes from around 49 days (7th week), and biliary epithelial cells (now expressing SOX9 and CK19), which by a process of selection and deletion around the ingrowing portal venous network initially form the ductal plate and then a more mature tubularising biliary network. Actual contact and interlacing with the extrahepatic duct occur at or around 12 weeks gestational age, just in time to transport newly formed bile from the hepatocytes into the gallbladder and duodenum.

As this biliary timeline is shared by the determination of visceral situs, spleen formation, evolution of the portal venous and caval venous system anomalies it is not too much to speculate that BASM is also an embryonic defect. The actual mechanism is still obscure though, and a genetic mutation has long been sought to explain BASM. Previous case reports suggested mutations in *CFC1*, *NODAL*, *FOXA2* and *ZIC3*, e.g., [17]. However, the first systematic search in a population was only recently carried out by Berauer et al. [18] using whole exome screening of 67 infants with the "BASM" phenotype and in 58 including their parents as a trio analysis. This being a good example of the benefits of a large multicentre biobank—the ChiLDReN network. It is worth noting, however, that only 60% of this group actually had a splenic malformation, with four being counted despite only having isolated renal anomalies—something not a part of the original definition [15]. Five children with "BASM" had rare biallelic variants in the gene, polycystin 1-like 1 (*PKD1L1*) found on chromosome 7. There is also a biologically plausible pathogenic mechanism, at least in the mouse, as *Pkd1l1* heterodimerizes with *Pkd2l1* in primary cilia, to form a transmembrane ciliary calcium channel that ultimately influences downstream Hedgehog signalling. Such heterodimers are required to establish normal left–right asymmetry and are an obvious fit for the genesis of situs inversus.

If not genetic then what? Well, the original BASM series also identified a link with maternal diabetes and possibly other first trimester 'insults', which influence the embryonic environment though these still remain poorly defined [10,15]. The National Birth Defects Prevention study from the USA also recently identified a significant association between first trimester use of bronchodilators and anti-inflammatory medication and subsequent biliary atresia in their offspring. Whether the cases identified were syndromic in any way is not known [19].

The Cat-eye syndrome (CES) or at least, aneuploidy of chromosome 22, is less well described, but its association with BA seems clear [20]. We originally described five infants (4 with BA) from a combined London and Paris series with a range of genetic anomalies including classical Cat-eye syndrome, partial duplication of chromosome 22 (supernumerary der(22) syndrome), and a mosaic for trisomy 22. Clinically, these infants typically have coloboma, cardiac anomalies and anorectal malformations. Some have even had neonatal surgical procedures before the biliary association was recognised.

There are also other defined syndromes which may have BA as a component though are much less frequently reported. Some examples from our National BA series of over 800 infants were Kabuki syndrome [21] (characteristic facial features, skeletal anomalies and mild developmental delay), Zimmermann–Laband syndrome (cranio-facial and oral abnormalities including gingival fibromatosis), Kartagener syndrome (ciliary motility pathology causing situs inversus, chronic sinusitis and bronchiectasis) and perhaps the much more common Hirschsprung disease (Table 2). In some of these, there were also overlapping features with BASM—both of the infants with Kartagener syndrome for instance.

There also appears to be a non-random association (i.e., more than would be expected by chance) with some other otherwise isolated anomalies such as oesophageal atresia, duodenal atresia, jejunal atresia, cleft palate, etc. (Table 1). Again, some showed an obvious overlap with BASM (e.g., duodenal atresia with 10/13 cases), while others did not (e.g., oesophageal atresia with 1/8 cases).

We have recently characterised another sub-group defined purely by its association with cardiac anomalies (cardiac-associated biliary atresia or CABA) [16]. While we do not claim that this has a uniform pathogenesis, it is clearly a high-risk subgroup and one of the main contributors for actual mortality in BA overall. As an aside, we have recommended a 'heart-first' strategy with restorative cardiac surgical physiology preceding KPE if possible, to improve both liver outcome and overall survival.

2.2. Cystic Biliary Atresia

Cystic changes, usually containing mucus, but sometimes bile, can also be found at the level of the otherwise obliterated extrahepatic biliary tree [22–24]. This is cystic BA (CBA), and care needs to be taken to avoid being misdiagnosed as a congenital choledochal cyst. Both may be antenatally detected on the maternal ultrasound, usually around the time of the feta anomaly scan at 18–20 weeks of gestation, though the former changes are usually consistently smaller [23]. This distinction is important, as they have a different clinical course. All those with CBA will remain jaundiced with pale stool, while some neonates with cystic choledochal malformations may actually clear the jaundice and have normally pigmented stool. Timely operative cholangiography is the key investigation in a jaundiced infant with a postnatally confirmed subhepatic cyst. In CBA, this may show a connection with the intrahepatic ducts or ductules and it is usually tenuous and clearly abnormal, often being described as "cloud-like" [22].

Table 2. Associated anomalies and structural biliary anomalies in the National England and Wales Biliary Atresia Registry (January 1999–December 2019) $n = 867$.

Anomaly	Total N (%)	Notes and Overlap
Recognised Syndromic Association		
BASM	122 (14.1%)	
Cat-Eye/Emanuel syndrome	7 (0.8%)	
Possible Syndromic Association		
Kabuki syndromic	3	
Kartagener's syndrome	2	BASM ($n = 2$)
Hirschsprung's disease	2	Cat-eye syndrome ($n = 1$)
Zimmermann-Laband syndrome	1	
Gastrointestinal Anomalies		
Duodenal atresia	13 (1.5%)	BASM ($n = 10$)
Ano-rectal anomalies	5	BASM ($n = 1$)
Oesophageal atresia	8 (1%)	BASM ($n = 1$)
Jejunal/ileal atresia	4	BASM ($n = 3$)
Pyloric stenosis	1	Ch6p deletion
Other Anomalies		
Cardiac anomalies (isolated)	6	Ring Chromosome18 ($n = 1$)
Cleft lip/palate	6	
Isolated Anomalies		
Exomphalos	1	
Gastroschisis	1	
Spina bifida	1	
Choanal atresia	1	

This, at least, implies an onset beyond 12 weeks (to allow bile to come into the common duct), which is completely developed by 16–18 weeks, the earliest point at which antenatal detection might be made. This phase is co-incident with the arterialisation of the liver, and one could speculate that there may have been some ischaemic event affecting the distal extrahepatic duct with consequential proximal dilatation.

Early studies showed that it was possible to reproduce the key features of CBA in experimental models: by ligation of the common bile duct in foetal lambs at about 80 days of gestation, and by ligation of the hepatic artery in foetal rabbits [25–27]. Not only can this produce cystic extrahepatic change, but also in a proportion impairment of the intrahepatic bile ducts as well [27]. More recently, a group from Porto Allegre, Brazil have looked at the possible role of ischaemia in reproducing the cholangiopathy of (isolated, not necessarily CBA) BA by hepatic arterial morphometry and expression of angiogenesis mediators. BA specifically seems to be characterised by an increase in arterial medial layer thickness at the time of portoenterostomy compared to controls and becoming progressive in those requiring liver transplant [28]. Furthermore, gene expression of hypoxia-inducible factors (HIF), HIF1a and HIF2a were increased in BA cases, while vascular endothelial growth factors (VEGFA) (VEGFR1 and VEGFR2) were decreased suggesting reduced angiogenesis [29]. Whether these observations are indicative of an aetiological factor or in some way secondary to the inevitable changes wrought by fibrogenesis is not known.

Most CBA cases, even those with bile-filled cysts, should still come to a radical resection and wide portoenterostomy rather than attempt to preserve any part of the cyst. Post-operatively, these infants have >75% chance of clearance of jaundice and native liver preservation, though their prognosis does appear to have a marked relationship with age at surgery [30]. Certainly by comparison with the other variants, these children have a better long-term prognosis [31], though our recent review of 20 year follow-up in the national BA registry showed that a significant proportion of these seemed to decompensate requiring liver replacement during their transition to adulthood (unpublished observation).

2.3. Cytomegalovirus-Associated BA [See Also Fischler et al. CMV and BA in Same Issue]

In 1974, the American paediatrician, Benjamin Landing, proposed that a perinatal viral infection might be one of the origins of BA [32]. Nevertheless, he was not too specific in this pronouncement, and also proposed the same for choledochal cysts and neonatal hepatis as well. Several candidate viruses have been suggested over the years, with the original being REO-virus Type 3 both by serological [33] and PCR studies [34], though this has been disputed by more recent Japanese evidence involving a much bigger numbers of patients [35] and a review of published studies [36]. Indeed, the relevance of any viral identification was questioned by Rauschenfels et al. from Hannover who, using multiple viral PCR primers, identified viral genetic material in a significant proportion, but felt this was more likely to be a secondary phenomenon [37].

Of all the candidate hepatotropic viruses, perinatal cytomegalovirus (CMV) infection, a double-stranded DNA virus from the Herpesviridae family, has received most attention. The relationship was first suggested by Bjorn Fischler and a Swedish group in 1998 observing a high proportion of their cohort of BA with signs of CMV infection [38].

It is clear that this virus can be detected in a variable proportion of cases of BA, but this too has shown marked global variation. Therefore, using CMV IgM antibodies as a marker of infection up to 30% of Chinese BA series have been positive [39] compared to about 10% in a UK series [40]. Furthermore, in a series from Denver, CO, 55% of BA cases were shown to have CMV-specific T cell responses at the time of surgery also suggesting early exposure [41].

What is not known is the timing of exposure of the virus in these infants. We have no additional data of their CMV status—i.e., antenatal maternal CMV serology or whether for instance their neonatal screening blood spot tests were also IgM positive.

In our experience, CMV IgM positive infants do have distinct clinical and histological features compared to those with IBA, such as: an older age at diagnosis; larger ultrasound-measured spleen sizes and a greater degree of histological liver inflammation and fibrosis, even when that is corrected for post-natal age [40]. Interestingly it can also be shown that they have a Th1 predominant mononuclear cell infiltrate, again compared to those with IBA and even the syndromic BA infants [42].

At least at Kings College Hospital, these infants, by comparison to CMV IgM negative controls, have a poorer outcome with a reduced clearance of jaundice and native liver survival together with a demonstrable increase in actual mortality [40]. A more recent systematic analysis of published evidence also seemed to support CMV as a negative prognostic factor [43].

The actual mechanism of the cholangiopathy in such infants is intriguing and may not be simple direct cholangiocyte damage by the virus. Rather, it is believed to be a more subtle auto-immune process with the virus triggering self-damage, allowing perpetuation of a pro-inflammatory immune response driven by macrophages, NK cells, Th1 and Th17 cells and unrestrained by a postulated deficit in regulatory T cells. The details of this aspect are outside the remit of this article, but the concepts are illustrated by Figure 3, based on Kilgore and Mack [44] and Ortiz-Perez et al. [45].

2.4. Isolated BA

The term "isolated" BA is used when there are no other defining characteristics, and unfortunately, this is the largest clinical grouping with no real hint as to its aetiological mechanism. Nevertheless, these still might include genetic [9,10], developmental [10], ischaemic [28], environmental [46] and other viral causes [34,35,38,40,44,45].

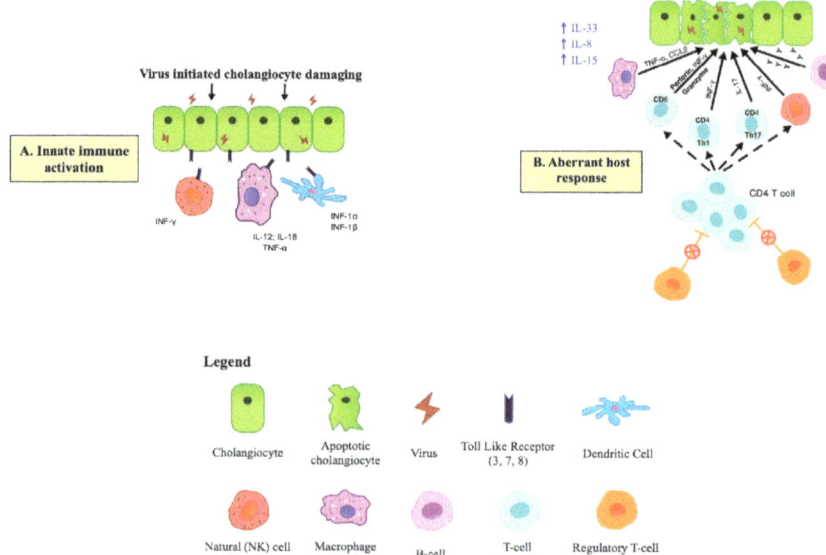

Figure 3. Suggested immunopathogenesis of Biliary Atresia. (**A**) Transient virus infection of cholangiocytes results in upregulation of Toll-Like Receptors (TLR) and a broad-based activation of the innate immune system involving macrophages, dendritic cells and NK cells. (**B**) Adaptive T cell proliferation (Th2 and Th17 predominant), supported by B cells and activated macro-phages cause cholangiocyte damage, possibly unrestrained by the absence of Tregs. Dissection of the Porta Hepatis. The bile duct remnant has been transected and is lying on segment 4 of the retracted liver. The white dotted area outlines the extent of the porta hepatis which will then be anastomosed to the Roux jejunal loop.

There may well be some kind of non-Mendelian genetic predisposition to the development of isolated BA, although the scale of this is completely unknown. The relationship between *ADD3* and *XPNPEP1* mutations has been mentioned before [9], though more recent studies involving genome-wide association studies (GWAS) in various discrete populations have also implicated *GPC-1* [47]. The latter is expressed in biliary epithelial cells and is involved in inflammatory mediators making a contribution to biliary pathology plausible. Other recent studies have used whole exome sequencing (WES) in small cohorts of clinically diagnosed BA cases throwing up candidate genes that have included those involved in the ABC superfamily, and the Notch signalling pathway (JAG1) [48]. Finally, there may be mutations which can modify the response to treatment (i.e., Kasai portoenterostomy). Mezina and Karpen [49] reported a greater frequency of variants (e.g., p.A934T) in the gene encoding the phospholipid floppase, *ABCB4* in those who required early liver transplant compared to those with a good outcome. Whether these are really significant either as predisposing or modifying elements remains to be seen. Clearly, there may be overlap, at least genetic, with a variety of other, more distinct, neonatal cholestasis syndromes such as Alagille's syndrome and PFIC.

3. Pathological Classification

At surgery, and essentially unrelated to the foregoing descriptions, the pathological type of BA is defined by the most proximal level of biliary obstruction. Type 1 BA (5–10%) is where obstruction to bile flow is at the level of common bile duct, and typically bile is found in the gallbladder. The proximal biliary tract is often cystic in these. In Type 2 BA, the obstruction is at the level of the common hepatic duct and dissection within the porta hepatis will show two distinct, albeit thick-walled and abnormal, hepatic ducts. This is exceedingly rare in most series (1–2%). By contrast, Type 3 BA, is by far the most common (>90%) with its obstruction level high within the porta hepatis and in these there are no visible macroscopic ductules present—the transected porta presenting a fairly uniform bland appearance.

BASM is somewhat of an exception to the foregoing, as there is a characteristic appearance of the remnant extrahepatic bile duct. There is usually a small solid gallbladder and absent common bile duct, with often quite defined proximal segmental branching in and around the abnormal portal vasculature.

4. Timing of Disease Onset

This is an important principle in trying to identify when BA actually occurs. We have already made the case for intrauterine onset in BASM, and the other syndromic and non-syndromic associations; and for cystic biliary atresia, but for the largest grouping of isolated and indeed viral-association BA we really have little actual evidence. Is isolated BA truly a congenital anomaly present at birth or is it acquired somewhat later? The pendulum has swung on this over the years, as initially it was felt to be mostly perinatal in onset with a period of normal pigmented stools and later onset of jaundice.

Still there are two important areas of study which might tilt the balance of opinion. The first arose from obstetric observations initially made by a French group [50]. γ-glutamyl transpeptidase (GGT) is specifically secreted by biliary epithelial cells and is normally found in high levels in amniotic fluid during the second trimester due to passage of bile into the foetal intestine. Its level normally tails off during the third trimester as the foetal anal sphincter closes. In cases that were later shown to be BA, this second trimester rise does not happen suggesting that the bile flow had already ceased. A more recent series of clinical experience with amniotic fluid GGT measurement has been reported by an Israeli group and combined with non-visualisation of the foetal gallbladder [51,52]. Perhaps surprisingly, this latter observation is not usually associated with BA. However, amniotic fluid GGT was measured in 32 cases with the non-visualisation in this series and found to be low in five. In three of these, a postnatal diagnosis of BA was made.

The second key evidential observation for the isolated form comes from the work of Sanjiv Harpavat's group in Houston, Texas [53]. Initially, they retrospectively screened fractionated bilirubin levels in BA infants and showed that their direct conjugated bilirubin was abnormally elevated in all 34 BA patients at day 1 and 2 of life [54]. Subsequent studies from the same group have confirmed this key observation [55] and also raised considerable expectations for neonatal screening for BA at least in North America.

5. Conclusions

BA is still a fascinating enigma of a disease with much to unravel as far as its clinical manifestation. It seems unlikely we will uncover a universal hypothesis to explain its aetiology sometime soon and appropriate caution should accompany those laboratory findings which assume insight, particularly when based on experimental animal models without parallel in the natural world. It seems far more likely that the infants that we see both in the operating room and the clinic have arrived there by a multiplicity of possible pathways.

Author Contributions: M.D. conceived and designed the review and wrote the first draft; A.M. contributed to the final draft and drew Figure 3; N.H. contributed to the final draft. All authors have read and agreed to the published version of the manuscript.

Funding: This research received no external funding.

Acknowledgments: We acknowledge the key contribution made by EP Ong and K Sharif (Birmingham Children's Hospital) and N Alizai and M Dawrant (Leeds Children's Hospital) in the formation and maintenance of the National (England and Wales) Biliary Atresia Registry.

Conflicts of Interest: The authors declare no conflict of interest.

Abbreviations

BA	biliary atresia,
BASM	biliary atresia splenic malformation,
CES	cat-eye syndrome
CHD	congenital heart disease,
IVC	inferior vena cava,
AST	aspartate aminotransferase,
CMV	cytomegalovirus,
GGT	γ-glutamyl transpeptidase
IBAT	Ileal bile acid transporters,
KPE	Kasai's portoenterostomy,
MMP-7	Serum matrix metalloproteinase-7.

References

1. Petersen, C.; Davenport, M. Aetiology of biliary atresia: What is actually known? *Orphanet J. Rare Dis.* **2013**, *8*, 128. [CrossRef]
2. Lin, Y.-C.; Chang, M.-H.; Liao, S.-F.; Wu, J.-F.; Ni, Y.-H.; Tiao, M.-M.; Lai, M.-W.; Lee, H.-C.; Lin, C.-C.; Wu, T.-C.; et al. Decreasing rate of biliary atresia in Taiwan: A survey, 2004–2009. *Pediatrics* **2011**, *128*, 2004–2009. [CrossRef]
3. Wada, H.; Muraji, T.; Yokoi, A.; Okamoto, T.; Sato, S.; Takamizawa, S.; Tsugawa, J.; Nishijima, E. Insignificant seasonal and geographical variation in incidence of biliary atresia in Japan: A regional survey of over 20 years. *J. Pediatr. Surg.* **2007**, *42*, 2090–2092. [CrossRef] [PubMed]
4. Chardot, C.; Carton, M.; Spire-Bendelac, N.; Pommelet, C.L.; Golmard, J.L.; Auvert, B. Epidemiology of biliary atresia in France: A national study 1986–96. *J. Hepatol.* **1999**, *31*, 1006–1013. [CrossRef]
5. Livesey, E.; Cortina Borja, M.; Sharif, K.; Alizai, N.; McClean, P.; Kelly, D.; Hadzic, N.; Davenport, M. Epidemiology of biliary atresia in England and Wales (1999–2006). *Arch. Dis. Child. Fetal Neonatal Ed.* **2009**, *94*, 451–456. [CrossRef]
6. Hopkins, P.C.; Yazigi, N.; Nylund, C.M. Incidence of Biliary Atresia and Timing of Hepatoportoenterostomy in the United States. *J. Pediatr.* **2017**, *187*, 253–257. [CrossRef] [PubMed]
7. Schreiber, R.A.; Barker, C.C.; Roberts, E.A.; Martin, S.R.; Alvarez, F.; Smith, L.; Butzner, J.D.; Wrobel, I.; Mack, D.; Moroz, S.; et al. Biliary Atresia: The Canadian Experience. *J. Pediatr.* **2007**, *151*, 659–665. [CrossRef] [PubMed]
8. Evans, H.M.; Asher, M.I.; Cameron-Christie, S.; Farthing, S.; McCall, J.; Robertson, S.P.; Wong, H.; Morreau, P.N. Ethnic Disparity in the Incidence and Outcome of Biliary Atresia in New Zealand. *J. Pediatr. Gastroenterol. Nutr.* **2018**, *66*, 218–221. [CrossRef]
9. Garcia-Barceló, M.M.; Yeung, M.Y.; Miao, X.P.; Tang, C.S.M.; Chen, G.; So, M.T.; Ngan, E.S.W.; Lui, V.C.H.; Chen, Y.; Liu, X.L.; et al. Genome-wide association study identifies a susceptibility locus for biliary atresia on 10q24.2. *Hum. Mol. Genet.* **2010**, *19*, 2917–2925. [CrossRef] [PubMed]
10. Lama, W.Y.; Tang, C.S.-M.; So, M.-T.; Yue, H.; Hsu, J.S.; Chung, P.H.-Y.; Nichlls, J.M.; Yeung, F.; Lee, C.-W.D.; Ngo, D.N.; et al. Identification of a wide spectrum of ciliary gene mutations in nonsyndromic biliary atresia patients implicates ciliary dysfunction as a novel disease mechanism. *EBioMedicine* **2021**, *71*, 103530. [CrossRef]
11. Davenport, M.; Tizzard, S.A.; Underhill, J.; Mieli-Vergani, G.; Portmann, B.; Hadžić, N. The biliary atresia splenic malformation syndrome: A 28-year single-center retrospective study. *J. Pediatr.* **2006**, *149*, 393–400. [CrossRef]
12. Fanna, M.; Masson, G.; Capito, C.; Girard, M.; Guerin, F.; Hermeziu, B.; Lachaux, A.; Roquelaure, B.; Gottrand, F.; Broue, P.; et al. Management of Biliary Atresia in France 1986 to 2015: Long-term Results. *J. Pediatr. Gastroenterol. Nutr.* **2019**, *69*, 416–424. [CrossRef] [PubMed]
13. Zhan, J.; Feng, J.; Chen, Y.; Liu, J.; Wang, B. Incidence of biliary atresia associated congenital malformations: A retrospective multicenter study in China. *Asian J. Surg.* **2017**, *40*, 429–433. [CrossRef] [PubMed]
14. Nio, M.; Wada, M.; Sasaki, H.; Tanaka, H.; Watanabe, T. Long-term outcomes of biliary atresia with splenic malformation. *J. Pediatr. Surg.* **2015**, *50*, 2124–2127. [CrossRef] [PubMed]
15. Davenport, M.; Savage, M.; Mowat, A.P.; Howard, E.R. Biliary atresia splenic malformation syndrome: An etiologic and prognostic subgroup. *Surgery* **1993**, *113*, 662–668.
16. Aldeiri, B.; Giamouris, V.; Pushparajah, K.; Miller, O.; Baker, A.; Davenport, M. Cardiac-associated biliary atresia (CABA): A prognostic subgroup. *Arch. Dis. Child.* **2021**, *106*, 68–72. [CrossRef]
17. Tsai, E.A.; Grochowski, C.M.; Falsey, A.M.; Rajagopalan, R.; Wendel, D.; Devoto, M.; Krantz, I.D.; Loomes, K.M.; Spinner, N.B. Heterozygous Deletion of FOXA2 Segregates with Disease in a Family with Heterotaxy, Panhypopituitarism, and Biliary Atresia. *Hum. Mutat.* **2015**, *36*, 631–637. [CrossRef]
18. Berauer, J.P.; Mezina, A.I.; Okou, D.T.; Sabo, A.; Muzny, D.M.; Gibbs, R.A.; Hegde, M.R.; Chopra, P.; Cutler, D.J.; Perlmutter, D.H.; et al. Identification of Polycystic Kidney Disease 1 Like 1 Gene Variants in Children With Biliary Atresia Splenic Malformation Syndrome. *Hepatology* **2019**, *70*, 899–910. [CrossRef]
19. Howley, M.M.; Papadopoulos, E.A.; Van Bennekom, C.M.; Van Zutphen, A.R.; Carmichael, S.L.; Munsie, J.P.W.; Herdt, M.L.; Browne, M.L. Asthma Medication Use and Risk of Birth Defects: National Birth Defects Prevention Study, 1997-2011. *J. Allergy Clin. Immunol. Pract.* **2020**, *8*, 3490–3499.e9. [CrossRef]

20. Allotey, J.; Lacaille, F.; Lees, M.M.; Strautnieks, S.; Thompson, R.J.; Davenport, M. Congenital bile duct anomalies (biliary atresia) and chromosome 22 aneuploidy. *J. Pediatr. Surg.* **2008**, *43*, 1736–1740. [CrossRef]
21. McGaughran, J.M.; Donnai, D.; Clayton-Smith, J. Biliary atresia in Kabuki syndrome. *Am. J. Med. Genet.* **2000**, *91*, 157–158. [CrossRef]
22. Caponcelli, E.; Knisely, A.S.; Davenport, M. Cystic biliary atresia: An etiologic and prognostic subgroup. *J. Pediatr. Surg.* **2008**, *43*, 1619–1624. [CrossRef] [PubMed]
23. Yu, P.; Dong, N.; Pan, Y.K.; Li, L. Comparison between cystic biliary atresia and choledochal cyst: A clinical controlled study. *Pediatr. Surg. Int.* **2021**, in press. [CrossRef]
24. Tsuchida, Y.; Kawarasaki, H.; Iwanaka, T.; Uchida, H.; Nakanishi, H.; Uno, K. Antenatal diagnosis of biliary atresia (type I cyst) at 19 weeks' gestation: Differential diagnosis and etiologic implications. *J. Pediatr. Surg.* **1995**, *30*, 697–699. [CrossRef]
25. Holder, T.M.; Ashcraft, K.W. Production of experimental biliary atresia by ligation of the common bile duct in the fetus. *Surg. Forum* **1966**, *17*, 356–357.
26. Spitz, L. Ligation of the common bile duct in the fetal lamb: An experimental model for the study of biliary atresia. *Pediatr. Res.* **1980**, *14*, 740–748. [CrossRef]
27. Morgan, W.W., Jr.; Rosenkrantz, J.C.; Hill, R.B., Jr. Hepatic arterial interruption in the fetus—An attempt to simulate biliary atresia. *J. Pediatr. Surg* **1966**, *1*, 342–346. [CrossRef]
28. dos Santos, J.L.; da Silveira, T.R.; da Silva, V.D.; Cerski, C.T.; Wagner, M.B. Medial thickening of hepatic artery branches in biliary atresia. A morphometric study. *J. Pediatr. Surg.* **2005**, *40*, 637–642. [CrossRef]
29. Fratta, L.X.S.; Hoss, G.R.W.; Longo, L.; Uribe-Cruz, C.; Da Silveira, T.R.; Vieira, S.M.G.; Kieling, C.O.; Dos Santos, J.L. Hypoxic-ischemic gene expression profile in the isolated variant of biliary atresia. *J. Hepatobiliary Pancreat. Sci.* **2015**, *22*, 846–854. [CrossRef] [PubMed]
30. Davenport, M.; Caponcelli, E.; Livesey, E.; Hadzic, N.; Howard, E. Surgical outcome in biliary atresia etiology affects the influence of age at surgery. *Ann. Surg.* **2008**, *247*, 694–698. [CrossRef]
31. Davenport, M.; Ong, E.; Sharif, K.; Alizai, N.; McClean, P.; Hadzic, N.; Kelly, D.A. Biliary atresia in England and Wales: Results of centralization and new benchmark. *J. Pediatr. Surg.* **2011**, *46*, 1689–1694. [CrossRef]
32. Landing, B.H. Considerations of the pathogenesis of neonatal hepatitis, biliary atresia and choledochal cyst–the concept of infantile obstructive cholangiopathy. *Prog. Pediatr. Surg.* **1974**, *6*, 113–139. [PubMed]
33. Morecki, R.; Glaser, J.H.; Cho, S.; Balistreri, W.F.; Horwitz, M.S. Biliary atresia and Reovirus Type 3 infection. *N. Engl. J. Med.* **1982**, *307*, 481–484. [CrossRef] [PubMed]
34. Tyler, K.L.; Sokol, R.J.; Oberhaus, S.M.; Le, M.; Karrer, F.M.; Narkewicz, M.R.; Tyson, R.W.; Murphy, J.R.; Low, R.; Brown, W.R. Detection of reovirus RNA in hepatobiliary tissues from patients with extrahepatic biliary atresia and choledochal cysts. *Hepatology* **1998**, *27*, 1475–1482. [CrossRef]
35. Saito, T.; Shinozaki, K.; Matsunaga, T.; Ogawa, T.; Etoh, T.; Muramatsu, T.; Kawamura, K.; Yoshida, H.; Ohnuma, N.; Shirasawa, H. Lack of evidence for reovirus infection in tissues from patients with biliary atresia and congenital dilatation of the bile duct. *J. Hepatol.* **2004**, *40*, 203–211. [CrossRef]
36. Saito, T.; Terui, K.; Mitsunaga, T.; Nakata, M.; Ono, S.; Mise, N.; Yoshida, H. Evidence for viral infection as a causative factor of human biliary atresia. *J. Pediatr. Surg.* **2015**, *50*, 1398–1404. [CrossRef]
37. Rauschenfels, S.; Krassmann, M.; Al-Masri, A.N.; Verhagen, W.; Leonhardt, J.; Kuebler, J.F.; Petersen, C. Incidence of hepatotropic viruses in biliary atresia. *Eur. J. Pediatr.* **2009**, *168*, 469–476. [CrossRef]
38. Fischler, B.; Ehrnst, A.; Forsgren, M.; Orvell, C.; Nemeth, A. The viral association of neonatal cholestasis in Sweden: A possible link between cytomegalovirus infection and extrahepatic biliary atresia. *J. Pediatr. Gastroenterol. Nutr.* **1998**, *27*, 57–64. [CrossRef]
39. Zhao, D.; Gong, X.; Li, Y.; Sun, X.; Chen, Y.; Deng, Z.; Zhang, Y. Effects of cytomegalovirus infection on the differential diagnosis between biliary atresia and intrahepatic cholestasis in a Chinese large cohort study. *Ann. Hepatol.* **2021**, *23*, 100286. [CrossRef]
40. Zani, A.; Quaglia, A.; Hadzić, N.; Zuckerman, M.; Davenport, M. Cytomegalovirus-associated biliary atresia: An aetiological and prognostic subgroup. *J. Pediatr. Surg.* **2015**, *50*, 1739–1745. [CrossRef] [PubMed]
41. Brindley, S.M.; Lanham, A.M.; Karrer, F.M.; Tucker, R.M.; Fontenot, A.P.; Mack, C.L. Cytomegalovirus-specific T-cell reactivity in biliary atresia at the time of diagnosis is associated with deficits in regulatory T cells. *Hepatology* **2012**, *55*, 1130–1138. [CrossRef] [PubMed]
42. Hill, R.; Quaglia, A.; Hussain, M.; Hadzic, N.; Mieli-Vergani, G.; Vergani, D.; Davenport, M. Th-17 cells infiltrate the liver in human biliary atresia and are related to surgical outcome. *J. Pediatr. Surg.* **2015**, *50*, 1297–1303. [CrossRef]
43. Zhao, Y.; Xu, X.; Liu, G.; Yang, F.; Zhan, J. Prognosis of biliary atresia associated with cytomegalovirus: A meta-analysis. *Front. Pediatr.* **2021**, *9*, 710450. [CrossRef] [PubMed]
44. Kilgore, A.; Mack, C.L. Update on investigations pertaining to the pathogenesis of biliary atresia. *Pediatr. Surg. Int.* **2017**, *33*, 1233–1241. [CrossRef]
45. Ortiz-Perez, A.; Donnelly, B.; Temple, H.; Tiao, G.; Bansal, R.; Mohanty, S.K. Innate immunity and pathogenesis of biliary atresia. *Front. Immunol.* **2020**, *11*, 1–14. [CrossRef] [PubMed]
46. Lorent, K.; Gong, W.; Koo, K.A.; Waisbourd-Zinman, O.; Karjoo, S.; Zhao, X.; Sealy, I.; Kettleborough, R.N.; Stemple, D.L.; Windsor, P.A.; et al. Identification of a plant isoflavonoid that causes biliary atresia. *Sci. Transl. Med.* **2015**, *7*, 286ra67. [CrossRef]

47. Cui, S.; Leyva-Vega, M.; Tsai, E.A.; Eauclaire, S.F.; Glessner, J.T.; Hakonarson, H.; Devoto, M.; Haber, B.A.; Spinner, N.B.; Matthews, R.P. Evidence from human and zebrafish That GPC1 is a biliary atresia susceptibility gene. *Gastroenterology* **2013**, *144*, 1107–1115.e3. [CrossRef]
48. Sangkhathat, S.; Laochareonsuk, W.; Maneechay, W.; Kayasut, K.; Chiengkriwate, P. Variants associated with infantile cholestatic syndromes detected in extrahepatic biliary atresia by whole exome studies: A 20-case series from Thailand. *J. Pediatr. Genet.* **2018**, *7*, 67–73.
49. Mezina, A.; Karpen, S.J. Genetic contributors and modifiers of biliary atresia. *Dig. Dis.* **2015**, *33*, 408–414. [CrossRef]
50. Muller, F.; Gauthier, F.; Laurent, J.; Schmitt, M.; Boué, J. Amniotic fluid GGT and congenital extrahepatic biliary damage. *Lancet* **1991**, *337*, 232–233. [CrossRef]
51. Dreux, S.; Boughanim, M.; Lepinard, C.; Guichet, A.; Rival, J.M.; de Becdelievre, A.; Dugueperoux, I.; Muller, F. Relationship of non-visualization of the fetal gallbladder and amniotic fluid digestive enzymes analysis to outcome. *Prenat. Diagn.* **2012**, *32*, 423–426. [CrossRef] [PubMed]
52. Bardin, R.; Ashwal, E.; Davidov, B.; Danon, D.; Shohat, M.; Meizner, I. Nonvisualization of the fetal gallbladder: Can levels of gamma-glutamyl transpeptidase in amniotic fluid predict fetal prognosis? *Fetal Diagn. Ther.* **2016**, *39*, 50–55. [CrossRef] [PubMed]
53. Mysore, K.R.; Shneider, B.L.; Harpavat, S. Biliary atresia as a disease starting in utero: Implications for treatment, diagnosis, and pathogenesis. *J. Pediatr. Gastroenterol. Nutr.* **2019**, *69*, 396–403. [CrossRef] [PubMed]
54. Harpavat, S.; Finegold, M.J.; Karpen, S.J. Patients with biliary atresia have elevated direct/conjugated bilirubin levels shortly after birth. *Pediatrics* **2011**, *128*, e1428–e1433. [CrossRef] [PubMed]
55. Harpavat, S.; Garcia-Prats, J.A.; Shneider, B.L. Newborn bilirubin screening for biliary atresia. *N. Engl. J. Med.* **2016**, *375*, 605–606. [CrossRef]

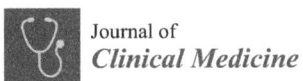

Article

Adjuvant Therapy with Budesonide Post-Kasai Reduces the Need for Liver Transplantation in Biliary Atresia

Joachim F. Kuebler [1], Omid Madadi-Sanjani [1], Eva D. Pfister [2], Ulrich Baumann [2], David Fortmann [1], Johannes Leonhardt [3], Benno M. Ure [1], Michael P. Manns [4], Richard Taubert [4] and Claus Petersen [1,*]

[1] Department of Pediatric Surgery, Hannover Medical School, 30625 Hannover, Germany; kuebler.joachim@mh-hannover.de (J.F.K.); madadi-sanjani.omid@mh-hannover.de (O.M.-S.); fortmann.david@mh-hannover.de (D.F.); ure.benno@mh-hannover.de (B.M.U.)
[2] Department of Paediatric Gastroenterology and Hepatology, Hannover Medical School, 30625 Hannover, Germany; pfister.eva-doreen@mh-hannover.de (E.D.P.); baumann.u@mh-hannover.de (U.B.)
[3] Clinic for Pediatric Surgery, Klinikum Braunschweig, 38118 Braunschweig, Germany; j.leonhardt@klinikum-braunschweig.de
[4] Department of Gastroenterology, Hepatology and Endocrinology, Hannover Medical School, 30625 Hannover, Germany; manns.michael@mh-hannover.de (M.P.M.); taubert.richard@mh-hannover.de (R.T.)
* Correspondence: petersen.claus@mh-hannover.de; Tel.: +49-511-532-9047; Fax: +49-511-532-9059

Abstract: Based on the hypothesis that autoimmunological factors coregulate the pathomechanism in biliary atresia (BA), adjuvant therapy with steroids has become routine, although its efficacy has never been proven. In 2010, a study on the advantages of budesonide compared to prednisolone in autoimmune hepatitis gave rise to experimental therapy using budesonide as an adjuvant BA treatment. Ninety-five BA patients prospectively received a budesonide 2 mg/dose rectal foam daily for three months (SG). A case-matched control group (CG: 81) was retrospectively recruited. The outcome measures were survival with native liver (SNL), determined at six months and two years after the Kasai procedure. The follow-up rate was 100%. At six months, SNL was statistically not different but became so after two years (SG: 54%; CG: 32%; $p < 0.001$). No steroid-related side effects were observed, except for eight patients with finally caught-up growth retardation. This study demonstrates for the first time a significantly longer survival with native liver in patients with BA after adjuvant therapy. However, indication, dosage, and duration of any budesonide application is not given in neonates with BA. Hence, we suggest extending the postoperative use of budesonide in a multicenter observational study with a clearly defined follow-up protocol, particularly in terms of potentially underestimated side effects.

Keywords: biliary atresia; budesonide; adjuvant therapy; liver transplantation

1. Introduction

The most frequent indication of pediatric liver transplantation (LTx) is given in patients with biliary atresia (BA) within the course of an unfavorable outcome after the Kasai procedure [1]. Even under the best circumstances and after early referral to pediatric liver units, the overall outcome remains unsatisfying and the survival with native liver (SNL) drops below 30% over the long term [2,3]. As long as the etiology and the pathomechanism of BA are not yet understood, Kasai portoenterostomy (KPE) per se or sequential surgery by KPE and LTx remain the only therapeutic options and provide an overall survival rate of about 90% [1,4].

On the basis of the hypothesis that BA is a triggered inflammatory process, following (auto)immunological patterns [5–7], the perioperative administration of corticosteroids has become routine. Despite the fact that this treatment has no beneficial effect on LTx incidence, which has been demonstrated in several well-designed studies, postoperative steroids are still used by most pediatric surgeons [8–10].

In 2010, Manns et al. reported that the induction of biochemical remission in patients with autoimmune hepatitis (AIH) would be more effective using budesonide instead of prednisolone, both in combination with azathioprine [11]. Salvage therapy with budesonide was also capable of doubling remission rate in difficult to treat AIH patients [12,13]. Likewise, when added to standard therapy with ursodesoxycholic acid [14–16], budesonide improved the therapeutic effects on primary biliary cholangitis (PBC), an autoimmune liver disease manifesting mostly in adults. Although it was a highly speculative idea that the pathomechanism could be in any way comparable in AIH, PBC and BA, this paper gave reason to consider potentially similar effects in biliary atresia. Following a thorough interdisciplinary discussion and detailed consideration, a clinical trial protocol was prepared. From 2011 onward, when the Kasai procedure was scheduled, we offered this experimental adjuvant therapy to parents. After reviewing the first cases, we were already observing an increasing number of patients whose bilirubin turned normal, which encouraged us to pursue this attempt. This trend stabilized during the following years and, from an ethical point of view, we realized that we could not deprive future cases of this option. On the other hand, patients with rare diseases, for whom mid- and long-term observation is inevitable, require a longer follow-up period in order to obtain statistically sound results. Hence, we continued with the protocol of rectally applied budesonide after KPE until passing the number of more than 120 patients. We then reviewed their data in the context of survival with a native liver and the need for liver transplantation at defined and reproducible reference dates.

2. Materials and Methods

2.1. Diagnostics and Treatment

From May 2011 onward we informed all parents of BA-patients about the option of an experimental treatment with budesonide. During a reflection period lasting until the fifth postoperative day, scheduled for the beginning of the treatment, the team was consistently available for discussing further details. After another extensive medical briefing, the parents then signed their informed consent for the off-label use of budesonide, which included details of the patients' age, the indication, the dosage, and the application. They were also informed about any potential side effects and assured that they could stop the treatment by tapering the dosage at any time without giving reasons. The parents also agreed that patients would be closely followed-up and that their data would be prospectively registered. A retrospective analysis of this data has been approved by the ethical committee of Hannover Medical School (No. 9429_BO_K_2020).

With being a tertiary referral center, all patients with neonatal cholestasis—and particularly those who are suspected to have BA—undergo a diagnostic process developed in an interdisciplinary manner. Biliary atresia is confirmed or excluded by endoscopic retrograde cholangiography (ERC) and/or intraoperative visualization of the extrahepatic bile ducts [17]. Portoenterostomies were performed according to the original Kasai procedure in a standardized technique along with the following surgical key points: small transverse center right laparotomy, mobilization of the liver, intraoperative cholangiography (if necessary), preparation of the hepatoduodenal ligament and extensive dissection of the porta hepatis using magnification, preparing of a 40 to 50 cm Roux-Y-loop without valve creation, performing a funnel-shaped KPE, wedge liver biopsy, and no drainage.

Postoperatively, the patients were monitored via intermediate care and oral feeding (with breast milk and/or a medium-chain triglycerides formula) was restarted within 24 h. The perioperatively given prophylaxis of antibiotics (trimethoprim) was continued for 10 to 14 days and then switched to oral for a minimum of six months. Fat-soluble vitamins and also ursodeoxycholic acid were prescribed with long-term intentions with respect to the clinical course. Post-Kasai, a budesonide 2 mg/dose rectal foam (Budenofalk™) was started on day five and with a continued daily application for three months. Patients of the control group were not treated by other steroids alternatively because we stopped anti-inflammatory adjuvant therapy since our high dosage study revealed no benefit in terms of jaundice free survival with native liver [18].

The follow-up of the patients was determined by the course of the disease. Babies with an uneventful development (colored stools, no jaundice, no ascites, decreasing bilirubin, age-appropriate weight gain) were initially followed up every three months, then with increasing intervals at 6 and 12 months, respectively. Patients with unfavorable outcomes were scheduled for LTx evaluation according to their individual course. Most of the patients were followed up in our own liver unit, although others did return to their local hospitals. Any healthcare colleagues involved were informed about the budesonide treatment and were asked to observe the patients thoroughly and to report any unexpected observations, particularly with regards to potential corticoid-induced symptoms.

2.2. Patients and Data Management

From the turn of the millennium, BA patients' data were prospectively recorded in EBAR (European Biliary Atresia Registry) [18], which was incorporated in 2013 into the newly-established internet-based BARD-registry (Biliary Atresia and Related Diseases, www.BARD-online.com, accessed on 15 October 2021) [1]. The registry includes each patient's initial entry dataset, a second data entry six months after the Kasai, then continued by infinite annual follow-ups or until the moment of LTx or death. Seamless data entry is supported by an e-mail reminder, which is automatically sent out to the user when follow-up data entries are due. The provider declares that the registry is in compliance with German data protection guidelines. Parents and patients of all BA patients since 2000 are informed that their pseudonymized data is used for scientific purposes exclusively and they can request the erasure of their data at any time without giving reasons.

Patients who changed to other centers were asked to agree with the same follow-up procedures. For these patients, data acquisition sometimes required active contact with the families, the pediatricians, and the liver units or transplant centers, respectively. In cases where the follow-up data was not completely recorded to the BARD-registry, traveling to participating centers for on-site data collection was necessary (D.F.).

The study group (SG) was built from patients born between February 2011 and October 2019, consisting of those whose parents agreed with an adjuvant budesonide treatment as described above. The controls were retrospectively recruited from our own patient cohort, born between March 2002 and October 2019, including those patients whose parents refused the budesonide treatment. Patients in the control group (CG) were also documented in the BARD-registry and the seamless follow-up procedure was the same as for the SG. The criteria for the case-matched CG were sex and age at the time of the KPW. Additionally, the following variables were included: gestational age, syndromic vs. non-syndromic form as well as bilirubin (total), AST, ALT, GGT, and liver fibrosis (calculated according to the Ishak classification) at the time of KPE. Cases that had been involved in other studies [17,19,20] were excluded.

As an outcome measurement, our definitions included the survival over all (SOA), survival with native liver (SNL) and jaundice-free survival with native liver, bilirubin < 20 µmol/L (jfSNL), determined at six months, two years after the KPE and October, 2021 (when the observation period was closed).

Neither of the registries routinely collect the parameters for steroid side effects. Therefore, we reviewed the files of those 82 patients separately, which are followed up in our pediatric liver unit for certain key parameters: percentile-related physical growth, the appearance of Cushing's symptoms, elevated blood glucose, infections that require antibiotic treatment, and skeleton conspicuities like reduced bone mineral density (when X-rays were indicated).

2.3. Statistics

We analyzed quantitative data using SPSS V.24.0, considering results statistically significant when $p < 0.05$. Differences in survival rates were analyzed using Kaplan–

Meier survival curves and significance was determined by log-rank test. To describe factors affecting survival, we used descriptive statistics, χ^2 tests and multivariate analysis of variance.

3. Results

As of the reporting date of this still ongoing observational study, 95 BA patients born between 2011 and 2019 could be included (SG) while 81 patients born between 2002 and 2019 were matched for the CG. Twenty-two newborns, which have also been operated by the Kasai procedure during this period could not be considered because their parents did not agree to the experimental treatment with budesonide. However, they could only partially be included into the control group because only eight of them met the matching criteria. The follow-up of all 176 patients was truncated by the end of October 2021 with 100% completeness and no drop-off.

Concerning the inclusion criteria, no considerable difference could be found between both groups. A mild predominance was given for females (SG 62%/38% and CG 58%/42%), while the average age at KPE was 60 days (range 26–142) in the SG and 65 days (range 16–150) in the CG. None of the parameters were statistically different between both groups, except for preoperative bilirubin (SG: 136 µmol; CG 156 µmol). On the other hand, two parameters had a predictive value for all patients in terms of SOA: the survival with native liver was worse in patients with the syndromic form of BA, but the jfSNL was higher in those patients who had been operated on between days 31 and 60 (Supporting Information Tables S1 and S2). In addition, the following study group characteristics had been gathered: seven patients had congenital heart defects (e.g., hemodynamically significant ASD in five patients, tetralogy of Fallot, and hypoplastic left heart syndrome with a congenitally absent inferior vena cava in one patient each). Also, five patients had been tested positive for CMV. None of these parameters gave ground for exclusion – neither with respect to the budesonide treatment nor to the cause of death post-Kasai.

Survival with native liver at the defined reference dates was the main outcome objective. Six months after KPE, 78% of the SG survived without LTx as opposed to 73% of the controls. This difference becomes statistically significant after two years when 54% of the patients with budesonide live with their own liver in contrast to 32% of the control group—with the same being true for the jfSNL ($p < 0.001$). Our results, therefore, show a difference for six months after KPE as 55% in the SG vs. 35% in the CG, and 45% vs. 28% two years later (Table 1).

Table 1. Outcome after Kasai procedure with and without adjuvant budesonide therapy at six months and two years after the Kasai portoenterostomy (KPE).

	Study/Control Group	SOA	*p*-Value n.s.	SNL	*p*-Value n.s.	jfSNL	*p*-Value
6 months post KPE N = 176	SG	99% (94/95)	n.s.	78% (74/95)	n.s.	55% (52/95)	n.s.
	CG	100% (81/81)		73% (60/81)		35% (29/81)	
2 years post KPE N = 176	SG	92% (87/95)	n.s.	54% (51/95)	$p < 0.001$	45% (43/95)	$p < 0.001$
	CG	88% (73/81)		32% (26/81)		28% (23/81)	

Study group (SG) and control group (CG), survival over all (SOA), survival with native liver (SNL) and jaundice-free survival with native liver (jfSNL). n.s., nonsignificant.

Overlooking the whole observation period of 20 years, the SOA of all patients was 89% and no difference could be found between both groups at any of the target points (Supporting Information Figure S1). In both groups, three patients died before the first measurement point at six months and in period up to two years after KPE, another five patients deceased in the SG, and nine in the CG. In the latter group another one died on the waiting list. These patients were not excluded from any statistical analysis. However, long-term survival with their native liver (130 months) was found to be 49% in the SG, with 48% even being jaundice free. In the control group, the SNL dropped after 229 months to 20% and to 18% for jfSNL, respectively, as shown in Figure 1.

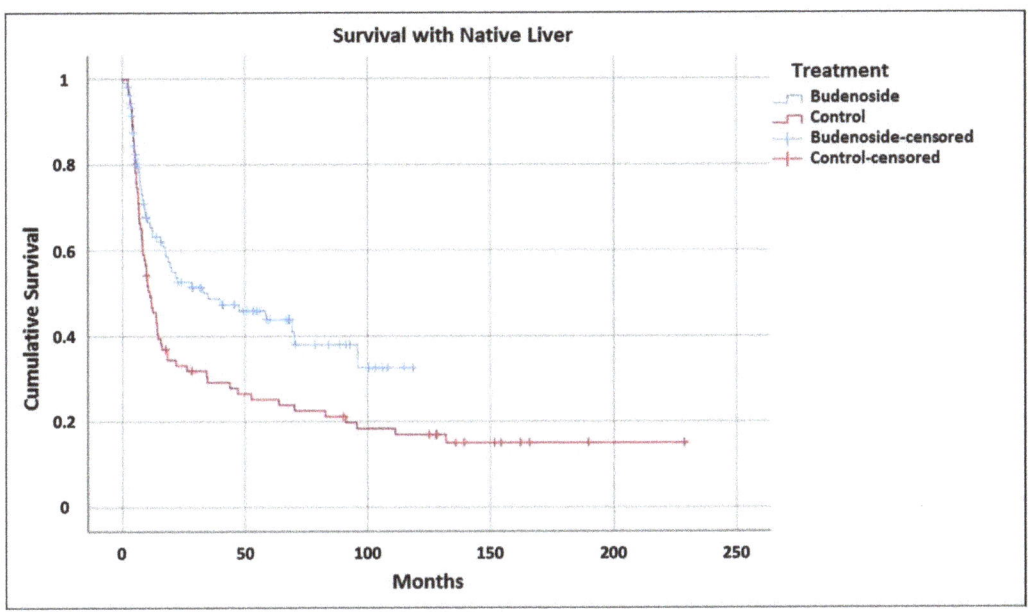

Figure 1. After two years, survival with native liver was 54% in the study and 32% in the control group ($p < 0.001$).

At the end of the observation period, 12 additional BA patients with budesonide therapy, who already passed the six-month evaluation date after KPE, showed identical outcome in terms of SNL and jfSnL.

With regard to steroid side effects, none of the 72 patients from the study group followed-up by our clinic showed a Cushing-like appearance or had elevated blood sugar levels. The physical development was reviewed only in those patients, who survived with their native liver for at least two years. In eight of these patients, the bodyweight six months after KPE was documented as either at or below the third percentile. All but one of them had a catch-up to the 15th or 50th percentile. Six months after KPE, six patients already presented as overweight at the 85th percentile, which did not decrease within the following 18 months.

4. Discussion

The first clinical corticosteroid trials after Kasai procedures date from the 1980s and are followed by numerous other studies and meta-analyses [10]. Consistently, they conclude that no benefit has been shown so far in terms of mid- or long-term improved survival with native liver. In this context, a recently published Cochrane review also stated that "further randomized, placebo-controlled trials are required to be able to determine if glucocorticosteroids may be of benefit in the postoperative management of infants with biliary atresia treated with Kasai portoenterostomy" [21,22].

Our series doesn't fulfill these requirements but reveals for the first time that, according to long-term evaluation, BA patients with adjuvant therapy survive significantly longer with their native liver. Nevertheless, our clinical trial needs to be critically reviewed and inevitably requires a check for whether the study group is representative of all biliary atresia patients. In accordance with the literature, the patients in our SG are predominantly female and the syndromic form of BA was documented for 11% of patients, while other associated diseases, like congenital heart defects, were diagnosed in 7%. In addition, a 5% CMV positivity corresponds with other series. Summarizing the SG parameters and the control inclusion criteria, this study's patients could be considered as representative of BA.

Another crucial factor concerns the outcome objectives of adjuvant therapy series in BA in general. Indeed, one may ask why the 2-year SNL and jfSNL of our study group is higher than in our controls but not different from other series reported by renowned liver units. This alleged inconsistency is explainable by the following arguments. Firstly, studies from East Asian centers cannot be directly compared to Caucasian series because the incidence of BA is different in both regions and a potentially diverging pathomechanism of postoperatively developing liver fibrosis is a matter for discussion. Secondly, BA studies in general use diverging outcome measures in terms of follow-up periods and nonuniform definition of jaundice-free SNL [23]. Finally, no other study provides a 100% follow-up of BA patients over a period of nearly 10 years in the SG and nearly 19 years in the CG (Supporting Information Table S3). Herein, we explicitly refer to long-term survival, shown in Figure 1, where the jfSNL rate in the SG remains stable beyond 65 months. In the control group, the number of SNL patients drops continuously and falls below the 20% line, which is slightly lower than recorded in other long-term reports. However, particularly for this period, the indication and optimal timing of LTx are not regulated and depend upon many factors, which limits the comparability of long-term series. In principle, therefore, a strict one-to-one comparison of BA studies should be handled with great care and caution.

Besides the considerations of the comparability and reliability of diverging BA studies, two key aspects also need to be addressed.

The first aspect concerns the question of why our regime of rectally-applied budesonide appeared to be more efficient than high dose prednisolone. The advantages of budesonide over commonly-used steroids like prednisolone might result from the approximately 15 times higher affinity to the steroid receptor and the 90% hepatic first-pass effect. The dose of rectal budesonide given (2 mg) to our patients is roughly equivalent to a dose of 10 mg/kg/d of prednisolone. This is comparable to high dose regimens of glucocorticoids used after Kasai portoenterostomy in former studies (Supporting Information Table S3). Both characteristics allow a higher topical steroid concentration with less systemic steroid specific side effects (SSSE). In combination with the longer treatment, these factors might contribute to budesonide´s higher efficacy.

Budesonide was administered orally in AIH and PBC studies [11–16] leading to a complete portal venous drainage with topic effect on the liver. A similar effect was observed in adult patients with primary biliary cholangitis, whose biochemical disease markers improved after oral treatment with budesonide [GH]. We chose the rectal application due to its ease of application and based on the assumption that a higher dosage of budesonide in the rectum and colon versus the upper gastrointestinal tract could be achieved. Additionally, recent studies demonstrate the role of gut microbiota in experimental [24] and clinical [25] BA, as well as in the regulation of liver immunity [26]. However, only a little is known about the role of the gut liver axis in biliary atresia [27].

Besides the strong activity on the classic glucocorticoid receptor, budesonide has also been shown to have stronger noncanonical effects compared to corticoids, such as predniso(lo)ne. This includes rapid nongenomic effects via a receptor located in the cell membrane, which has been shown to contribute significantly to its action [28,29]. Furthermore, glucocorticoids are able to bind to and activate other receptors, while budesonide has less cross-reactivity with the mineralocorticoid receptor. However, budesonide is also known to be an agonist on the pregnane x receptor—a potential target for the treatment of cholestatic liver diseases [30,31]. Research activity in this broad field is still very new and little is known yet about the effects of a noncanonical pathway in human hepatobiliary diseases, while there are reports from animal studies about the effects of this pathway on hepatocytes [32].

The second aspect concerns indications for the use of budesonide, which, in principle, does not differ between pediatric patients and adults. The leading diagnoses are eosinophilic esophagitis, autoimmune hepatitis, active ulcerative colitis, and a mild to moderate course of Crohn's disease. The most frequently reported adverse events are aphthous stomatitis, acne vulgaris, moon face, headache after oral administration, burning pain in the rectum, anal fissure, frequent urge to defecate, and bleeding after rectal use. These side effects depend on the steroid dosage and duration, while reduced glucose tolerance, growth retardation, increased appetite following weight gain, increased risk of infection and osteopenia can occur with long-term administration [33]. The critical aspect of this study is that the indication, dosage, and duration of any budesonide application are not given to neonates with BA. For this reason, we observed the study group patients with a particular emphasis on steroid-related side effects, which usually have no part in any BA follow-up protocol. Only eight out of 72 patients were documented as having growth retardation that had finally caught up, which could be considered as a steroid-related side effect. However, a more meticulous follow-up protocol is mandatory when budesonide is used routinely in BA patients.

5. Conclusions and Perspectives

In the history of biliary atresia treatment, there are two milestones to be highlighted: firstly, Kasai portoenterostomy and, secondly, liver transplantation achievements, namely, split liver Tx and living-related Tx. Apart from these two surgical procedures, no progress has been made in decades, particularly regarding the different protocols of adjuvant therapy post-KPE. The majority of studies report on corticosteroids in various dosages but all of them have failed to identify evidence in terms of longer survival with the patients' own livers. New studies with antiviral therapy, the administration of immunoglobulins, N-acetylcysteine, intestinal bile salt transport inhibitors, obeticholic acid [8], the Chinese herbs mixture "Inchinko-to" [34] and other treatments are on the way. Currently, however, our work on rectally-administered budesonide after KPE is the only existing study demonstrating a significant decrease of the need for liver transplantation in BA in respect of both mid- and long-term objectives. In light of these results, we advocate for a prospective observational multicenter study with a long follow-up and a major focus on steroid-related side effects, as well as clinical and basic research on the gut–liver axis factors (41) in biliary atresia.

Supplementary Materials: The following are available online at https://www.mdpi.com/article/10.3390/jcm10245758/s1, Figure S1: Kaplan-Meier curves: survival over all, Table S1: Demographic and laboratory features of the study population, Table S2: Outcome related to the age in days, when the Kasai procedure was performed, Table S3: Compilation of 14 adjuvant therapy studies after Kasai portoenterostomy.

Author Contributions: C.P., J.L., U.B., B.M.U. and M.P.M. conceived the study; C.P., E.D.P., J.F.K. and U.B. conceived the analysis plan; C.P., U.B., J.F.K. and B.M.U. designed the study; C.P., J.F.K., D.F. and O.M.-S. collected and analyzed the data; J.F.K., O.M.-S., R.T. and C.P. drafted the initial manuscript. All authors analyzed and interpreted the results, critically edited the manuscript, approved the final work, and agree to be accountable for the accuracy and integrity of the work. All authors have read and agreed to the published version of the manuscript.

Funding: This observational study received no external funding.

Institutional Review Board Statement: The study protocol is in accordance to the declaration of Helsinki and was approved by the ethic committee of the Hannover Medical School (No. 9429_BO_K_2020).

Informed Consent Statement: Informed consent was obtained from all subjects involved in the study.

Data Availability Statement: Not applicable.

Acknowledgments: Hannover Medical School is full member of the European Reference Network on Rare Hepatological Diseases (https://rare-liver.eu/) and coordinator for biliary atresia in Pillar 2: Metabolic, Biliary Atresia & Related Diseases.

Conflicts of Interest: C.P. reports relationship of medical advisory board with Intercept Pharmaceuticals, Mallinckrodt Pharmaceuticals and Medxpert; E.D.P. is member of the advisory board of GMPorphan and Univar, and has received grants from Mirum, Albireo and Alexion; U.B. is a consultant for Albireo, Mirum Pharma, Alnylam, Vivet and Nestlé; M.P.M. is member of scientific advisory boards and and consultant for Falk Pharma GmbH on autoimmune and cholestatic liver diseases, all of which are unrelated to the submitted work; J.F.K., O.M.-S., D.F., J.L., B.M.U., R.T. declare no competing interest to the report.

Abbreviations

AIH	Autoimmune Hepatitis
ALT	Alanine Aminotransferase
ASD	Atrial Septal Defect
AST	Aspartate Aminotransferase
BA	Biliary Atresia
BARD	Biliary Atresia and Related Diseases
CG	Control Group
CMV	Cytomegalovirus
EBAR	European Biliary Atresia Registry
ERC	Endoscopic Retrograde Cholangiography
GGT	Gamma Glutamyl Transferase
jfSNL	Jaundice-free Survival with Native Liver
KPE	Kasai Portoenterostomy
LTx	Liver Transplantation
PBC	Primary Biliary Cholangitis
SG	Study Group
SNL	Survival with Native Liver
SSSE	Systemic Steroid Specific Side Effects

References

1. Verkade, H.J.; Bezerra, J.A.; Davenport, M.; Schreiber, R.A.; Mieli-Vergani, G.; Hulscher, J.B.; Sokol, R.J.; Kelly, D.A.; Ure, B.; Whitington, P.F.; et al. Biliary atresia and other cholestatic childhood diseases: Advances and future challenges. *J. Hepatol.* **2016**, *65*, 631–642. [CrossRef]
2. Fanna, M.; Masson, G.; Capito, C.; Girard, M.; Guerin, F.; Hermeziu, B.; Lachaux, A.; Roquelaure, B.; Gottrand, F.; Broue, P.; et al. Management of Biliary Atresia in France 1986 to 2015: Long-term Results. *J. Pediatr. Gastroenterol. Nutr.* **2019**, *69*, 416–424. [CrossRef] [PubMed]
3. Parolini, F.; Boroni, G.; Milianti, S.; Tonegatti, L.; Armellini, A.; Magne, M.G.; Pedersini, P.; Torri, F.; Orizio, P.; Benvenuti, S.; et al. Biliary atresia: 20–40-year follow-up with native liver in an Italian centre. *J. Pediatr. Surg.* **2019**, *54*, 1440–1444. [CrossRef] [PubMed]
4. Petersen, C.; Davenport, M. Aetiology of biliary atresia: What is actually known? *Orphanet J. Rare Dis.* **2013**, *8*, 128. [CrossRef]
5. Mack, C.L. What Causes Biliary Atresia? Unique Aspects of the Neonatal Immune System Provide Clues to Disease Pathogenesis. *Cell. Mol. Gastroenterol. Hepatol.* **2015**, *1*, 267–274. [CrossRef]
6. Kilgore, A.; Mack, C.L. Update on investigations pertaining to the pathogenesis of biliary atresia. *Pediatr. Surg. Int.* **2017**, *33*, 1233–1241. [CrossRef]
7. Klemann, C.; Schröder, A.; Dreier, A.; Möhn, N.; Dippel, S.; Winterberg, T.; Wilde, A.; Yu, Y.; Thorenz, A.; Gueler, F.; et al. Interleukin 17, Produced by gammadelta T Cells, Contributes to Hepatic Inflammation in a Mouse Model of Biliary Atresia and Is Increased in Livers of Patients. *Gastroenterology* **2016**, *150*, 229–241. [CrossRef]
8. Burns, J.; Davenport, M. Adjuvant treatments for biliary atresia. *Transl. Pediatr.* **2020**, *9*, 253–265. [CrossRef]
9. Pietrobattista, A.; Mosca, A.; Liccardo, D.; Alterio, T.; Grimaldi, C.; Basso, M.; Saffioti, M.C.; Della Corte, C.; Spada, M.; Candusso, M. Does the Treatment After Kasai Procedure Influence Biliary Atresia Outcome and Native Liver Survival? *J. Pediatr. Gastroenterol. Nutr.* **2020**, *71*, 446–451. [CrossRef] [PubMed]
10. Zhang, M.Z.; Xun, P.C.; He, K.; Cai, W. Adjuvant steroid treatment following Kasai portoenterostomy and clinical outcomes of biliary atresia patients: An updated meta-analysis. *World J. Pediatr.* **2016**, *13*, 20–26. [CrossRef]
11. Manns, M.P.; Woynarowski, M.; Kreisel, W.; Lurie, Y.; Rust, C.; Zuckerman, E.; Bahr, M.J.; Günther, R.; Hultcrantz, R.W.; Spengler, U.; et al. Budesonide induces remission more effectively than prednisone in a controlled trial of patients with autoimmune hepatitis. *Gastroenterology* **2010**, *139*, 1198–1206. [CrossRef]
12. Manns, M.P.; Jaeckel, E.; Taubert, R. Budesonide in Autoimmune Hepatitis: The Right Drug at the Right Time for the Right Patient. *Clin. Gastroenterol. Hepatol.* **2017**, *16*, 186–189. [CrossRef] [PubMed]

13. Peiseler, M.; Liebscher, T.; Sebode, M.; Zenouzi, R.; Hartl, J.; Ehlken, H.; Pannicke, N.; Weiler-Normann, C.; Lohse, A.W.; Schramm, C. Efficacy and Limitations of Budesonide as a Second-Line Treatment for Patients With Autoimmune Hepatitis. *Clin. Gastroenterol. Hepatol.* **2018**, *16*, 260–267. [CrossRef] [PubMed]
14. Leuschner, M.; Maier, K.P.; Schlichting, J.; Strahl, S.; Herrmann, G.; Dahm, H.H.; Ackermann, H.; Happ, J.; Leuschne, U. Oral budesonide and ursodeoxycholic acid for treatment of primary biliary cirrhosis: Results of a prospective double-blind trial. *Gastroenterology* **1999**, *117*, 918–925. [CrossRef]
15. Rautiainen, H.; Kärkkäinen, P.; Karvonen, A.-L.; Nurmi, H.; Pikkarainen, P.; Nuutinen, H.; Färkkilä, M. Budesonide combined with UDCA to improve liver histology in primary biliary cirrhosis: A three-year randomized trial. *Hepatology* **2005**, *41*, 747–752. [CrossRef] [PubMed]
16. Hirschfield, G.M.; Beuers, U.; Kupcinskas, L.; Ott, P.; Bergquist, A.; Färkkilä, M.; Manns, M.P.; Parés, A.; Spengler, U.; Stiess, M.; et al. A placebo-controlled randomised trial of budesonide for PBC following an insufficient response to UDCA. *J. Hepatol.* **2021**, *74*, 321–329. [CrossRef]
17. Petersen, C.; Meier, P.N.; Schneider, A.; Turowski, C.; Pfister, E.D.; Manns, M.P.; Ure, B.M.; Wedemeyer, J. Endoscopic retrograde cholangiopancreaticography prior to explorative laparotomy avoids unnecessary surgery in patients suspected for biliary atresia. *J. Hepatol.* **2009**, *51*, 1055–1060. [CrossRef]
18. Petersen, C.; Madadi-Sanjani, O. Registries for Biliary Atresia and Related Disorders. *Eur. J. Pediatr. Surg.* **2015**, *25*, 469–473. [PubMed]
19. Petersen, C.M.; Harder, D.; Melter, M.; Becker, T.; Von Wasielewski, R.; Leonhardt, J.; Ure, B.M. Postoperative high-dose steroids do not improve mid-term survival with native liver in biliary atresia. *Am. J. Gastroenterol.* **2008**, *103*, 712–719. [CrossRef]
20. Ure, B.M.; Kuebler, J.F.; Schukfeh, N.; Engelmann, C.; Dingemann, J.; Petersen, C. Survival with the native liver after laparoscopic versus conventional kasai portoenterostomy in infants with biliary atresia: A prospective trial. *Ann. Surg.* **2011**, *253*, 826–830. [CrossRef]
21. Tyraskis, A.; Parsons, C.; Davenport, M. Glucocorticosteroids for infants with biliary atresia following Kasai portoenterostomy. *Cochrane Database Syst. Rev.* **2016**, *5*. [CrossRef]
22. Karrer, F.; Lilly, J.R. Corticosteroid therapy in biliary atresia. *J. Pediatr. Surg.* **1985**, *20*, 693–695. [CrossRef]
23. Petersen, C. Biliary atresia: Unity in diversity. *Pediatr. Surg. Int.* **2017**, *33*, 1255–1261. [CrossRef]
24. Jee, J.; Mourya, R.; Shivakumar, P.; Fei, L.; Wagner, M.; Bezerra, J.A. Cxcr2 signaling and the microbiome suppress inflammation, bile duct injury, and the phenotype of experimental biliary atresia. *PLoS ONE* **2017**, *12*, e0182089. [CrossRef]
25. Tessier, M.E.M.; Cavallo, L.; Yeh, J.; Harpavat, S.; Hoffman, K.L.; Petrosino, J.F.; Shneider, B.L. The Fecal Microbiome in Infants With Biliary Atresia Associates With Bile Flow After Kasai Portoenterostomy. *J. Pediatr. Gastroenterol. Nutr.* **2020**, *70*, 789–795. [CrossRef] [PubMed]
26. Ma, C.; Han, M.; Heinrich, B.; Fu, Q.; Zhang, Q.; Sandhu, M.; Agdashian, D.; Terabe, M.; Berzofsky, J.A.; Fako, V.; et al. Gut microbiome-mediated bile acid metabolism regulates liver cancer via NKT cells. *Science* **2018**, *360*, eaan5931. [CrossRef] [PubMed]
27. Albillos, A.; de Gottardi, A.; Rescigno, M. The gut-liver axis in liver disease: Pathophysiological basis for therapy. *J. Hepatol.* **2020**, *72*, 558–577. [CrossRef] [PubMed]
28. Krogsgaard, L.R.; Munck, L.K.; Bytzer, P.; Wildt, S. An altered composition of the microbiome in microscopic colitis is driven towards the composition in healthy controls by treatment with budesonide. *Scand. J. Gastroenterol.* **2019**, *54*, 446–452. [CrossRef] [PubMed]
29. Nunez, G.J.; Johnstone, T.B.; Corpuz, M.L.; Kazarian, A.G.; Mohajer, N.N.; Tliba, O. Glucocorticoids rapidly activate cAMP production via G αs to initiate non-genomic signaling that contributes to one-third of their canonical genomic effects. *FASEB J.* **2020**, *34*, 2882–2895. [CrossRef]
30. Zimmermann, C.; van Waterschoot, R.A.B.; Harmsen, S.; Maier, A.; Gutmann, H.; Schinkel, A.H. PXR-mediated induction of human CYP3A4 and mouse Cyp3a11 by the glucocorticoid budesonide. *Eur. J. Pharm. Sci.* **2009**, *36*, 565–571. [CrossRef]
31. Goldsetin, J.; Levy, C. Novel and emerging therapies for cholestatic liver diseases. *Liver Int.* **2018**, *38*, 1520–1535. [CrossRef] [PubMed]
32. Dindia, L.; Murray, J.; Faught, E.; Davis, T.L.; Leonenko, Z.; Vijayan, M.M. Novel nongenomic signaling by glucocorticoid may involve changes to liver membrane order in rainbow trout. *PLoS ONE* **2012**, *7*, e46859.
33. Alonso, E.M.; Ye, W.; Hawthorne, K.; Venkat, V.; Loomes, K.M.; Mack, C.L.; Hertel, P.M.; Karpen, S.J.; Kerkar, N.; Molleston, J.P.; et al. Impact of Steroid Therapy on Early Growth in Infants with Biliary Atresia: The Multicenter Steroids in Biliary Atresia Randomized Trial. *J. Pediatr.* **2018**, *202*, 179–185. [CrossRef] [PubMed]
34. Tamura, T.; Kobayashi, H.; Yamataka, A.; Lane, G.J.; Koga, H.; Miyano, T. Inchin-ko-to prevents medium-term liver fibrosis in postoperative biliary atresia patients. *Pediatr. Surg. Int.* **2007**, *23*, 343–347. [CrossRef] [PubMed]

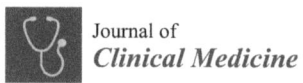
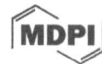

Article

Cholangitis Definition and Treatment after Kasai Hepatoportoenterostomy for Biliary Atresia: A Delphi Process and International Expert Panel

Ana M. Calinescu [1,*,†], Omid Madadi-Sanjani [2,†], Cara Mack [3], Richard A. Schreiber [4], Riccardo Superina [5], Deirdre Kelly [6,†], Claus Petersen [2,†] and Barbara E. Wildhaber [1,†]

1 Division of Child's and Adolescent's Surgery, Swiss Pediatric Liver Center, Geneva University Hospitals, University of Geneva, 1205 Geneva, Switzerland; barbara.wildhaber@hcuge.ch
2 Department of Pediatric Surgery, Hannover Medical School, 30625 Hannover, Germany; madadi-sanjani.omid@mh-hannover.de (O.M.-S.); Petersen.Claus@mh-hannover.de (C.P.)
3 Section of Gastroenterology, Hepatology and Nutrition, Digestive Health Institute, Children's Hospital Colorado, University of Colorado School of Medicine, Aurora, CO 80011, USA; cara.mack@childrenscolorado.org
4 Division of Gastroenterology, Hepatology and Nutrition, BC Children's Hospital, University of British Columbia, Vancouver, BC V5Z 4H4, Canada; rschreiber@cw.bc.ca
5 Division of Transplant Surgery, Ann and Robert H. Lurie Children's Hospital of Chicago, Northwestern University Feinberg School of Medicine, Chicago, IL 60611, USA; RSuperina@luriechildrens.org
6 Liver Unit, Birmingham Women's and Children's Hospital, Birmingham B15 2TG, UK; deirdrekelly@nhs.net
* Correspondence: ana-maria.calinescu@hcuge.ch; Tel.: +41-22-382-46-62
† Partners of the European Reference Network Rare-Liver.

Abstract: (1) Background: Acute cholangitis during the first year after Kasai hepatoportoenterostomy (HPE) has a negative impact on patient and native liver survival. There are no consistent guidelines for the definition, treatment, and prophylaxis of cholangitis after HPE. The aim of this study was to develop definition, treatment, and prophylaxis guidelines to allow for expeditious management and for standardization in reporting. (2) Methods: the Delphi method, an extensive literature review, iterative rounds of surveys, and expert panel discussions were used to establish definition, treatment, and prophylaxis guidelines for cholangitis in the first year after HPE. (3) Results: Eight elements (pooled into two groups: clinical and laboratory/imaging) were identified to define cholangitis after HPE. The final proposed definitions for suspected and confirmed cholangitis are a combination of one element, respectively, two elements from each group; furthermore, the finding of a positive blood culture was added to the definition of confirmed cholangitis. The durations for prophylaxis and treatment of suspected and confirmed cholangitis were uniformly agreed upon by the experts. (4) Conclusions: for the first time, an international consensus was found for guidelines for definition, treatment, and prophylaxis for cholangitis during the first year after Kasai HPE. Applicability will need further prospective multicentered studies.

Keywords: biliary atresia; cholangitis; Kasai; hepatoportoenterostomy

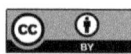

1. Introduction

Acute cholangitis after Kasai hepatoportoenterostomy (HPE) is known to have a negative impact on prognosis; it predicts liver failure [1] and is associated with earlier liver transplantation [2]. Furthermore, repeated cholangitis episodes are thought to be an important factor contributing to the progression of liver cirrhosis, ultimately leading to liver transplantation in biliary atresia patients and to decreased survival rates [3–7].

Reports on the incidence of cholangitis in biliary atresia patients vary between 40% and 93% [8]. Most of the cholangitis episodes develop within the first two years of life, and especially within the first year of life [9–12]. Despite improvements in postoperative management over the last decades, the incidence of cholangitis remains stable over time [13]. Hypotheses about the etiology of cholangitis includes intestinal bacterial migration, translocation from lymphatics, hematogenous spread via portal vein as well as an immune inflammatory response [14]. While attempts have been made to standardize the diagnosis of cholangitis after Kasai HPE, there are still no clear guidelines as to how to define the disease [15]. The Tokyo Guidelines, developed for adult patients, are clearly not applicable to diagnose cholangitis in children during the first year after Kasai HPE [16,17].

The use of prophylactic antibiotics has been shown to be beneficial to decrease the rate of recurrent cholangitis [18]. However, prophylaxis must be balanced against the possibility of lethal cholangitis secondary to resistant organisms [4]. This said, it is almost impossible to compare the existing body of literature due to the wide variety in practices of cholangitis prophylaxis and, again, the lack of a unanimous thus comparable definition of cholangitis [5,19].

Quick and effective treatment of cholangitis after Kasai HPE is paramount. The threshold for suspecting cholangitis must be low, allowing for the introduction of a prompt and effective treatment to avoid further liver damage as well as potentially lethal septicemia. For prophylaxis, antibiotic regimens and durations are widely variable in the pediatric literature [10,20,21].

The aim of this work was to propose unambiguous criteria for the diagnosis and treatment of cholangitis after Kasai HPE for biliary atresia patients during the first year after Kasai HPE, based on a systematic review of the literature and the consensus of international experts, reached within the Biliary Atresia and Related Disorders (BARD) community (http://www.bard-online.com/, accessed on 15 December 2021) and during a Webinar held in July 2021.

2. Materials and Methods

2.1. Systematic Literature Review

We systematically reviewed the following databases: Embase, PubMed, Web of Science, and the Cochrane Database from the beginning of each database through November 2019. We used the search terms: "Cholangitis"(Mesh:noexp) OR Cholangitis(Title/Abstract) AND ("Portoenterostomy, Hepatic"(Mesh) OR "Biliary Atresia"(Mesh) OR "Hepatic Portoenterostomy"(Title/Abstract) OR "Hepatic Portoenterostomies"(Title/Abstract) OR hepatoportoenterostomies(Title/Abstract) OR hepatoportoenterostomy(Title/Abstract) OR "Kasai Procedure"(Title/Abstract) OR "Kasai portoenterostomy"(Title/Abstract) OR "Post-Kasai"(Title/Abstract) OR "Kasai operation"(Title/Abstract) OR biliary atresia(Title/Abstract)). Two authors (AMC and OMS) completed the search strategy independently. Selected titles and abstracts were reviewed to identify suitable articles that gave information about definition and/or antibiotic prophylaxis and/or antibiotic treatment of cholangitis after Kasai HPE. Whether studies met the eligible criteria was determined based on author consensus. Language was restricted to English. Systematic literature review set the base for the 1st Delphi questionnaire for the definition and treatment of cholangitis.

2.2. Formatting and Pretesting of the 1st Delphi Questionnaire

To establish the different consensus, the well-structured Delphi method was used as proposed by Dalkey N.C. [22,23].

Study design 1st Delphi questionnaire: self-administered, web-based survey using the online tool SurveyMonkey (http://www.surveymonkey.com, accessed on 13 June 2021).

Study outcomes 1st Delphi questionnaire: Study outcomes were stated as: (i) to define items included in the cholangitis definition (primary outcome) and (ii) to identify current practices for primary prophylaxis after HPE and treatment of cholangitis occurring in biliary atresia patients within the first year after HPE (secondary outcomes). Of note, the terms cholangitis and acute cholangitis were used interchangeably throughout the questionnaires and the manuscript.

Study population 1st Delphi questionnaire: The survey targeted pediatric surgeons and hepatologists working in Europe, North America, Asia, and Australia. The questionnaire was electronically distributed to the 34 faculty members of BARD and 28 centers of the European Reference Network—Rare Liver.

Development of the 1st Delphi questionnaire: The variables assessed in the 1st Delphi questionnaire (regarding cholangitis definition, primary prophylaxis after Kasai HPE, and treatment) were selected with the help of the systematic literature review and by consulting international experts in biliary atresia. The questionnaire was initiated using a semi-structured interview, separately run with two experienced pediatric surgeons, with the aim of identifying redundant, irrelevant, or poorly worded questions [24]. Clinical sensibility testing of the questionnaire, aiming to assess its comprehensiveness, clarity, and validity was then conducted by running the questions to 10 other pediatric surgeons and hepatologists to be answered with a 7 point Likert scale. Finally, the reliability of the questionnaire was assessed with a test re-test: the questionnaire was given to the same 10 pediatric surgeons and hepatologists after a 2 week interval, and the reproducibility of their answers was assessed with a Spearman correlation coefficient (0.73). The survey was held in English. No questions were mandatory; each participant could advance in the survey after skipping a question. The questionnaire is depicted in Supplementary Materials Document S1.

Distribution of the 1st Delphi questionnaire: The survey was distributed by e-mail, with a cover letter stating the objectives of the survey and providing an estimate of the completion time, according to the principles of Dillman and recommendations of Burns and coworkers [24]. The first e-mail was sent in August 2020, and two reminder e-mails were sent two and four weeks later.

2.3. Format of the 2nd Delphi Questionnaire

Study design 2nd Delphi questionnaire: idem. 1st questionnaire.

Study outcomes 2nd Delphi questionnaire: While the 1st questionnaire allowed for identification of criteria to use in the definition of acute cholangitis, this 2nd questionnaire aimed at (i) confirming the weighting of individual criteria in order to provide consensus for a cholangitis definition after Kasai HPE and (ii) to define the regimen and duration of primary prophylaxis after Kasai HPE and treatment of cholangitis. Thus, study outcomes were stated as: (i) to define biliary atresia-associated cholangitis (primary outcome) and (ii) to define biliary atresia-associated cholangitis prophylaxis and treatment (secondary outcomes).

Study population 2nd Delphi questionnaire: The survey targeted pediatric surgeons and hepatologists of the 34 faculty members of BARD only.

Development of the 2nd Delphi questionnaire: Criteria that achieved a consensus of more than 50% of the Delphi 1 participants (1st questionnaire) were taken into consideration for the 2nd Delphi questionnaire. As in clinical practice we often suspect cholangitis in infants after HPE and start treatment even if cholangitis is not yet confirmed, we stratified definitions of cholangitis in (i) suspected and (ii) confirmed, each of them with a respective duration of antibiotic treatment. Further, regimen and duration of primary prophylaxis after Kasai HPE was addressed. The questionnaire was administered to three experienced pediatric surgeons with the aim of identifying redundant, irrelevant, or poorly worded questions [24]. The questionnaire is available in Supplementary Materials Document S2.

Distribution of the 2nd Delphi questionnaire: idem. 1st questionnaire.

Administration of the 2nd Delphi questionnaire: idem. 1st questionnaire. The first e-mail was sent in April 2021, with a reminder e-mail two weeks later.

2.4. Pre-Meeting Working Group

A working group of 3 hepatologists (CM, RSc, and DK) and 5 surgeons (AMC, OMS, RSu, CP, and BEW) analyzed the results from the 2nd Delphi questionnaire and unanimously agreed on a proposed definition for suspected and confirmed cholangitis, treatment of suspected and confirmed cholangitis, and for prophylaxis of primary cholangitis after Kasai HPE. This process took place from 18 June through 22 June 2021.

2.5. Expert Panel Meeting

The proposed definitions of suspected and confirmed cholangitis, primary prophylaxis after Kasai HPE, and treatment of suspected and confirmed cholangitis were discussed within an expert panel meeting during the BARD Webinar held on 1 July 2021 as well as with the other participants in the webinar through a live chat. Panelists were provided with a summary depicting the rankings from the 1st and 2nd Delphi survey as well as the pre-meeting working group proposal. BEW served as moderator of the meeting. Approximatively 10 min of open-ended discussion was allotted for each of the three matters. The chat discussions and the recording of the webinar were used to capture the key elements and the discussion topics.

2.6. Statistical Analysis

The Pearson correlation coefficient was used to indicate correlation between the 1st and 2nd Delphi questionnaires.

3. Results

3.1. Literature Search

The literature search identified 615 scientific papers, and 109 publications finally met the inclusion criteria and were selected for full article review.

The clinical definition of cholangitis used in the literature varied largely (Appendix A, Table A1). The following items were used to define cholangitis: fever in 73.3% (80/109) of the studies; new or increasing jaundice was used in 55% (60/109); fever *and* new or increasing jaundice in 33.9% (37/109); stool color change in 44.9% (49/109); some form of abdominal discomfort in 6.4% (7/109) of the selected articles.

The laboratory elements for defining cholangitis were elevated bilirubin in 60.5% (66/109); white blood cells and elevated liver tests in 32.1% (35/109); two laboratory criteria (elevated white blood cells (WBCs) and elevated bilirubin) in 29.3% (32/109), elevated inflammatory parameters (C-reactive protein (CRP) and/or procalcitonin (PCT)) in 16.5% (18/109); positive blood cultures required to define cholangitis in 13.7% (15/109) of the articles.

The presence of bile lakes was included in the definition of cholangitis for 12.8% (14/109) of the authors.

The most frequently administered antibiotic prophylaxis was sulfamethoxazole and trimethoprim in 39.4% (15/38) of the articles (Table 1). Primary antibiotic prophylaxis (after the immediate postoperative period) was given between 6 and 12 months in 29.4% (5/17) of the reviewed articles.

Table 1. Overview of reported (2000–2021) cholangitis prophylaxis after Kasai hepatoportoenterostomy and cholangitis rates. Bid, bis in die; Qid, quater in die.

Authors	Nr. px	Cholangitis Prophylaxis	Cholangitis Prophylaxis Duration	Cholangitis Rates
Chuang J., et al., 2000 [13]	39	Sulfamethoxazole	3 months	46%
Lally K.P., et al., 1989 [25]	41	Sulfamethoxazole; Ampicillin; Cephalosporins	1 to several months	21.9%
Wu E.T., et al., 2001 [10]	37	Sulfamethoxazole 4 mg/kg or Neomycin 25 mg/kg 4×/week	Unknown	75%
Bu L.N., et al., 2003 [9]	19	Sulfamethoxazole 20 mg/kg/d bid or Neomycin 25 mg/kg/d qid, 4 days/week	6–7 months	-
Meyers R.L., et al., 2003 [26]	28	Piperacillin/Tazobactam 300 mg/kg/d qid + Gentamycin 5 mg/kg/d or Cefoperazone 150 mg/kg/d divided into 3 doses followed by Sulfamethoxazole 10 mg/kg/d bid	First regimen given 2–3 months and then unknown	34.4%

Table 1. Cont.

Authors	Nr. px	Cholangitis Prophylaxis	Cholangitis Prophylaxis Duration	Cholangitis Rates
Lai H.S., et al., 2006 [18]	163	Sulfamethoxazole 20 mg/kg/d bid or Neomycin 25 mg/kg/d, qid, 4 days/week	3 years	72.3%
Hung P.Y., et al., 2006 [4]	185	Oral antibiotics	1–6 months	54.6%
Kelly D.A., et al., 2007 [27]	-	Amoxicillin or Cephalexin or Sulfamethoxazole	Alternate every 2–3 months for 1 year minimum	-
Stringer M.D., et al., 2007 [28]	71	Cephalexin 25 mg/kg 2×/day oral	1 month	46%
Vejchapipat P., et al., 2007 [29]	53	Cotrimoxazole	1 year	45.2%
Petersen C., et al., 2008 [21]	49	Cefaclor 45 mg/kg/d oral	1 year	-
De Vries W., et al., 2012 [30]	214	Sulfamethoxazole or Neomycin/Colistin/Nystatin or Ciprofloxacin	-	55.1%
Wang B., et al., 2014 [31]	25	-	6 months	35%
Tyraskis A., et al., 2016 [32]	104	Cefalexin 25 mg/kg/d	1 month	-
Webb N.L., et al., 2016 [33]	29	-	>1 year	75%
Lee W.S., et al., 2017 [34]	52	-	3 months	36%
Pang W., et al., 2019 [19]	218	3rd generation Cephalosporin, oral	6 months	27%
Parolini F., et al., 2019 [35]	174	Sulfamethoxazole and Cephalosporin, 1 year if good bile drainage	1 year	32%
Ramachandran P., et al., 2019 [36]	62	Alternating Amoxicillin–Clavulanic Acid 40 mg/kg/d bid and Cefpodoxime 10 mg/kg/d bid, alternating	6 months	43.5%
Baek S.H., 2020 [37]	160	None	None	78.8%
Chen G., et al., 2021 [38]	180	Sulfamethoxazole 25 mg/kg/d bid for 2 weeks then Cefaclor 40 mg/kg/d bid for 2 weeks, alternating every 2 weeks	6 months	66.1%
Goh L., et al., 2021 [39]	54	Cotrimoxazole	1 year minimum	72%

The most common antibiotic for the treatment of cholangitis was ceftriaxone in 51.6% (16/31) of the studies for a duration of 2 weeks in 46.1% (6/13) of the reviewed articles (Table 2).

3.2. 1st Delphi Questionnaire

The 1st Delphi questionnaire was answered by 62 surgeons and hepatologists. Clinical elements defining cholangitis were answered as follows: fever/shivering 96.7% (60/62), stool color change 67.4% (42/62), new or increasing jaundice 91.9% (57/62), and abdominal distension/abdominal pain 66.1% (41/62) (Figure 1a). Laboratory elements defining cholangitis included increased levels of WBCs 95.1% (59/62), CRP 90.3% (56/62), PCT 54.8% (34/62), bilirubin 96.7% (60/62), gamma-glutamyl transferase (GGT) 90.3% (56/62), transaminases 85.4% (53/62), and positive blood cultures 79% (49/62). Bile lakes were included in the definition of cholangitis by 63.3% of the participants (43/62) (Figure 1b).

Table 2. Overview of reported (2000–2021) cholangitis treatment after Kasai hepatoportoenterostomy and native liver survival rates if available. NLS, native liver survival; CRP, C-reactive protein.

Authors	Number of Patients	Cholangitis Treatment	Cholangitis Treatment Duration	Native Liver Survival
Chuang J., et al., 2000 [13]	39	Cephalosporin and Aminoglycoside	7–10 days or till negative CRP	-
Wu E.T., et al., 2001 [10]	37	Ceftriaxone	At least 5 days	-
Van Heurn E., et al., 2003 [14]	77	3rd generation Cephalosporin	1 week	-
Wong K.K., et al., 2004 [20]	19	Cefoperazone 25 mg/kg 3×/day or Meropenem 20 mg/kg 3×/day	2 weeks	-
Petersen C., et al., 2008 [21]	49	3rd generation Cephalosporin and Aminoglycoside	3 weeks	6 month, NLS 63% 2 year, NLS 31%
Lee J Y., et al., 2014 [12]	27	Ampicillin, Gentamycin, and Metronidazole or Unasyn	14 days	-
Lien T., et al., 2015 [40]	20	Ceftriaxone	14 days	-
Chiang L.W., et al., 2017 [41]	58	Ceftriaxone 100 mg/kg/day or Piperacilline–Tazobactam 320 mg/kg/day recently	-	Overall NLS, 48.3% 2 year NLS, 72% 5 year NLS, 45.7%
Lee W.S., et al., 2017 [34]	52	-	10–14 days	NLS, 37%
Li Z., et al., 2017 [42]	80	Meropenem or Cefoperazone	-	-
Li D., et al., 2018 [5]	113	Meropenem 20 mg/kg 3×/j	5 days	-
Calinescu A.M., et al., 2019 [43]	62	Piperacillin–Tazobactam	3 weeks	4 year NLS for cholangitis patients, 36%
Ramachandran P., et al., 2019 [36]	62	Piperacillin–Tazobactam	-	1 year NLS for cholangitis patients, 33%
Chung P.H.Y., et al., 2020 [44]	128	Meropenem Cefoperazone	2 weeks 2 weeks	1 year NLS, 85.7% 1 year NLS, 69%

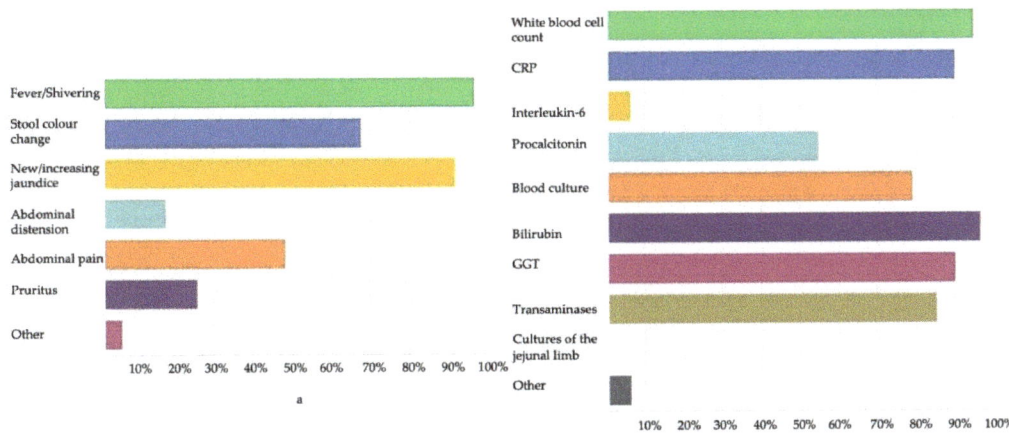

Figure 1. First Delphi questionnaire (a) Clinical signs following Kasai hepatoportoenterostomy included in the definition of cholangitis according to the 1st Delphi questionnaire. (b) Laboratory and imaging elements following Kasai hepatoportoenterostomy included in the definition of cholangitis according to the 1st Delphi questionnaire.

Of the participants, 89.6% (52/62) answered affirmatively with regard to primary antibiotic prophylaxis to prevent cholangitis after HPE; 53.8% (28/62) declared using sulfamethoxazole–trimethoprim.

The duration of cholangitis treatment was answered as 3 weeks according to 29% (16/62) of the participants, with piperacillin–tazobactam in 70.9% (39/62) of the answers.

3.3. 2nd Delphi Questionnaire

The response rate of the 2nd Delphi questionnaire was 44.1% (15/34).

The clinical elements included in the definition of cholangitis showed a Pearson correlation coefficient of 0.9 ($p = 0.004$) between the 1st and 2nd Delphi questionnaires. We did not correlate the laboratory and imaging elements between the two surveys, as items from the 1st Delphi survey were merged into fewer elements in the 2nd Delphi survey.

In the 1st Delphi survey, eight elements were identified as defining cholangitis and were pooled in two groups: (A) clinical elements—fever without extrahepatic source and/or shivering, stool color change, new/increasing jaundice, abdominal discomfort (vomiting, poor feeding, and irritability); (B) laboratory and imaging elements—inflammatory response (WBCs and/or CRP and/or PCT), increased/increasing transaminases, increased/increasing GGT and/or bilirubin, and bile lakes.

As for the definition of suspected cholangitis, the participants identified mainly one or more elements from A 5/15 (33.3%) and one element from A and one element from B 4/15 (26.67%) (Figure 2).

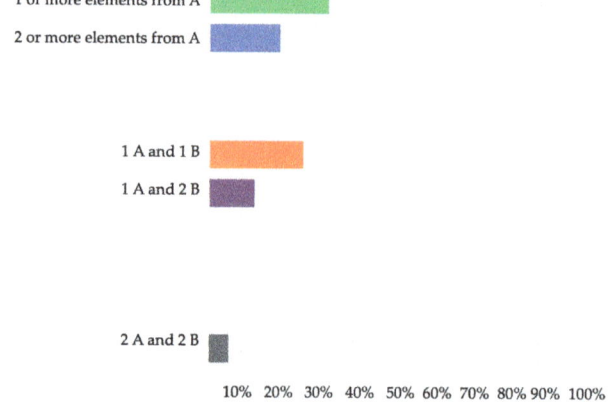

Figure 2. Definition of suspected cholangitis according to the 2nd Delphi questionnaire.

The treatment duration of a suspected cholangitis was selected to be 1 or 2 weeks by 6/15 (40%) of the participants (Figure 3).

As for the definition of confirmed cholangitis, the participants identified equally one element from A and one element from B and two elements from A and two elements from B, 4/15 (26.67%) both choices (Figure 4).

The treatment duration of a confirmed cholangitis was selected to be 10 days for 8/15 (53.3%) and 3 weeks for 5/15 (33.3%) (Figure 5).

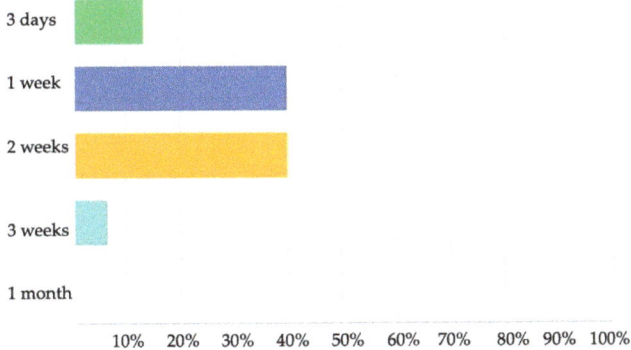

Figure 3. Treatment duration of suspected cholangitis according to the 2nd Delphi questionnaire.

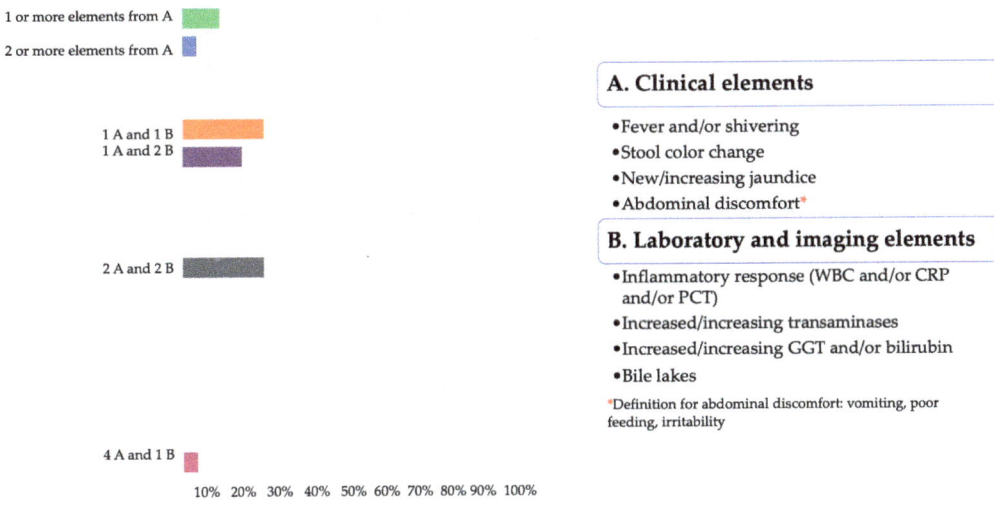

Figure 4. Definition of confirmed cholangitis according to the 2nd Delphi questionnaire.

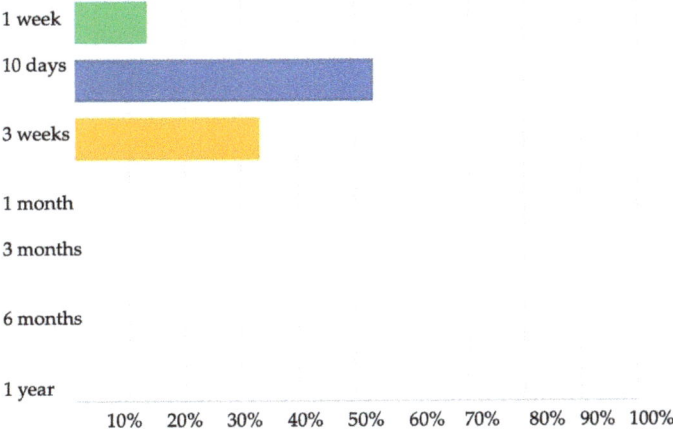

Figure 5. Treatment duration of confirmed cholangitis according to the 2nd Delphi questionnaire.

The duration of the peroral primary prophylaxis after HPE was most frequently answered to be 1 year by 5/15 (33.3%) of the participants and 3 months by 4/15 (26.6%) (Figure 6).

None
1 week or less
10 days
2 weeks
3 weeks
1 month
3 months
6 months
1 year
Other
10%
20%
30%
40%
50%
60%
70%
80%
90%
100%

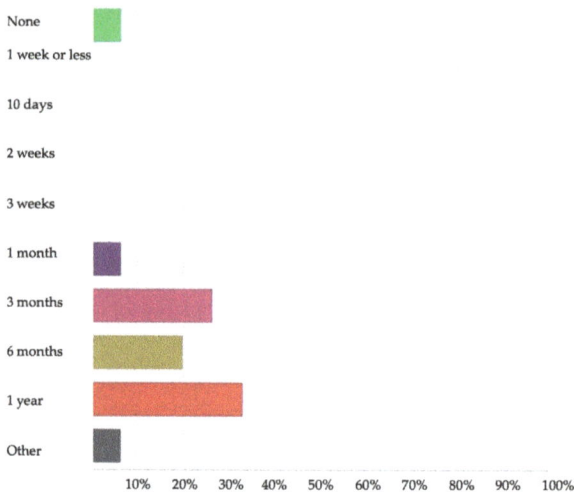

Figure 6. Peroral prophylaxis duration after Kasai hepatoportoenterostomy according to the 2nd Delphi questionnaire.

For both treatment duration and prophylaxis, the correlation coefficient was not applicable due to the modified subgroups between the two Delphi surveys.

3.4. Pre-Meeting Working Group

The working group analyzed the results from the 1st and 2nd Delphi surveys and an agreement was found as described in Figure 7. The chosen definitions for suspected and confirmed cholangitis were based on a combination of the eight clinical, laboratory, and imaging items. Of note, the working group added that a suspected cholangitis having a positive blood culture transformed into a confirmed cholangitis.

A. Clinical elements
•Fever and/or shivering
•Stool color change
•New/increasing jaundice
•Abdominal discomfort*
B. Laboratory and imaging elements
•Inflammatory response (WBC and/or CRP and/or PCT)
•Increased/increasing transaminases
•Increased/increasing GGT and/or bilirubin
•Bile lakes
*Definition for abdominal discomfort: vomiting, poor feeding, irritability
Suspected Cholangitis**:
- Definition: one item in A + one item in B
- Treatment: 10 – 14 days
Confirmed Cholangitis**:
- Definition: two items in A + two items in B
or
"suspected cholangitis" + positive blood culture
- Treatment: 14 – 21 days
Peroral prophylaxis of cholangitis: 6 – 12 months
**Cholangitis within 1st year after Kasai

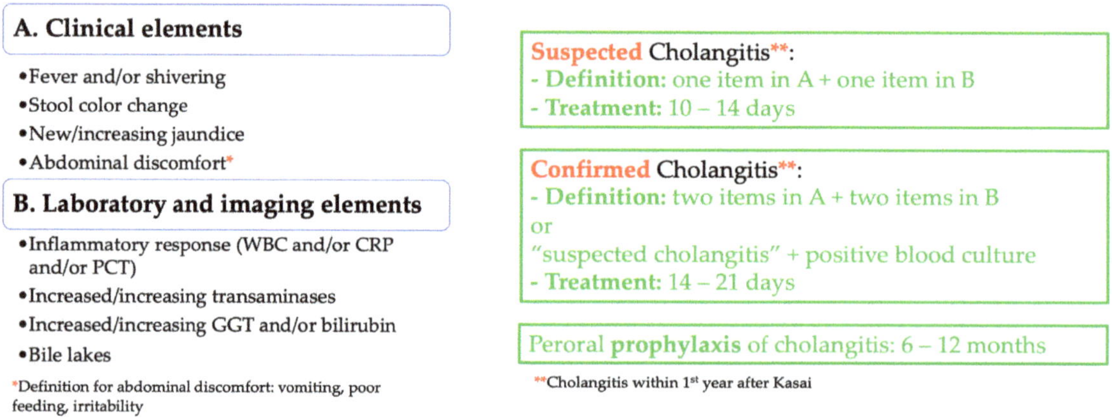

Figure 7. Working group proposal for cholangitis definitions, prophylaxis, and treatment.

3.5. Expert Panel

Comments from the expert panel meeting are summarized in Section 4.

4. Discussion

Cholangitis, a potentially life-threatening condition after the Kasai HPE, is defined as inflammation or infection of the bile duct system [45]. Although the definition of the pathological picture of cholangitis is unequivocal, diagnostic criteria are far from clear-cut, and many different definitions exist to delineate the clinical diagnosis. Whereby some clinicians suspect post-Kasai cholangitis in any situation where the patient is "not well", others need a clearly febrile baby to feel in line with the diagnosis. When reviewing the literature on the topic, this discrepancy between different definitions is immediately depictable, mirroring the difficulties clinicians have to diagnose their patients. This study aimed to find, via the Delphi method and an expert panel, a consensus on the criteria that have diagnostic importance for cholangitis after Kasai HPE, thus defining suspected and confirmed cholangitis. Further, we established recommendations for cholangitis prophylaxis and a treatment plan for each suspected and confirmed cholangitis.

4.1. Definitions of Suspected and Confirmed Cholangitis

In the pediatric literature few authors discuss the concept of a suspected or presumed cholangitis [21,46], but terms such as *suspected* and *definite* diagnosis appear within the Tokyo guidelines, which guide the clinician to the diagnosis of cholangitis [16]. Yet, regarding the clinical applicability of the Tokyo guidelines, it is important to note that they have been tested only in adult cohorts [47]. Thus, there is a consensus among experts that these guidelines clearly do not seem suitable for small children. Based on the Tokyo guidelines our pediatric expert panel intensively discussed the weight of the included items for a definition in young children. Although some items were unanimously supported, such as fever or shivering and sudden stool color change as well as inflammatory laboratory elements, some needed extensive discussions. This said, the Delphi method clearly helped to weigh the different opinions and to come to a consensus. Of note, the idea to create a score by attributing a value for each item and to define cholangitis when a certain total value is reached was rapidly rejected due to the (1) lack of evidence and (2) the more difficult implementation and, thus, the less likelihood to be used in the everyday clinical practice.

Of note, the following definitions are proposed for first episode(s) of cholangitis within the first year after Kasai HPE and are not thought to be used to define refractory and/or recurrent cholangitis 1 year after Kasai HPE.

Suspected cholangitis: The definition for *suspected* cholangitis that was finally chosen was **one** item from the list A (fever and/or shivering, *or* stool color change, *or* new/increasing jaundice, *or* abdominal discomfort) and **one** item from the list B (inflammatory response, *or* increased/increasing transaminases, *or* increased/increasing GGT or bilirubin, *or* the presence of bile lakes) to define this clinical picture needing the related treatment (Figure 5). Both the working group and expert panel agreed to have a very low threshold to suspect cholangitis in order for babies not to be missed and potentially evolve towards severe, life-threatening confirmed cholangitis. Swift and prompt cholangitis treatment in this circumstance might avoid liver deterioration.

Confirmed cholangitis: The proposed definition for *confirmed* cholangitis included **two** items from list A and **two** items from list B (Figure 5). Further, the expert panel proposed that a baby with *suspected* cholangitis revealing a positive blood culture should shift the diagnosis to confirmed cholangitis. Of note, reported rates of positive blood cultures in cholangitis were variable: according to the published series, they ranged from 25.8% to 43.6% [12,48]. A further consideration from the panelists was to include the treatment response of a suspected cholangitis into the definition of a confirmed cholangitis but decided that this should finally be up to the discretion of the treating clinician and should not be included in the definition. Although participants and experts initially were positive to include fever *without* an extrahepatic source as a mandatory criterion for a confirmed cholangitis, we concluded that two *other* additional clinical criteria from the list A, associated with two laboratory elements, can also confirm cholangitis. Some experts and participants also proposed liver biopsy (percutaneous or laparoscopic) to confirm cholangitis. Although the risk for major complications associated with liver biopsy has been reported to be less than 1% [49], the procedure is invasive, and should be limited to specific clinical situations such as intractable cholangitis without positive blood cultures or recurrent cholangitis [48,50]. The item was therefore not included in the definition of confirmed cholangitis in the discussed setting, i.e., children within the 1st year after Kasai HPE who present with a first episode of cholangitis.

4.2. Treatment of Suspected and Confirmed Cholangitis

Suspected cholangitis: The treatment duration for a suspected cholangitis was unanimously preferred to be 10–14 days. This recommendation is in line with the shorter antibiotic treatment duration for post Kasai HPE cholangitis reported in the literature [5,10,13,40]. Both working group and expert panel agreed that this proposed treatment duration is adequate for patients with the diagnosis of suspected cholangitis, but also agreed that a treatment duration of only 7–10 days seems too short and risks leading to episodes of recurrent or refractory cholangitis. Whether 10 or 14 day therapy is chosen is up to the discretion of the treating clinician and the level of suspicion for suspected cholangitis.

Confirmed cholangitis: The treatment duration for confirmed cholangitis was chosen to be 14–21 days, corresponding to the reported longer treatment duration for cholangitis after Kasai HPE [21,43]. The choice between a 14 and 21 day treatment regimen is up to the clinician, who will decide based on the patient's clinical condition and treatment response. The working group and panel participants both readily agreed on this treatment duration and there was no debate on this subject.

4.3. Cholangitis Prophylaxis

In the literature, there is uncertainty regarding long-term prescription of antibiotics to prevent cholangitis after Kasai HPE; little published data support the use of one antibiotic over another [51] or a specific duration of antibiotic prophylaxis [8]. Further, the fact that antibiotic prophylaxis might induce antibiotic resistance must also be taken into consideration. Yet, as outlined by the overwhelming majority of the respondents of our surveys and the expert panel, clinical practice favors antibiotic administration to prevent cholangitis after Kasai HPE. Weighing the benefits and risks, the participants and expert panel chose the duration of prophylaxis to be 6–12 months. Of note, no differentiation was suggested to be made between draining and non-draining HPE.

5. Conclusions

We herein have developed standardized definitions for suspected and confirmed cholangitis after Kasai HPE. The definitions include the most important clinical, laboratory, and imaging criteria for cholangitis, identified through a group of international experts using the Delphi method. These definitions can not only be easily applied in the clinical setting of non-specialized, general pediatric clinics, but may also be used as an outcome measure in studies reporting on complications after Kasai HPE and/or the impact of cholangitis on native liver survival and patient survival. The duration of antibiotic prophylaxis and treatment was identified in the literature review and confirmed by both Delphi survey participants and panelists. Preliminary applicability will be further tested in a multicentered prospective study.

Supplementary Materials: The following are available online at https://www.mdpi.com/article/10.3390/jcm11030494/s1, Supplementary Document S1: Cholangitis definition and management after Kasai hepatoportoenterostomy for biliary atresia questionnaire—1st Delphi questionnaire; Supplementary Document S2: Definition of cholangitis and management after Kasai hepatoportoenterostomy for biliary atresia—2nd Delphi questionnaire.

Author Contributions: Conceptualization, A.M.C., O.M.-S., C.M., R.A.S., R.S., D.K., C.P. and B.E.W.; methodology, A.M.C., O.M.-S., C.P. and B.E.W.; software, A.M.C. and O.M.-S.; validation, A.M.C., O.M.-S., C.M., R.A.S., R.S., D.K., C.P. and B.E.W.; formal analysis, A.M.C.; investigation, A.M.C. and O.M.-S.; writing—original draft preparation, A.M.C. and B.E.W.; writing—review and editing, A.M.C., O.M.-S., C.M., R.A.S., R.S., D.K., C.P. and B.E.W.; visualization, A.M.C., O.M.-S., C.M., R.A.S., R.S., D.K., C.P. and B.E.W.; supervision, B.E.W. All authors have read and agreed to the published version of the manuscript.

Funding: This research received no external funding.

Institutional Review Board Statement: Ethical review and approval were waived for this study, due to the Delphi methodology.

Informed Consent Statement: Not applicable.

Acknowledgments: We would like to thank all of our colleagues who participated in the preliminary versions of the surveys as well as the librarian for her help with the systematic literature review.

Conflicts of Interest: The authors declare no conflict of interest.

Appendix A

Table A1. Overview of cholangitis definition after Kasai hepatoportoenterostomy and reported (2000–2021) rates of cholangitis, native liver survival (NLS), and patient survival (PS). ALT, alanine aminotransferase; AST, aspartate aminotransferase; CRP, C reactive protein; GGT, gamma-glutamyl transpeptidase; NLS, native liver survival; PA, alkaline phosphatase; PS, patient survival; WBC, white blood cell count.

Authors	Number of Patients	Cholangitis Definition	Cholangitis Rates	NLS/PS
Chuang J., et al., 2000 [13]	39	Fever > 38 °C without obvious extrahepatic source with an elevated serum bilirubin	46%	-
Wu E.T., et al., 2001 [10]	45	Fever, acholic stools, and/or increasing jaundice +/− positive blood cultures	75%	PS, 67.5%
Selvalingam S., et al., 2002 [52]	61	Fever and leukocytosis (no other cause) + increase direct bilirubin or AST or ALT or paler stools +/− positive blood culture	57%	1 year PS, 90%
Bu L.N., et al., 2003 [9]	19	Unexplained fever ≥ 38 °C, acholic stools, increased jaundice or positive blood culture	100%	-
Van Heurn E., et al., 2003 [14]	77	Fever > 38 °C, not explained otherwise or abrupt recurrence or increase of clinical jaundice with increased bilirubin levels or acholic stools		
Ogasawara Y., et al., 2003 [53]	21	Fever > 38 °C and elevated bilirubin and leukocytosis	52.3%	PS, 100%
Wong K.K., et al., 2004 [20]	19	Fever > 38.5 °C of unknown origin more than 48 h, progressive jaundice and derangement of liver function, passage of acholic stools	-	-
Kobayashi H., et al., 2005 [54]	63	Fever > 38 °C, with elevated serum bilirubin and leukocytosis	15.8%	-
Shinohara T., et al., 2005 [55]	18	Unexplained fever > 38 °C, with elevated CRP and bilirubin.	44.4%	-
Hung P., et al., 2006 [4]	22	High fever with no other obvious focus with acholic stools, increased jaundice, or positive blood culture	54.6%	2 year NLS, 53.2% 5 year NLS, 34.7% 10 year NLS, 30.5%
Lai H.S., 2006 [18]	163	Recurrent clay colored stool, icterus, or hyperbilirubinemia	72.3%	-

Table A1. *Cont.*

Authors	Number of Patients	Cholangitis Definition	Cholangitis Rates	NLS/PS
Stringer M.D., et al., 2007 [28]	71	Deteriorating liver function + pale stools and fever	46%	NLS, 67.5% PS, 93.3%
Vejchapipat P., et al., 2007 [29]	53	Fever > 38.5 °C, change of stool color, leukocytosis (>12 G/L) with polymorphonuclear leukocytes predominance	45.2%	-
Petersen C., et al., 2008 [21]	49	Suspected cholangitis: any of fever, recurrence of acholic stools, leukocytosis, elevated liver function tests, increasing bilirubin	-	6 month, NLS 63% 2 year, NLS 31% 6 month, PS 90% 2 year, PS 78%
Sanghai S.R., et al., 2009 [56]	88	Fever with clay colored stool, leukocytosis and/or vomiting, abdominal distension and bacteriemia	33.3%	-
Suzuki T., et al., 2010 [57]	53	Fever, blood biochemistry and the decrease of bile secretion (fecal color change)	13.2% (early)	NLS, 73.6% PS, 88.7%
Kumagi T., et al., 2011 [46]	22	Presumed cholangitis: fever and chills with or without jaundice, nausea or abdominal pain and abnormal biliary imaging: stricture, dilatation and/or stone, with or without evidence of an acute rise in liver tests or improvement upon administration of antibiotics	50%	PS, 95.5% NLS, 81.8%
Lee J.Y., et al., 2014 [12]	27	Fever > 37.5 °C or worsening jaundice, transaminitis or acholic stools +/− positive blood cultures	64.3%	-
Ng V., et al., 2014 [58]	219	Fever > 38 °C without other obvious source, new onset of acholic stools, right upper quadrant pain or tenderness and both elevation of direct bilirubin by 25% and at least 1 mg/dL above baseline, positive blood culture not required	62.1%	-
Wada M., et al., 2014 [59]	36	Elevated serum bilirubin > 2.5 mg/dL, leukocytosis with left shift and normal to acholic stools in a febrile patient (>38 °C)	48.8%	-
Lien T., et al., 2015 [40]	20	Unexplained fever > 38 °C, acholic stools, increased jaundice or positive blood cultures	20%	-
Qiao G., et al., 2015 [60]	262	Fever > 38 °C, without other reason, recurrence or increased jaundice, increased bilirubin, acholic stools	54.9%	5 year PS, 43.3% 5 year NLS, 75.8%
Webb N.L., et al., 2016 [33]	29	Fever > 38.5 °C, and elevated liver transaminases in the absence of other cause for febrile illness	75%	5 year NLS, 45.8%
Chiang L.W., et al., 2017 [41]	58	Fever without other attributable cause, acholic stool and/or deepening jaundice	30.5%	Overall NLS, 48.3% 2 year NLS, 72% 5 year NLS, 45.7%
Kelay A., et al., 2017 [61]	-	Fever, abdominal pain, worsening or recurring jaundice with acholic stools, changes in bilirubin and liver enzymes level together with acute changes in WBC and inflammatory markers such as CRP	-	-
Lee W.S., et al., 2017 [34]	52	Fever > 38 °C without other source, abdominal pain and new onset of acholic stools, and elevation of conjugated bilirubin and/or GGT from previous baseline	52%	NLS, 37% PS, 51%
Stagg H., et al., 2017 [15]	-	Fever and/or jaundice, altered liver biochemistry, blood cultures (96%) and liver biopsy (26%)	-	-

Table A1. *Cont.*

Authors	Number of Patients	Cholangitis Definition	Cholangitis Rates	NLS/PS
Chen S., et al., 2018 [3]	366	Fever ≥ 38 °C and acholic stool, increase of jaundice and bilirubin or positive blood cultures	67.7%	NLS, 74%
Chung P., et al., 2018 [48]	192	Fever ≥ 38.5 °C, with either increased bilirubin ≥ 20 μmol/L or acholic stool.	35.4%	-
Jiang H., et al., 2018 [62]	-	High fever, bile discharge reduced or stopped, abdominal distention, vomiting and reduced liver function, worsening jaundice, elevated levels of Bilirubin and ALAT, pale or clay-colored stools, dark yellow colored urine, WBC and neutrophils elevated	-	-
Li D., et al., 2018 [5]	113	Fever without identifiable source and 1. Reappearance of jaundice or acholic stools; 2. Sudden elevation of bilirubin > 2.5 mg/dL or AST or 3. Positive blood culture	-	-
Nakajima H., et al., 2018 [63]	66	Fever > 38 °C, elevated serum bilirubin > 2.5 mg/dL, leukocytosis with left shift and normal to acholic stools	55%	NLS, 74%
Xiao H., et al., 2018 [64]	166	Fever > 38 °C, unexplained by other reasons, abrupt recurrence or increased clinical jaundice with increased bilirubin levels, acholic stools, significantly increased serum WBC and neutrophil	44.5%	2 year NLS, 79.5%
Ginstrom D., et al., 2019 [65]	61	Fever > 38 °C without any other identifiable source, treated with intravenous antibiotics	79%	-
Liu J., et al., 2019 [6]	180	At least 2 of: 1. Unexplained fever > 38 °C, 2. Recurrence or exacerbation of jaundice with increased bilirubin or changes from yellow to acholic stools, 3. Elevated CRP	66.1%	NLS, 53.9% PS, 80%
Pang W., et al., 2019 [19]	218	Fever and/or altered stool or refractory jaundice, CRP and/or WBC elevation and sudden elevation of bilirubin or ALT or AST	27%	-
Parolini F., et al., 2019 [35]	174	Fever, abdominal pain, worsening or recurrent jaundice, change in stool color associated with rise in bilirubin and liver enzyme levels, white cell count and inflammatory markers	32%	20 year NLS, 18.3%
Ramachandran P., et al., 2019 [36]	62	1. Fever, pale stools. 2. Elevated WBC and CRP. 3. Elevation of bilirubin and/or liver enzymes	43.5%	-
Baek S.H., et al., 2020 [37]	160	Fever > 38 °C or elevated inflammatory markers and evidence of cholestasis or abnormal liver function tests in accordance with Tokyo guidelines	78.8%	5 year PS, 93.3%
Madadi-Sanjani O., et al., 2020 [66]	26	Acholic stools or increase in serum bilirubin + fever or increase in inflammatory parameters	34.6%	-
Chen G., et al., 2021 [38]	180	1. Fever ≥ 38 °C or elevated CRP and 2. Recurrent acholic stool or jaundice with elevated bilirubin	66.1%	NLS, 84.4%
Chung P.H.Y., et al., 2021 [67]	231	Fever > 38.5 °C and bilirubin > 20 μmol/L on 2 consecutive blood samples; severe cholangitis if more than 2 weeks of antibiotics.	25.7%	NLS, 66.2%
Goh L., et al., 2021 [39]	54	1. Systemic inflammation: fever or elevated inflammatory markers CRP and WBC and 2 evidence of cholestasis or abnormal liver function tests—PA, GGT, AST, ALT > 1.5 normal ranges and/or elevation from baseline levels	72%	NLS, 79.4%

References

1. Nio, M.; Wada, M.; Sasaki, H.; Tanaka, H.; Okumura, A. Risk factors affecting late-presenting liver failure in adult patients with biliary atresia. *J. Pediatr. Surg.* **2012**, *47*, 2179–2183. [CrossRef]
2. Koga, H.; Wada, M.; Nakamura, H.; Miyano, G.; Okawada, M.; Lane, G.J.; Okazaki, T.; Yamataka, A. Factors influencing jaundice-free survival with the native liver in post-portoenterostomy biliary atresia patients: Results from a single institution. *J. Pediatr. Surg.* **2013**, *48*, 2368–2372. [CrossRef] [PubMed]
3. Chen, S.Y.; Lin, C.C.; Tsan, Y.T.; Chan, W.C.; Wang, J.D.; Chou, Y.J.; Lin, C.H. Number of cholangitis episodes as a prognostic marker to predict timing of liver transplantation in biliary atresia patients after Kasai portoenterostomy. *BMC Pediatr.* **2018**, *18*, 119. [CrossRef]
4. Hung, P.Y.; Chen, C.C.; Chen, W.J.; Lai, H.S.; Hsu, W.M.; Lee, P.H.; Ho, M.C.; Chen, T.H.; Ni, Y.H.; Chen, H.L.; et al. Long-term prognosis of patients with biliary atresia: A 25 year summary. *J. Pediatr. Gastroenterol. Nutr.* **2006**, *42*, 190–195. [CrossRef] [PubMed]
5. Li, D.; Chen, X.; Fu, K.; Yang, J.; Feng, J. Preoperative nutritional status and its impact on cholangitis after Kasai portoenterostomy in biliary atresia patients. *Pediatr. Surg. Int.* **2017**, *33*, 901–906. [CrossRef] [PubMed]
6. Liu, J.; Dong, R.; Chen, G.; Dong, K.; Zheng, S. Risk factors and prognostic effects of cholangitis after Kasai procedure in biliary atresia patients: A retrospective clinical study. *J. Pediatr. Surg.* **2019**, *54*, 2559–2564. [CrossRef] [PubMed]
7. Ryon, E.L.; Parreco, J.P.; Sussman, M.S.; Quiroz, H.J.; Willobee, B.A.; Perez, E.A.; Sola, J.E.; Thorson, C.M. Drivers of Hospital Readmission and Early Liver Transplant after Kasai Portoenterostomy. *J. Surg. Res.* **2020**, *256*, 48–55. [CrossRef] [PubMed]
8. Decharun, K.; Leys, C.M.; West, K.W.; Finnell, S.M. Prophylactic Antibiotics for Prevention of Cholangitis in Patients With Biliary Atresia Status Post-Kasai Portoenterostomy: A Systematic Review. *Clin. Pediatr.* **2016**, *55*, 66–72. [CrossRef]
9. Bu, L.N.; Chen, H.L.; Chang, C.J.; Ni, Y.H.; Hsu, H.Y.; Lai, H.S.; Hsu, W.M.; Chang, M.H. Prophylactic oral antibiotics in prevention of recurrent cholangitis after the Kasai portoenterostomy. *J. Pediatr. Surg.* **2003**, *38*, 590–593. [CrossRef]
10. Wu, E.T.; Chen, H.L.; Ni, Y.H.; Lee, P.I.; Hsu, H.Y.; Lai, H.S.; Chang, M.H. Bacterial cholangitis in patients with biliary atresia: Impact on short-term outcome. *Pediatr. Surg. Int.* **2001**, *17*, 390–395. [CrossRef]
11. Gunadi; Gunawan, T.A.; Widiyanto, G.; Yuanita, A.; Mulyani, N.S.; Makhmudi, A. Liver transplant score for prediction of biliary atresia patients' survival following Kasai procedure. *BMC Res. Notes* **2018**, *11*, 381. [CrossRef]
12. Lee, J.Y.; Lim, L.T.; Quak, S.H.; Prabhakaran, K.; Aw, M. Cholangitis in children with biliary atresia: Health-care resource utilisation. *J. Paediatr. Child Health* **2014**, *50*, 196–201. [CrossRef]
13. Chuang, J.H.; Lee, S.Y.; Shieh, C.S.; Chen, W.J.; Chang, N.K. Reappraisal of the role of the bilioenteric conduit in the pathogenesis of postoperative cholangitis. *Pediatr. Surg. Int.* **2000**, *16*, 29–34. [CrossRef]
14. Van Heurn, L.W.E.; Saing, H.; Tam, P.K. Cholangitis after hepatic portoenterostomy for biliary atresia: A multivariate analysis of risk factors. *J. Pediatr.* **2003**, *142*, 566–571. [CrossRef]
15. Stagg, H.; Cameron, B.H.; Ahmed, N.; Butler, A.; Jimenez-Rivera, C.; Yanchar, N.L.; Martin, S.R.; Emil, S.; Anthopoulos, G.; Schreiber, R.A.; et al. Variability of diagnostic approach, surgical technique, and medical management for children with biliary atresia in Canada—Is it time for standardization? *J. Pediatr. Surg.* **2017**, *52*, 802–806. [CrossRef]
16. Wada, K.; Takada, T.; Kawarada, Y.; Nimura, Y.; Miura, F.; Yoshida, M.; Mayumi, T.; Strasberg, S.; Pitt, H.A.; Gadacz, T.R.; et al. Diagnostic criteria and severity assessment of acute cholangitis: Tokyo Guidelines. *J. Hepatobiliary Pancreat. Surg.* **2007**, *14*, 52–58. [CrossRef]
17. Takada, T.; Strasberg, S.M.; Solomkin, J.S.; Pitt, H.A.; Gomi, H.; Yoshida, M.; Mayumi, T.; Miura, F.; Gouma, D.J.; Garden, O.J.; et al. TG13: Updated Tokyo Guidelines for the management of acute cholangitis and cholecystitis. *J. Hepatobiliary Pancreat. Sci.* **2013**, *20*, 1–7. [CrossRef] [PubMed]
18. Lai, H.S.; Chen, W.J.; Chen, C.C.; Hung, W.T.; Chang, M.H. Long-term prognosis and factors affecting biliary atresia from experience over a 25 year period. *Chang Gung. Med. J.* **2006**, *29*, 234–239.
19. Pang, W.B.; Zhang, T.C.; Chen, Y.J.; Peng, C.H.; Wang, Z.M.; Wu, D.Y.; Wang, K. Ten-Year Experience in the Prevention of Post-Kasai Cholangitis. *Surg. Infect.* **2019**, *20*, 231–235. [CrossRef] [PubMed]
20. Wong, K.K.; Fan, A.H.; Lan, L.C.; Lin, S.C.; Tam, P.K. Effective antibiotic regime for postoperative acute cholangitis in biliary atresia—An evolving scene. *J. Pediatr. Surg.* **2004**, *39*, 1800–1802. [CrossRef] [PubMed]
21. Petersen, C.; Harder, D.; Melter, M.; Becker, T.; Wasielewski, R.V.; Leonhardt, J.; Ure, B.M. Postoperative high-dose steroids do not improve mid-term survival with native liver in biliary atresia. *Am. J. Gastroenterol.* **2008**, *103*, 712–719. [CrossRef]
22. Graham, B.; Regehr, G.; Wright, J.G. Delphi as a method to establish consensus for diagnostic criteria. *J. Clin. Epidemiol.* **2003**, *56*, 1150–1156. [CrossRef]
23. Dalkey, N.C. An experimental application of the Delphi method to the use of experts. *Manag. Sci.* **1963**, *9*, 458–467. [CrossRef]
24. Burns, K.E.; Duffett, M.; Kho, M.E.; Meade, M.O.; Adhikari, N.K.; Sinuff, T.; Cook, D.J.; Group, A. A guide for the design and conduct of self-administered surveys of clinicians. *CMAJ* **2008**, *179*, 245–252. [CrossRef] [PubMed]
25. Lally, K.P.; Kanegaye, J.; Matsumura, M.; Rosenthal, P.; Sinatra, F.; Atkinson, J.B. Perioperative factors affecting the outcome following repair of biliary atresia. *Pediatrics* **1989**, *83*, 723–726. [CrossRef] [PubMed]
26. Meyers, R.L.; Book, L.S.; O'Gorman, M.A.; Jackson, W.D.; Black, R.E.; Johnson, D.G.; Matlak, M.E. High-dose steroids, ursodeoxycholic acid, and chronic intravenous antibiotics improve bile flow after Kasai procedure in infants with biliary atresia. *J. Pediatr. Surg.* **2003**, *38*, 406–411. [CrossRef]

27. Kelly, D.A.; Davenport, M. Current management of biliary atresia. *Arch. Dis. Child.* **2007**, *92*, 1132–1135. [CrossRef]
28. Stringer, M.D.; Davison, S.M.; Rajwal, S.R.; McClean, P. Kasai portoenterostomy: 12-year experience with a novel adjuvant therapy regimen. *J. Pediatr. Surg.* **2007**, *42*, 1324–1328. [CrossRef]
29. Vejchapipat, P.; Passakonnirin, R.; Sookpotarom, P.; Chittmittrapap, S.; Poovorawan, Y. High-dose steroids do not improve early outcome in biliary atresia. *J. Pediatr. Surg.* **2007**, *42*, 2102–2105. [CrossRef]
30. De Vries, W.; de Langen, Z.J.; Groen, H.; Scheenstra, R.; Peeters, P.M.; Hulscher, J.B.; Verkade, H.J.; Netherlands Study Group of Biliary Atresia and Registry (NeSBAR). Biliary atresia in the Netherlands: Outcome of patients diagnosed between 1987 and 2008. *J. Pediatr.* **2012**, *160*, 638–644.e2. [CrossRef]
31. Wang, B.; Feng, Q.; Ye, X.; Zeng, S. The experience and technique in laparoscopic portoenterostomy for biliary atresia. *J. Laparoendosc. Adv. Surg. Tech. A* **2014**, *24*, 350–353. [CrossRef]
32. Tyraskis, A.; Davenport, M. Steroids after the Kasai procedure for biliary atresia: The effect of age at Kasai portoenterostomy. *Pediatr. Surg. Int.* **2016**, *32*, 193–200. [CrossRef]
33. Webb, N.L.; Jiwane, A.; Ooi, C.Y.; Nightinghale, S.; Adams, S.E.; Krishnan, U. Clinical significance of liver histology on outcomes in biliary atresia. *J. Paediatr. Child Health* **2017**, *53*, 252–256. [CrossRef] [PubMed]
34. Lee, W.S.; Ong, S.Y.; Foo, H.W.; Wong, S.Y.; Kong, C.X.; Seah, R.B.; Ng, R.T. Chronic liver disease is universal in children with biliary atresia living with native liver. *World J. Gastroenterol.* **2017**, *23*, 7776–7784. [CrossRef]
35. Parolini, F.; Boroni, G.; Milianti, S.; Tonegatti, L.; Armellini, A.; Garcia Magne, M.; Pedersini, P.; Torri, F.; Orizio, P.; Benvenuti, S.; et al. Biliary atresia: 20-40-year follow-up with native liver in an Italian centre. *J. Pediatr. Surg.* **2019**, *54*, 1440–1444. [CrossRef] [PubMed]
36. Ramachandran, P.; Safwan, M.; Balaji, M.S.; Unny, A.K.; Akhtarkhavari, A.; Tamizhvanan, V.; Rela, M. Early Cholangitis after Portoenterostomy in Children with Biliary Atresia. *J. Indian Assoc. Pediatr. Surg.* **2019**, *24*, 185–188. [CrossRef]
37. Baek, S.H.; Kang, J.M.; Ihn, K.; Han, S.J.; Koh, H.; Ahn, J.G. The Epidemiology and Etiology of Cholangitis After Kasai Portoenterostomy in Patients With Biliary Atresia. *J. Pediatr. Gastroenterol. Nutr.* **2020**, *70*, 171–177. [CrossRef]
38. Chen, G.; Liu, J.; Huang, Y.; Wu, Y.; Lu, X.; Dong, R.; Shen, Z.; Sun, S.; Jiang, J.; Zheng, S. Preventive effect of prophylactic intravenous antibiotics against cholangitis in biliary atresia: A randomized controlled trial. *Pediatr. Surg. Int.* **2021**, *37*, 1089–1097. [CrossRef] [PubMed]
39. Goh, L.; Phua, K.B.; Low, Y.; Chiang, L.W.; Yong, C.; Chiou, F.K. Analysis of Cholangitis Rates with Extended Perioperative Antibiotics and Adjuvant Corticosteroids in Biliary Atresia. *Pediatr. Gastroenterol. Hepatol. Nutr.* **2021**, *24*, 366–376. [CrossRef]
40. Lien, T.H.; Bu, L.N.; Wu, J.F.; Chen, H.L.; Chen, A.C.; Lai, M.W.; Shih, H.H.; Lee, I.H.; Hsu, H.Y.; Ni, Y.H.; et al. Use of Lactobacillus casei rhamnosus to Prevent Cholangitis in Biliary Atresia After Kasai Operation. *J. Pediatr. Gastroenterol. Nutr.* **2015**, *60*, 654–658. [CrossRef]
41. Chiang, L.W.; Lee, C.Y.; Krishnaswamy, G.; Nah, S.A.; Kader, A.; Ong, C.; Low, Y.; Phua, K.B. Seventeen years of Kasai portoenterostomy for biliary atresia in a single Southeast Asian paediatric centre. *J. Paediatr. Child Health* **2017**, *53*, 412–415. [CrossRef] [PubMed]
42. Li, Z.; Ye, Y.; Wu, Z.; Wang, B. Learning Curve Analysis of Laparoscopic Kasai Portoenterostomy. *J. Laparoendosc. Adv. Surg. Tech. A* **2017**, *27*, 979–982. [CrossRef] [PubMed]
43. Calinescu, A.M.; Wilde, J.C.H.; Korff, S.; McLin, V.A.; Wildhaber, B.E. Perioperative Complications after Kasai Hepatoportoenterostomy: Data from the Swiss National Biliary Atresia Registry. *Eur. J. Pediatr. Surg.* **2020**, *30*, 364–370. [CrossRef]
44. Chung, P.H.Y.; Chok, K.S.H.; Wong, K.K.Y.; Tam, P.K.H.; Lo, C.M. Determining the optimal timing of liver transplant for pediatric patients after Kasai portoenterostomy based on disease severity scores. *J. Pediatr. Surg.* **2020**, *55*, 1892–1896. [CrossRef]
45. Sifri, C.D.; Madoff, L.C. Infections of the Liver and Biliary system (Liver abscess, cholangitis, cholecystitis). In *Mandell, Douglas and Bennett's Priciples and Practice of Infectious Diseases*, 8th ed.; WB Saunders: Philadelphia, PA, USA, 2015.
46. Kumagi, T.; Drenth, J.P.; Guttman, O.; Ng, V.; Lilly, L.; Therapondos, G.; Hiasa, Y.; Michitaka, K.; Onji, M.; Watanabe, Y.; et al. Biliary atresia and survival into adulthood without transplantation: A collaborative multicentre clinic review. *Liver Int.* **2012**, *32*, 510–518. [CrossRef] [PubMed]
47. Kiriyama, S.; Takada, T.; Hwang, T.L.; Akazawa, K.; Miura, F.; Gomi, H.; Mori, R.; Endo, I.; Itoi, T.; Yokoe, M.; et al. Clinical application and verification of the TG13 diagnostic and severity grading criteria for acute cholangitis: An international multicenter observational study. *J. Hepatobiliary Pancreat. Sci.* **2017**, *24*, 329–337. [CrossRef]
48. Chung, P.H.Y.; Tam, P.K.H.; Wong, K.K.Y. Does the identity of the bacteria matter in post-Kasai cholangitis? A comparison between simple and intractable cholangitis. *J. Pediatr. Surg.* **2018**, *53*, 2409–2411. [CrossRef]
49. Sandy, N.S.; Hessel, G.; Bellomo-Brandao, M.A. Major Complications of Pediatric Percutaneous Liver Biopsy Do Not Differ Among Physicians with Different Degrees of Training. *Am. J. Gastroenterol.* **2020**, *115*, 786–789. [CrossRef]
50. Luo, Y.; Zheng, S. Current concept about postoperative cholangitis in biliary atresia. *World J. Pediatr.* **2008**, *4*, 14–19. [CrossRef]
51. Pakarinen, M.P.; Rintala, R.J. Surgery of biliary atresia. *Scand. J. Surg.* **2011**, *100*, 49–53. [CrossRef]
52. Selvalingam, S.; Mahmud, M.N.; Thambidorai, C.R.; Zakaria, Z.; Mohan, N.; Isa, Sheila, M. Jaundice clearance and cholangitis in the first year following portoenterostomy for biliary atresia. *Med. J. Malays.* **2002**, *57*, 92–96.
53. Ogasawara, Y.; Yamataka, A.; Tsukamoto, K.; Okada, Y.; Lane, G.J.; Kobayashi, H.; Miyano, T. The intussusception antireflux valve is ineffective for preventing cholangitis in biliary atresia: A prospective study. *J. Pediatr. Surg.* **2003**, *38*, 1826–1829. [CrossRef] [PubMed]

54. Kobayashi, H.; Yamataka, A.; Koga, H.; Okazaki, T.; Tamura, T.; Urao, M.; Yanai, T.; Lane, G.J.; Miyano, T. Optimum prednisolone usage in patients with biliary atresia postportoenterostomy. *J. Pediatr. Surg.* **2005**, *40*, 327–330. [CrossRef]
55. Shinohara, T.; Muraji, T.; Tsugawa, C.; Nishijima, E.; Satoh, S.; Takamizawa, S. Efficacy of urinary sulfated bile acids for diagnosis of bacterial cholangitis in biliary atresia. *Pediatr. Surg. Int.* **2005**, *21*, 701–704. [CrossRef] [PubMed]
56. Sanghai, S.R.; Shah, I.; Bhatnagar, S.; Murthy, A. Incidence and prognostic factors associated with biliary atresia in western India. *Ann. Hepatol.* **2009**, *8*, 120–122. [CrossRef]
57. Suzuki, T.; Hashimoto, T.; Kondo, S.; Sato, Y.; Hussein, M.H. Evaluating patients' outcome post-Kasai operation: A 19-year experience with modification of the hepatic portoenterostomy and applying a novel steroid therapy regimen. *Pediatr. Surg. Int.* **2010**, *26*, 825–830. [CrossRef] [PubMed]
58. Ng, V.L.; Haber, B.H.; Magee, J.C.; Miethke, A.; Murray, K.F.; Michail, S.; Karpen, S.J.; Kerkar, N.; Molleston, J.P.; Romero, R.; et al. Medical status of 219 children with biliary atresia surviving long-term with their native livers: Results from a North American multicenter consortium. *J. Pediatr.* **2014**, *165*, 539–546.e2. [CrossRef]
59. Wada, M.; Nakamura, H.; Koga, H.; Miyano, G.; Lane, G.J.; Okazaki, T.; Urao, M.; Murakami, H.; Kasahara, M.; Sakamoto, S.; et al. Experience of treating biliary atresia with three types of portoenterostomy at a single institution: Extended, modified Kasai, and laparoscopic modified Kasai. *Pediatr. Surg. Int.* **2014**, *30*, 863–870. [CrossRef]
60. Qiao, G.; Li, L.; Cheng, W.; Zhang, Z.; Ge, J.; Wang, C. Conditional probability of survival in patients with biliary atresia after Kasai portoenterostomy: A Chinese population-based study. *J. Pediatr. Surg.* **2015**, *50*, 1310–1315. [CrossRef]
61. Kelay, A.; Davenport, M. Long-term outlook in biliary atresia. *Semin. Pediatr. Surg.* **2017**, *26*, 295–300. [CrossRef]
62. Jiang, H.; Gao, P.; Chen, H.; Zhong, Z.; Shu, M.; Zhang, Z.; She, J.; Liu, J. The Prognostic Value of CD8(+) and CD45RO(+) T Cells Infiltration and Beclin1 Expression Levels for Early Postoperative Cholangitis of Biliary Atresia Patients after Kasai Operation. *J. Korean Med. Sci.* **2018**, *33*, e198. [CrossRef]
63. Nakajima, H.; Koga, H.; Okawada, M.; Nakamura, H.; Lane, G.J.; Yamataka, A. Does time taken to achieve jaundice-clearance influence survival of the native liver in post-Kasai biliary atresia? *World J. Pediatr.* **2018**, *14*, 191–196. [CrossRef]
64. Xiao, H.; Huang, R.; Chen, L.; Diao, M.; Li, L. The Application of a Shorter Loop in Kasai Portoenterostomy Reconstruction for Ohi Type III Biliary Atresia: A Prospective Randomized Controlled Trial. *J. Surg. Res.* **2018**, *232*, 492–496. [CrossRef] [PubMed]
65. Ginstrom, D.A.; Hukkinen, M.; Kivisaari, R.; Pakarinen, M.P. Biliary Atresia-associated Cholangitis: The Central Role and Effective Management of Bile Lakes. *J. Pediatr. Gastroenterol. Nutr.* **2019**, *68*, 488–494. [CrossRef]
66. Madadi-Sanjani, O.; Schukfeh, N.; Uecker, M.; Eckmann, S.; Dingemann, J.; Ure, B.M.; Petersen, C.; Kuebler, J.F. The Intestinal Flora at Kasai Procedure in Children with Biliary Atresia Appears Not to Affect Postoperative Cholangitis. *Eur. J. Pediatr. Surg.* **2021**, *31*, 80–85. [CrossRef] [PubMed]
67. Chung, P.H.Y.; Chan, E.K.W.; Yeung, F.; Chan, A.C.Y.; Mou, J.W.C.; Lee, K.H.; Hung, J.W.S.; Leung, M.W.Y.; Tam, P.K.H.; Wong, K.K.Y. Life long follow up and management strategies of patients living with native livers after Kasai portoenterostomy. *Sci. Rep.* **2021**, *11*, 11207. [CrossRef] [PubMed]

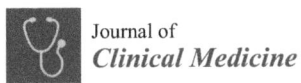 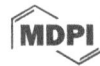

Article

Incidence, Impact and Treatment of Ongoing CMV Infection in Patients with Biliary Atresia in Four European Centres

Björn Fischler [1,*,†], Piotr Czubkowski [2,†,‡], Antal Dezsofi [3,†,‡], Ulrika Liliemark [1,†,‡], Piotr Socha [2,†,‡], Ronald J. Sokol [4,‡], Jan F. Svensson [5,†,‡] and Mark Davenport [6]

1. Astrid Lindgren Children's Hospital, Karolinska University Hospital, CLINTEC Karolinska Institutet, 171 64 Stockholm, Sweden; ulrika.liliemark@karolinska.se
2. The Children's Memorial Health Institute, 04 730 Warsaw, Poland; p.czubkowski@ipczd.pl (P.C.); p.socha@ipczd.pl (P.S.)
3. First Department of Pediatrics, Semmelweis University, 1085 Budapest, Hungary; dezsofi.antal@med.semmelweis-univ.hu
4. Pediatric Liver Center, Department of Pediatrics, University of Colorado School of Medicine, Children's Hospital Colorado, Aurora, CO 80045, USA; ronald.sokol@childrenscolorado.org
5. Astrid Lindgren Children's Hospital, Karolinska University Hospital, Department of Women's and Children's Health, Karolinska Institutet, 171 64 Stockholm, Sweden; jan.f.svensson@karolinska.se
6. Kings College Hospital, Department of Paediatric Surgery, London SE5 9RS, UK; markdav2@ntlworld.com
* Correspondence: bjorn.fischler@karolinska.se
† Full member of European Rare Network (ERN) for rare liver disease.
‡ Contributed equally, appear in alphabetical order.

Abstract: Cytomegalovirus (CMV) infection has been suggested to be of importance for the development and outcome of biliary atresia (BA). However, most data are only available from single centre studies. We retrospectively collected data on rates, outcomes, and treatments for ongoing CMV infection at the time of Kasai portoenterostomy (KPE) from four different tertiary centres in Europe. The rate of ongoing CMV infection varied between 10–32% in the four centres. CMV positive patients were significantly older and had higher levels of several liver biochemistries at the time of KPE ($p < 0.05$ for all comparisons). In the largest centre, CMV infection was more common in non-Caucasians, and CMV infected patients had poorer long-term survival with native liver than CMV negative patients ($p = 0.0001$). In contrast, survival with native liver in the subgroup of CMV infected patients who had received antiviral treatment was similar to the CMV negative group. We conclude that ongoing CMV infection at the time of KPE occurs in a significant proportion of BA patients and that these patients seem to differ from CMV negative patients regarding age and biochemistry at the time of KPE as well as long-term survival with native liver. The latter difference may be reduced by antiviral treatment, but randomized, controlled trials are needed before such treatment can be recommended routinely.

Keywords: biliary atresia; cytomegalovirus; survival native liver; antiviral treatment

1. Introduction

Cytomegalovirus (CMV) is a double-stranded DNA virus of the family *herpesviridae*. Though infection is normally mild in children and adults it can be serious in the immunocompromised host. Congenital CMV infection, in contrast, can be a significant cause of microcephaly, neurodevelopmental delay and hearing loss and is said to be present in 1–2% of all pregnancies [1].

The role of viruses in initiating or causing biliary atresia (BA) has been debated for at least 30 years but without a definitive consensus. Of all the possible viruses proposed, CMV appears to have the strongest evidence [1–3]. In an early Swedish study from 1998, CMV-IgM was detected in serum from 38% of BA patients at the time of Kasai portoenterostomy (KPE), which was significantly higher than the 6% found in age-matched controls without any liver disease [1]. Other studies have since suggested the rate of BA patients with ongoing CMV infection to be anywhere between 10 and 74% with Asian centres tending to have a higher prevalence [2–6]. In the largest European study to date, Zani et al. showed that infants with "CMV-IgM +ve BA" were older at the time of KPE and had distinctively different histopathological features in the liver, including more pronounced inflammation than BA patients without CMV infection [3]. It was also reported that CMV IgM +ve patients had a worse prognosis that was improved following anti-viral treatment (AVT) [7].

Currently, there is a lack of multicentre studies on the frequency, consequences and possible importance of CMV infection in BA. The aim of the present study was therefore to collect data from four European tertiary centres on the rate of ongoing CMV infection at the time of KPE, identify the differences between CMV infected and uninfected BA patients at the time of KPE and their outcomes, and to examine the possible effects of AVT.

2. Materials and Methods

Clinical and biochemical data were retrospectively collected from locally held databases and patient charts at the following centres in Europe: First Department of Pediatrics, Semmelweis University, Budapest; Kings College Hospital, London; Astrid Lindgren Children's Hospital, Karolinska University Hospital, Stockholm; and Children's Memorial Health Institute, Warsaw (Table 1).

Table 1. Description of the four participating centres with regard to treatment of biliary atresia.

	Budapest	London	Stockholm	Warsaw
National referral status	Only centre	Largest centre of three	Largest centre of two	Only major centre
Time period studied	2006–2021	2004–2021	2005–2018	1990–2019
Total national population (million)	10	65	10	38
Number of new BA patients/year	5	25	3	20
Rate of CMV testing in BA	67%	75%	100%	76%

CMV—cytomegalovirus; BA—biliary atresia.

Ongoing CMV infection (CMV positivity) detected before or at the time of KPE was defined by any of the following: a positive test for serum CMV-IgM, urine CMV-DNA by PCR or CMV-DNA in serum/plasma/whole blood by PCR.

CMV-positive BA patients were compared to CMV-negative patients with regard to ethnicity, associated anomalies, age and biochemical lab values at KPE and outcomes. For CMV-positive patients, treatment and outcome of antiviral treatment were recorded. For the largest centre (London), 50 CMV-positive patients were compared to 100 contemporaneous CMV-negative control BA patients. Two control patients were matched in time to one index CMV-positive case, to correct for practice and surgery at the time.

Data were reported as median (range) unless otherwise indicated. Differences were tested using non-parametric statistical tests and a p value of <0.05 was accepted as statistically significant.

In Stockholm and Warsaw, the study was approved by the local ethics committees. In Budapest and London, data collection was regarded as an audit of outcome and, thus, formal ethical approval was not required. Informed consent was waived in Stockholm and Warsaw since it was not required according to the ethical permit. Informed consent was obtained in Budapest.

3. Results

All four centres reported data from the past 15 years with one (Warsaw) dating back to 1990 (Table 1); the reported prevalence of CMV testing in BA patients was high in all four centres (67–100%) and was universal in one centre (Stockholm). The rate of ongoing CMV infection at the time of KPE varied between an estimated 10% in London to 32% in Stockholm and was associated with the age at KPE (Tables 2 and 3). In Budapest,

Stockholm and Warsaw, 81 out of a total of 407 BA patients (19.9%) had signs of ongoing CMV infection at the time of KPE. In London, an estimated 10% of all BA were CMV positive. For the purpose of further analysis 50 patients with ongoing CMV and 99 CMV-negative controls were chosen. Thus, altogether 180 CMV-positive BA patients from four centres were analysed.

Table 2. Rate of CMV positivity in tested patients in relation to age at Kasai portoenterostomy (KPE).

Rate CMV Positivity = Positive CMV/Total BA Cases (%) *	KPE < 30 days	KPE 31–70 days	KPE > 70 days
Budapest	0/7	0/22	9/23 (39%)
London	0/7	28/99 (28%)	22/43 (52%)
Stockholm	0	4/16 (25%)	8/21 (38%)
Warsaw	0	21/171 (12%)	39/147 (26%)
Total	0/14	53/308 (17%)	78/234 (33%)

KPE—Kasai portoenterostomy. * Total numbers presented for Budapest, Stockholm and Warsaw. For London patients each CMV positive matched with 2 CMV negative patients for time period.

Table 3. Comparison between CMV-positive and CMV-negative BA patients at time of Kasai portoenterostomy.

	Budapest	London	Stockholm	Warsaw
Age at KPE CMV pos/neg (days)	88/63 *	69/49 *	78/71 $p = 0.10$	79/71 *
Ethnic disparity	No	Yes	No	No
Other anomalies CMV pos/CMV neg	0%/23% $p = 0.18$	16%/18%	17%/12%	n/a
ALT (IU/L)	184/122	n/a	114/100	158/145
AST (IU/L)	295/173 *	n/a	221/175	n/a
Bilirubin total (micromoles/L)	171/144	169/141 *	152/154	168/160
Bilirubin conj (micromoles/L)	118/95	n/a	137/125	131/126
Gamma-GT (IU/L)	538/443	510/511	279/306	968/768 *
APRI	2.7/0.9 *	1.07/0.69 *	1.1/0.8	n/a

ALT—alanine aminotransferase; AST—aspartate aminotransferase; GT-glutamyl transpeptidase; APRI—AST to platelet ratio index; n/a—not available; * Difference statistically significant, $p \leq 0.05$. All biochemical values are medians.

Age at KPE was significantly higher in CMV positive than in CMV negative BA patients in three of the centres (all $p < 0.05$), with borderline significance in the fourth (Table 3). Available liver biochemistries at the time of KPE were often significantly higher in the CMV-positive group compared to the CMV-negative group although this was variable. For instance, CMV-positive infants were significantly more jaundiced in London than at the other three centres. APRi (a surrogate marker of liver fibrosis) was significantly elevated in two of the three centres where it was measured in infants with CMV-positive BA (Table 2).

In only one of the centres (London) was there an ethnic difference with CMV positivity being significantly more common among non-Caucasian patients than among Caucasians.

The effect of CMV on clinical outcomes was more difficult to delineate as two centres did not report jaundice clearance rates. Clearance was significantly lower in CMV-positive cases (37% vs. 71%; $p < 0.0001$) in London, while not statistically different in Stockholm (25% vs. 44%; $p = 0.26$) (Table 4). Any differences in native-liver survival were also unclear in some centres. However, it should be noted that there was no reported native-liver survival in CMV-positive infants in Budapest. Figure 1 illustrates a significant difference in native-liver survival according to CMV status in the London cohort with the largest number of patients; however, this was not consistently reported in the other centres.

Table 4. Rate and treatment of ongoing cytomegalovirus (CMV) infection in biliary atresia patients at the time of Kasai portoenterostomy.

	Budapest	London	Stockholm	Warsaw
Rate ongoing CMV at KPE, % (CMV positive/Total BA patient number)	17% (9/52)	10% [#]	32% (12/37)	19% (60/321)
Rate antiviral treatment in CMV pos, %	44	25	92	>50
Clearance of jaundice CMV neg/CMV pos (%)	n/a	71/37 *	44/26	n/a
Survival native liver CMV neg/CMV pos untreated/CMV pos treated (%)	28/0/0	60/20/60	40/n/a/26	30/30/30

[#] estimate (ref. [3]); * Difference statistically significant, $p \leq 0.05$; n/a not available.

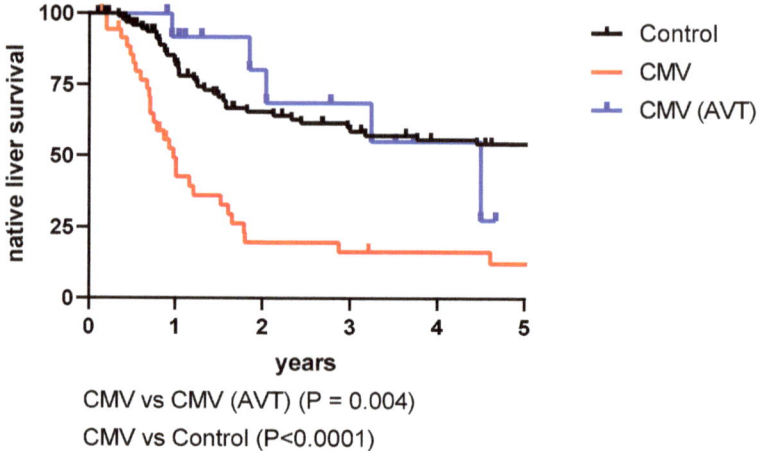

CMV vs CMV (AVT) (P = 0.004)
CMV vs Control (P<0.0001)

Figure 1. Native-liver survival in cytomegalovirus (CMV) positive patients with biliary atresia, with or without antiviral treatment (AVT) and CMV-negative controls in one of the participating centres (London). Log rank survival.

AVT (i.v. ganciclovir and/or oral valganciclovir) was widely used in CMV-positive patients in three centres (50–92% of CMV positive infants), but in only 25% of the London series. The London series showed a significant improved survival with native liver in those who were treated with AVT (Table 4, Figure 1); the median age at KPE was 64 days in treated versus 70 days in untreated ($p = 0.07$). Four AVT patients were older than 70 days at KPE; all cleared their jaundice.

4. Discussion

By collecting and comparing multicentre data from four tertiary centres we showed that the rate of CMV positivity in BA patients varies between centres, but that it is significantly higher than expected for age [1]. Overall, the numbers of CMV-positive BA infants from these European centres were somewhat lower than reported from other parts of the world, and we also noted an ethnic disparity in patients from the largest contributing centre [2–6].

The role of CMV in the pathogenesis of BA is still debated. It is therefore of interest to note that CMV-positive patients differed from CMV-negative patients with regard to age and levels of some biochemical parameters at KPE. This could suggest that CMV-positive patients constitute a specific subgroup, perhaps with later presentation and more pronounced hepatic and bile duct inflammation.

CMV has also been suggested to impact the outcome in BA patients with regard to clearance of jaundice and native-liver survival [3,8,9], and this was consistent with the data from London (Figure 1). Whether these reported differences in survival are due to effects of the viral infection or to the differences in age at KPE remains to be determined. However, the fact that AVT was associated with improved native-liver survival in the London series (Figure 1) suggests that ongoing CMV infection might affect long-term clinical outcomes.

A European survey on post-KPE practices by paediatric surgeons showed that almost 80% of the respondents routinely test for CMV serology and that half of those use AVT if ongoing infection is found [10]. However, there are few data on the effects of AVT in BA from other parts of the world and from the paediatric gastroenterologists/hepatologists who are often are responsible for the follow-up of these patients.

CMV can infect pre-, peri- and postnatally and for the patients reported here we could not determine the timing of transmission. This would clearly be of interest, since there is accumulating evidence to suggest that patients with BA are cholestatic at birth and that the underlying insult(s) occur in utero [11]. One way of advancing knowledge on this matter is to retrospectively analyse CMV-DNA on stored Guthrie cards, which are used for newborn screening of metabolic diseases. In a small study, CMV-DNA was detected on stored Guthrie cards, collected within three days of birth, in only one of 11 BA patients who had an ongoing CMV infection at the time of KPE [12]. That specific patient could therefore be defined as congenitally infected, whereas timing of infection in the remaining patients remained unclear.

Infections such as CMV could be of importance for the pathogenesis of BA not only through a direct viral hit but also by inducing an immune-mediated proinflammatory state causing cellular damage. In support of this hypothesis, Brindley et al. reported that "56% of BA patients had significant increases in interferon-gamma-producing liver T cells in response to cytomegalovirus (CMV), compared with minimal BA responses to other viruses or the control group CMV response. A positive correlation between BA plasma CMV immunoglobulin M (IgM) and liver T-cell CMV reactivity was identified" [13].

In a recently published meta-analysis including 784 patients from nine studies, BA patients with ongoing CMV infection had significantly poorer outcomes than CMV-negative patients, particularly regarding to clearance of jaundice [9]. Theoretically, this negative impact by CMV could be a result of infection at any time point before KPE and the underlying mechanism could either be due to direct viral infection or secondary immune activation [13]. Furthermore, it does highlight an opportunity to detect CMV infection and possibly treat it with AVT if this were found to be of clinical benefit. The data presented herein from London, although not from a randomized, double-blind trial, indicate that such treatment might be beneficial. However, these data need to be confirmed in a placebo-controlled randomized study. Given the overall low incidence of BA, such a study would require a multicentre effort, possibly involving existing disease specific networks, such as the European Rare disease Network (ERN) for rare liver diseases, of which 3 of the 4 participating centres herein are full members, and the Childhood Liver Disease Research Network (ChiLDReN) in North America [14,15].

This study has obvious limitations, one being the retrospective nature and the other being the difference in testing, treatment and follow-up practices between the participating centres. On the other hand, we did assemble data from centres in four European countries that add new information to the topic and also set the stage for future prospective studies.

We conclude that ongoing CMV infection occurs in a considerable proportion of BA patients in European centres of varying size, and that this group differed from CMV-negative patients with regard to age and certain biochemical parameters at KPE and clinical outcomes. We suggest to undertake prospective, multicentre based studies to examine the effects of CMV infection in BA patients and to perform clinical trials of AVT in a randomized placebo-controlled fashion.

Author Contributions: Conceptualization, B.F., P.C., P.S., R.J.S. and M.D.; methodology, B.F., P.C., P.S., R.J.S. and M.D.; validation, B.F., A.D., P.C., P.S., R.J.S. and M.D.; formal analysis, B.F., A.D., P.C., P.S., R.J.S. and M.D.; investigation, B.F., A.D., U.L., P.C., P.S., J.F.S., R.J.S. and M.D.; data curation, B.F., A.D., U.L., P.C., P.S., R.J.S., J.F.S. and M.D.; writing—original draft preparation, B.F.; writing—review and editing, B.F., A.D., U.L., P.C., P.S., R.J.S., J.F.S. and M.D. All authors have read and agreed to the published version of the manuscript.

Funding: This research received no external funding.

Institutional Review Board Statement: In Stockholm (permit number 2017/139-31) and Warsaw (permit number 293/KE/2001), the study was approved by the local ethics committee. In Budapest and London, data collection was regarded as an audit of outcomes and formal ethical approval was not required.

Informed Consent Statement: Informed consent was waived in Stockholm and Warsaw since it was not required according to the ethical permits. Written informed consent was obtained in Budapest.

Data Availability Statement: Data available on request due to restrictions eg privacy or ethical. The data presented in this study are available on request from the corresponding author. The data are not publicly available for ethical and legal reasons.

Conflicts of Interest: The authors declare no conflict of interest.

References

1. Fischler, B.; Ehrnst, A.; Forsgren, M.; Örvell, C.; Nemeth, A. The Viral Association of Neonatal Cholestasis in Sweden: A Possible Link between Cytomegalovirus Infection and Extrahepatic Biliary Atresia. *J. Pediatr. Gastroenterol. Nutr.* **1998**, *27*, 57–64. [CrossRef] [PubMed]
2. Xu, Y.; Yu, J.; Zhang, R.; Yin, Y.; Ye, J.; Tan, L.; Xia, H. The Perinatal Infection of Cytomegalovirus Is an Important Etiology for Biliary Atresia in China. *Clin. Pediatr.* **2011**, *51*, 109–113. [CrossRef] [PubMed]
3. Zani, A.; Quaglia, A.; Hadzić, N.; Zuckerman, M.; Davenport, M. Cytomegalovirus-associated biliary atresia: An aetiological and prognostic subgroup. *J. Pediatr. Surg.* **2015**, *50*, 1739–1745. [CrossRef] [PubMed]
4. Soomro, G.B.; Abbas, Z.; Hassan, M.; Luck, N.; Memon, Y.; Khan, A.W. Is there any association of extra hepatic biliary atresia with cytomegalovirus or other infections? *J. Pak. Med. Assoc.* **2011**, *61*, 281–283. [PubMed]
5. De Tommaso, A.M.; Andrade, P.D.; Costa, S.C.; Escanhoela, C.A.; Hessel, G. High frequency of Human Cytomegalovirus DNA in the Liver of Infants with Extrahepatic Neonatal Cholestasis. *BMC Infect. Dis.* **2005**, *5*, 108. [CrossRef] [PubMed]
6. Moore, S.W.; Zabiegaj-Zwick, C.; Nel, E. Problems related to CMV infection and biliary atresia. *S. Afr. Med J.* **2012**, *102*, 890. [CrossRef] [PubMed]
7. Parolini, F.; Hadzic, N.; Davenport, M. Adjuvant therapy of cytomegalovirus IgM + ve associated biliary atresia: Prima facie evidence of effect. *J. Pediatr. Surg.* **2019**, *54*, 1941–1945. [CrossRef] [PubMed]
8. Shen, C.; Zheng, S.; Wang, W.; Xiao, X.-M. Relationship between prognosis of biliary atresia and infection of cytomegalovirus. *World J. Pediatr.* **2008**, *4*, 123–126. [CrossRef] [PubMed]
9. Hao, Y.; Xu, X.; Liu, G.; Yang, F.; Zhan, J. Prognosis of Biliary Atresia Associated With Cytomegalovirus: A Meta-Analysis. *Front. Pediatr.* **2021**, *9*, 710450.
10. Wong, Z.H.; Davenport, M. What Happens after Kasai for Biliary Atresia? A European Multicenter Survey. *Eur. J. Pediatr. Surg.* **2018**, *29*, 001–006. [CrossRef] [PubMed]
11. Harpavat, S.; Finegold, M.J.; Karpen, S.J. Patients with Biliary Atresia Have Elevated Direct/Conjugated Bilirubin Levels Shortly After Birth. *Pediatrics* **2011**, *128*, e1428–e1433. [CrossRef] [PubMed]
12. Fischler, B.; Rodensjö, P.; Nemeth, A.; Forsgren, M.; Lewensohn-Fuchs, I. Cytomegalovirus DNA detection on Guthrie cards in patients with neonatal cholestasis. *Arch. Dis. Child.—Fetal Neonatal Ed.* **1999**, *80*, F130–F134. [CrossRef] [PubMed]
13. Brindley, S.M.; Lanham, A.M.; Karrer, F.M.; Tucker, R.M.; Fontenot, A.P.; Mack, C.L. Cytomegalovirus-specific T-cell reactivity in biliary atresia at the time of diagnosis is associated with deficits in regulatory T cells. *Hepatology* **2011**, *55*, 1130–1138. [CrossRef] [PubMed]
14. Bernts, L.H.P.; Jones, D.E.J.; Kaatee, M.M.; Lohse, A.W.; Schramm, C.; Sturm, E.; Drenth, J.P.H. Position statement on access to care in rare liver diseases: Advancements of the European reference network (ERN) RARE-LIVER. *Orphanet J. Rare Dis.* **2019**, *14*, 169. [CrossRef] [PubMed]
15. Venkat, V.; Ng, V.L.; Magee, J.C.; Ye, W.; Hawthorne, K.; Harpavat, S.; Molleston, J.P.; Murray, K.F.; Wang, K.S.; Soufi, N.; et al. Modeling Outcomes in Children with Biliary Atresia with Native Liver after 2 Years of Age. *Hepatol. Commun.* **2020**, *4*, 1824–1834. [CrossRef] [PubMed]

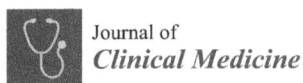

Article

Biliary Atresia in 2021: Epidemiology, Screening and Public Policy

Richard A. Schreiber [1,*], Sanjiv Harpavat [2], Jan B. F. Hulscher [3,†] and Barbara E. Wildhaber [4]

1. Division of Gastroenterology, Hepatology and Nutrition, Department of Pediatrics, Faculty of Medicine, University of British Columbia, Vancouver, BC V6T 1Z3, Canada
2. Division of Gastroenterology, Hepatology and Nutrition, Department of Pediatrics, Baylor College of Medicine and Texas Children's Hospital, Houston, TX 77030, USA; harpavat@bcm.edu
3. Department of Surgery, Division of Pediatric Surgery, University Medical Center Groningen, University of Groningen, 9713 GZ Groningen, The Netherlands; j.b.f.hulscher@umcg.nl
4. Swiss Pediatric Liver Center, Division of Pediatric Surgery, Department of Pediatrics, Gynecology, and Obstetrics, University of Geneva, 1205 Geneva, Switzerland; barbara.wildhaber@hcuge.ch
* Correspondence: rschreiber@cw.bc.ca; Tel.: +1-604-875-2332 (ext. 1); Fax: +1-604-875-3244
† Partners of the European reference network RARE-LIVER.

Abstract: Biliary atresia (BA) is a rare newborn liver disease with significant morbidity and mortality, especially if not recognized and treated early in life. It is the most common cause of liver-related death in children and the leading indication for liver transplantation in the pediatric population. Timely intervention with a Kasai portoenterostomy (KPE) can significantly improve prognosis. Delayed disease recognition, late patient referral, and untimely surgery remains a worldwide problem. This article will focus on biliary atresia from a global public health perspective, including disease epidemiology, current national screening programs, and their impact on outcome, as well as new and novel BA screening initiatives. Policy challenges for the implementation of BA screening programs will also be discussed, highlighting examples from the North American, European, and Asian experience.

Keywords: biliary atresia; pediatric liver disease; newborn screening; public health; epidemiology

Citation: Schreiber, R.A.; Harpavat, S.; Hulscher, J.B.F.; Wildhaber, B.E. Biliary Atresia in 2021: Epidemiology, Screening and Public Policy. *J. Clin. Med.* **2022**, *11*, 999. https://doi.org/10.3390/jcm11040999

Academic Editor: Claus Petersen

Received: 24 December 2021
Accepted: 9 February 2022
Published: 14 February 2022

Publisher's Note: MDPI stays neutral with regard to jurisdictional claims in published maps and institutional affiliations.

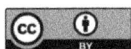

Copyright: © 2022 by the authors. Licensee MDPI, Basel, Switzerland. This article is an open access article distributed under the terms and conditions of the Creative Commons Attribution (CC BY) license (https:// creativecommons.org/licenses/by/ 4.0/).

1. Introduction

Biliary atresia (BA) is a rare orphan newborn liver disease that results from an idiopathic progressive fibrosclerosing obliteration of large bile ducts [1,2]. The condition is recognized as one of the most rapidly progressive liver diseases known to man. It is the leading cause of liver-related death in children and the foremost indication for liver transplantation in the pediatric population. BA clinically manifests in the first few weeks of life with jaundice and acholic pale stools, the prototypical clinical features of an obstructive-type jaundice, associated with the biochemical hallmark of serum conjugated (direct) hyperbilirubinemia. The current standard of care for BA is sequential surgery with an initial Kasai hepato-portoenterostomy (KPE), in which the obstructed bile duct is resected and a loop of the small bowel is brought to the porta hepatis of the liver to restore bile flow, followed by liver transplantation for those in whom the KP fails or who progress to cirrhosis and liver failure at a later pediatric age or into adulthood. Without any surgical intervention, all infants with BA will die by three years of age. The aims of this article are to provide up-to-date knowledge of the epidemiology of biliary atresia, to focus on the current clinically applicable BA screening strategies implemented in large populations or national programs, and to describe the challenges of BA screening in the context of public health policies.

2. Epidemiology and Pathogenesis

BA is a worldwide disease affecting multiple ethnicities. In a recent comprehensive review, the incidence of BA was shown to range widely among countries reporting population-based data, from approximately 1:5000 newborns in Taiwan to 1:20,000 in Europe, Canada, and areas in the USA [3,4]. The highest rates (1:3500) were reported from French Polynesia. Data from several Western countries and regions in the USA or from developing countries is sparse—if not absent—as depicted in Figure 1.

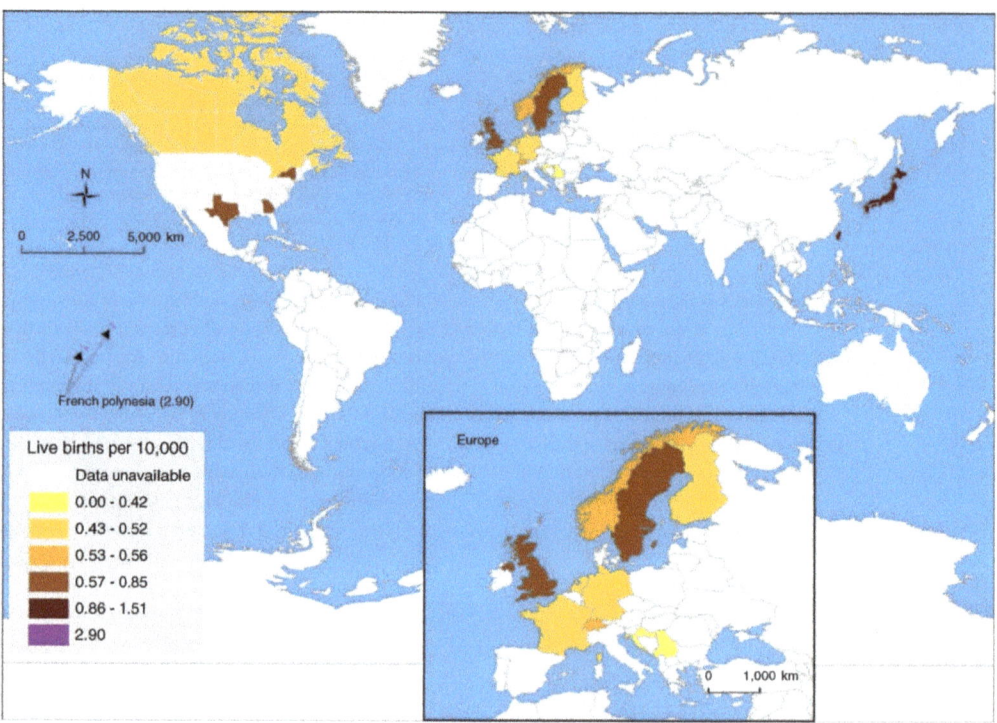

Figure 1. Worldwide incidences of biliary atresia (Jimenez–Rivera et al. [3], © 2013 reprinted by the permission of Wolters Kluwer Health).

BA is now recognized to have several clinical phenotypes, including isolated BA, syndromic BA with other malformations, cystic-type BA, and BA in association with the cytomegalovirus (CMV). Each of these may have differing etiologic and pathophysiologic mechanisms which could influence the regional frequency of the disease. For example, in Asia, only 2% of the BA cases have the syndromic phenotype, whereas in the West, up to 20% of BA cases are syndromic [4]. A recent Chinese report identified as many as 50% of BA cases being CMV-positive, whereas the UK found it was 10% in their series [5,6].

A "two-hit" theory has long been hypothesized for the pathogenesis of the isolated BA phenotype, with an initial viral infection followed by an exaggerated immune response inducing sclerosing cholangiopathy [7,8]. Several viruses have been shown to be implicated, including the rotavirus, reovirus, and CMV, but none has been conclusively linked to BA. Recently, the isoflavonoid "biliatresone" from the *Dysphania* plant has been invoked as a putative environmental factor in pathogenic disease models [9].

2.1. Seasonal Variability

If the origin of the isolated BA phenotype is attributable to an environmental/infectious insult during pregnancy or the perinatal period, one might expect case-clustering in time and space. In contrast, those with a syndromic BA phenotype might be more heavily influenced by genetic determinants. Reports on the epidemiology of BA are variable. In the recent comprehensive literature review by Jimenez–Rivera, 11 out of the 40 papers studied (27.5%) investigated seasonal variations in incidence [3]. Only two studies found significant seasonal variations: an increased incidence of BA from August to October in a southern US city and December to March in a southeastern US city, while the other papers did not find such seasonal variation, or at least, not any statistically significant clustering [10,11]. A recent paper from Korea which was not incorporated in the review supported clustering in summer, while on the other hand, recent results from the Netherlands, incorporating all BA cases in the country in the last three decades, did not observe any temporal clustering for isolated BA [12,13]. These contrasting results may be attributed to geographic or ethnic diversity, varying BA phenotypes, different pathogens, or other yet unknown factors. Interestingly, a weak yet statistically significant correlation between the incidence of maternal infection at the time of conception, including *Chlamydia trachomatis*, and the subsequent development of BA was observed in a recent Dutch study [13].

2.2. Geographic Variations

There clearly are worldwide differences in BA incidence. However, there might also be differences within one country or region. For instance, among the English and Welsh cohorts, geographical variations have been found along a northwest/southeast axis varying from 0.38 (northwest England) to 0.78 (southeast England)/10,000 live births [14]. In the Netherlands, there was a 68% increased incidence for isolated BA in rural areas when compared to urban areas, a difference not seen with syndromic BA [13]. This is in line with previous reports from Texas and Sweden, but in contrast to findings reported in the New York state [10,15,16]. Interestingly, several centers have observed a lower incidence of BA cases during the COVID-19 pandemic, when strict public health guidelines for social distancing, mask-wearing, and frequent handwashing were in place [17]. A study to evaluate BA incidence during the COVID-19 pandemic is currently underway in Europe (European Reference Network RARE LIVER). In conclusion, there is contradicting evidence regarding seasonal, as well as geographic clustering of BA, even within one area. Genetic and environmental factors may account for these observed epidemiologic variations, but these determinants are not well-defined. Large-scale international studies are needed to answer these epidemiological conundrums.

3. Early Intervention Is a Key Prognostic Indicator: The Need for Screening

The initial KPE operation, first reported in 1959 in Japan by Dr. Morio Kasai, was adopted as a realistic life-saving operation for affected infants in the Western world in the 1970s [18,19]. Further experience recognized that the success of the KPE, defined as the clearance of jaundice and normalization of the serum bilirubin by six months after surgery, correlated best with infant age at the time of surgery [20,21]. A successful KPE postpones the need for early urgent liver transplantation in infancy and gives the potential for longer native liver survival well into adulthood. For example, with surgery before 60 days of age, over 70% of patients become jaundice-free, and 75% of these cases have 10-year survival rates with their native liver [22–25]. In contrast, late KPE intervention after 90 days of age has a worse prognosis, with fewer than 25% of cases having 4- to 5-year native liver survival [26,27]. In these late-presenting cases, many centres instead defer the initial KPE and proceed directly to liver transplantation. However, reports from the UK and France gave evidence that the KPE could be successfully performed in infants older than 3 months of age, obviating the need for early liver transplantation, provided there are no preoperative signs of hepatic decompensation or severe portal hypertension [28,29].

3.1. KPE at Infant Age < 30 Days Is Optimal

Historically, several US and European experts advocated that a KPE performed at too early an age (<30 days) was ineffective [30]. The prevailing view suggested the optimal timing for the KPE was at 45–60 days of age. This 'old-school' dogma—that an age at KPE which is too young portends a much worse prognosis—has been conclusively disproven and should be abandoned. Recent studies have firmly demonstrated that KPE intervention at <30 days of age achieves best results and prolongs the native liver survival even into adulthood [26,27]. The largest series reported, including 1428 patients, showed that the 25-year survival rate with native liver was 38%, 27%, 22%, and 19% in patients who had their KPE in the first, second, and third months of life or later, respectively [25]. Japanese, Canadian, and French national studies have shown that optimal rates for native liver survival post-KPE were at a very young infant age, with the best outcomes in those who received the KPE at <30 days of age [22,26,27]. Importantly, an early KPE does not pose additional risks and is not associated with more complications compared with a KPE in older babies. Infant age and weight at the time of the operation are not significantly correlated with adverse events [31].

3.2. The Problem of 'Late' Referral

While all evidence points towards an operative KPE strategy of 'the sooner the better', children with BA often come to the attention of a pediatric gastroenterologist and/or a pediatric surgeon at a 'late' age. Over the last decade, the median age at KPE in Western countries has been at around 60 days, which implies that some 50% of cases do not have the KPE before that age and fail to meet the international quality criterium of <60 days of age [22,24–26,32]. The age of KPE has not improved over the last several decades [33]. The average age at KPE may be even older in some regions of Asia, South Asia, Africa, and South America, although comprehensive data are lacking.

There are several major obstacles to early disease recognition. Jaundice in newborns is considered a benign process most often associated with "breast milk jaundice", and further investigations are not pursued by newborn health care providers. This practice persists despite guideline recommendations by global expert panels and pediatric societies worldwide to test serum total and direct or conjugated bilirubin in all infants with persistent jaundice for more than two to three weeks. The monitoring for pale stools by health care providers or parents is not routine to standard well-baby care. Additionally, in several jurisdictions, the schedule for routine well-baby visits (within two weeks after birth and then at the first vaccination at two months of age) misses the 'window of opportunity' for early case identification.

4. Newborn Screening for Biliary Atresia

One solution to address the problem of late referral for BA is newborn screening. BA satisfies disease-specific criteria for newborn screening, as elaborated by the WHO guidelines. The condition is an important public health problem for infants, families, and the community at large. Without early detection and intervention, there is a likelihood for significant morbidity and mortality at a young age, with the potential need for urgent liver transplantation in infancy. This trajectory has a significant impact on the child and family, as well as caregivers and health-care resources. BA has a recognizable latent or early symptomatic stage. There are well-established BA care pathways with clearly defined diagnostic features and acceptable treatment regimens. Timely intervention improves outcomes with proven cost-effectiveness. What is lacking is a single diagnostic screening laboratory test. Moreover, the incorporation of a BA screening test into current newborn dried blood spot cards has been hindered by the lack of an acceptable biomarker. It is not possible to measure direct or conjugated bilirubin from the dried blood spot cards that are currently used in newborn screening programs. The measurement of glycocholic acid, chenodeoxycholic acid, or other bile acids on blood spot cards have poor sensitivity and specificity and lack sufficient screening performance [34].

4.1. The UK "Yellow Alert" Educational Campaign

The first attempt towards early BA detection was the "Yellow Alert" educational program introduced in the UK in 1993 by the late Professor Alex Mowat at King's College Hospital, in association with the UK Children's Liver Disease Foundation and the Department of Health [35]. The aim of this national campaign was to ensure direct or conjugated bilirubin testing in all babies with persistent jaundice after two weeks of age. Despite worldwide efforts to raise awareness through educational programs directed towards health care professionals and the public, the laboratory investigation of newborns with prolonged jaundice has not been well-integrated into standard care practice for neonates.

4.2. BA Screening Using a Stool Color Card

In 1994, Matsui introduced a seven-colour panel stool colour card (SCC) (three abnormal stool colours) to the Maternal and Child Health Handbook that was distributed to all pregnant women in the Tochigi Prefecture in Japan (Figure 2, Matsui A. [36]). Before or at the routine 1-month newborn follow-up, mothers returned the completed SCC card to the attending physician, and all suspected cases were then referred for further examination. Between 1994 and 2011, a total of 313,230 newborns were screened and 34 cases of BA were diagnosed [37]. The card return rate was 84%. The SCC screening performed well (Table 1). The mean infant age at KPE was 60 days through the 19-year screening period, having decreased significantly from 70 days in the 1987–1992 historic cohort prior to screening. Of the eight patents who were missed by SCC screening at 1 month, two had been in the NICU, and abnormal stool colour was overlooked; three patients were recognized to have a pale stool colour, but their caregivers did not pursue further examination because the babies were not visibly jaundiced; one patient had not used the SCC; one patient had reportedly normal stool colour at the 1 month follow-up; and one patient was identified outside of the program.

Following a regional pilot study in 2002–2003, Taiwan was the first country to introduce a national universal screening program for BA in 2004 using the SCC [38]. Their first iteration of the SCC, a six-colour panel card with three abnormal stool colours, was later changed to a nine-panel card with six abnormal stool colours. The SCC is integrated into the Taiwan child health care booklet given to every neonate in the country. Mothers are asked to contact the screening centre by phone or fax when concerned about their infant's stool colour. The SCC is checked by a physician at the routine 1 month health visit at the time of HBV vaccine delivery. During the Taiwan universal program of 2004–2005, there were a total of 422,273 births, and 75 BA cases were reported nationally [39]. In 2004 and 2005, 73% (29/40) and 97% (34/35) of the BA cases were successfully screened by the SCC before 60 days of age, respectively (Table 1). There were 187 false-positive cases reported with a transient pale stool colour. In 2004, 15 of the 40 BA cases had a KPE >60 days of age: eight patients had not used the SCC, one case had a delayed diagnosis by the health care professional, two suffered an erroneous judgment of stool colour, two had delayed identification of pale stool colour, and two had a delayed visit to the physician. In 2005, 9/35 cases had delayed surgery >60 days of age: three with delayed identification of pale coloured stool, three with delayed physician visits, one with incorrect judgment of stool colour, and one with a delay in diagnosis. In a five-year follow-up outcome study, the age >90-day KPE cohort had been virtually eliminated, and both the 3-month post-KPE jaundice-free rate and the 3-year jaundice-free native liver survival rate had improved from 35% to 68% and 32% to 57%, respectively, between the pre- and post-screening eras [40].

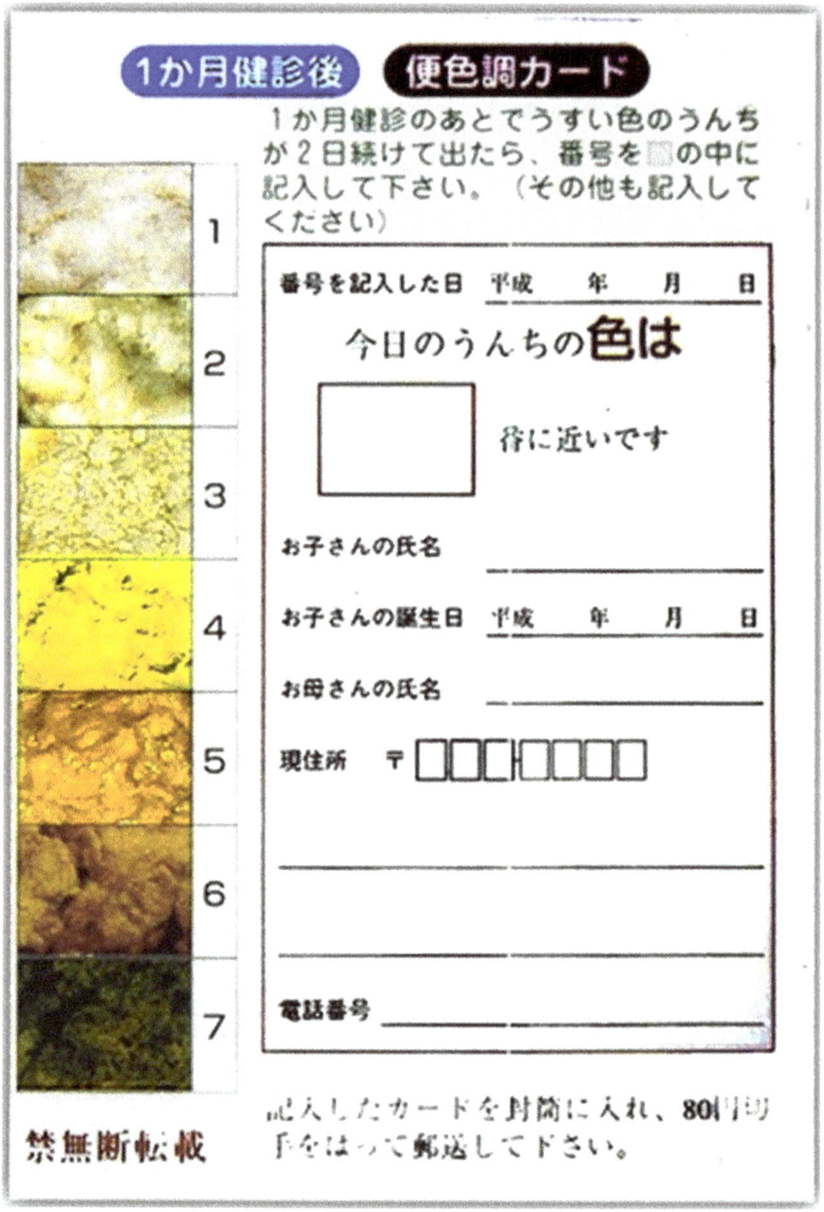

Figure 2. The Matsui stool colour card. This is the first version of SCC in Tochigi Prefecture, Japan. It was delivered to all pregnant women together with a "Maternal and Child Health Handbook". Stool colors were numbered. Images 1–3 were pale-pigmented, and images 4–7 were bile-pigmented stools. A mother is asked to compare the colour of her infant's stool to that of the card, to fill in a corresponding number just before the 1-month health checkup, and to hand it to the attending doctor. When pale-pigmented stools were suspected, the doctor reported to the SCC office by telephone or fax immediately; otherwise SCC were returned to the office by post weekly. The figure is provided to respectfully acknowledge the ground-breaking work of Professor Akira Matsui who passed away in 2020. There are now several versions of the SCC in many languages that are used for BA screening around the world. (Matsui [36], © 2013 reprinted by the permission of Springer Nature).

Table 1. BA screening performance.

Stool Colour Card Screening

Country	Year	# Screened Patients	BA Cases	Sensitivity (%)	Specificity (%)	PPV (%)	NPV (%)	KPE Age Pre-/Post Screening
Taiwan * [39] Universal national program	2004–2005	422,273	75	84	99.9	22.5	99.9	<60 days: 47%/67% 0>91 days post screening
Japan # [37] Tochigi Prefecture	1994–2011	313,230	34	76.5 (62.2–90.7)	99.9 (99.9–100.0)	12.7 (8.2–7.3)	99.9 (99.9–99.9)	67/56 (median days) 25%/11%>80 days
Chaoyang District Beijing † [41]	2013–2014	29,799	4	50	99.9	4.5	99.9	n/a
Canada § [42] British Columbia	2014–2016	87,583	6	83	99.9	6	99.9	n/a

* Diagnostic accuracy statistics for detecting BA by 60 days of life; # Diagnostic accuracy statistics for detecting BA by 1 month of life; † Diagnostic accuracy statistics for detecting BA by 4 months of life; § Diagnostic accuracy statistics for detecting BA by 1 month of life; n/a = not available.

Fractionated Bilirubin Screening

Country	Year	# Screened Patients	BA Cases	Sensitivity	Specificity	PPV	NPV	KPE Age Pre-/Post Screening
UK * [43]	1995–1997	23,214		100.0 (76–100)	99.5 (99.5–99.6)	10.3 (5–16)	n/a	n/a
US # [44]	2013–2014	11,636	2	100.0 (20–100)	99.9 (99.8–99.9)	18 (3–52)	n/a	n/a
US # [45]	2015–2018	123,279	7	100.0 (56–100)	99.9 (99.9–99.9)	5.9 (3–12)	100 (100–100)	56/36

* Diagnostic accuracy statistics for detecting BA by 28 days of life (last follow-up test for BA patients performed on day of life 22); # Diagnostic accuracy statistics for detecting BA by 2 weeks of life in a two-stage screening approach (first test in newborn period, second test at 2 weeks of life if first test abnormal); n/a = not available.

A recent SCC screening program in Sapporo, Japan in 2012 and in the Chao Yang district in Beijing, China in 2013 reported that both centers used a seven-colour panel card while having three abnormal coloured stools [46]. In Beijing, the SCC was distributed directly at maternity, and the family was advised to bring the stools and their infant to the SCC screening centre if abnormal stool colour was detected. Stool data were also verified directly with the family where the infant was aged 2 weeks, one month, and 1–4 months through a combination of mobile phone calls and text messaging, as well as the routine 42-day health check-up by pediatricians through the city's neonatal screening system. In Sapporo, the SCC is integrated into the Maternal and Child Health Handbook that is distributed together with postcards and maternal health check-up tickets to all women during their pregnancy. If abnormal stools are detected, the families are instructed to bring the stools and their infant to the local hospital. For each infant, a completed postcard with the SCC data was collected at the one-month health checkup.

A large-scale prospective Canadian cohort study in the province of British Columbia (BC) found that distribution of the SCC at maternity was the most effective and highly cost-effective screening strategy [47]. The findings were confirmed at another care centre in Montreal, Quebec [48]. The BC provincial screening program was implemented in 2014. The SCC was initially a six-panel colour card with three abnormal stool colours identical to the Taiwan colour stool photos. Currently, a nine-colour panel card analogous to the Taiwan SCC is used. The SCC is given to families at the time of discharge from the maternity unit. In the case of home delivery, the SCC is given by the midwife to the family. Babies admitted to a NICU are excluded from the program and not issued a SCC. Parents are instructed to regularly monitor their infant stool colour at home using the SCC for the first 30 days after birth, and to contact the screening centre by phone or email with any concerns about their infant's stool colour. All follow-ups are provided by a pediatric hepatologist. From 2014–2016, there were 87,583 births in British Columbia, and six cases of BA were identified [42]. The SCC screening successfully identified abnormal stool colour in 5/6 cases. In the one case of unsuccessful SCC screening, abnormal stool colour was not consistently recognized by the family and contact was not made with the screening centre. The family was instead seen by a physician because of prolonged jaundice, but no testing was done. The screening program instigated timely case referral to specialty care (defined as program screen success) in 3/6 BA cases. Of the three program screen failures, two families who correctly identified pale stools sought immediate consultation with their care providers; however, they were reassured and no further timely action was taken. In the third case, the infant was taken to the physician with complaints of jaundice but not of abnormal stool colour, and no investigations were performed. Most of these cases had late referral and delayed diagnosis with a median age of KPE of 116 days (49–184 days). The performance of the SCC screening was comparable to other national reports (Table 1). A new SCC is now utilized, having a highlighted statement to instruct physicians to order a fractionated bilirubin test for newborns who present with parental concerns about their infant's stool colour.

National BA screening programs using an SCC have been introduced in Switzerland and Japan [36,49]. Small pilot studies with the SCC have been conducted in regions or municipalities in Brazil [50], Cairo, Egypt [51], Shenzen (China) [52], Northern Portugal [53], and Lower Saxony Germany [54]. However, to our knowledge, comprehensive feasibility and performance studies of the SCC in these locales have not yet been reported.

4.3. BA Screening Using a Stool Colour Smartphone App

Several centers have developed mobile smartphone applications designed to help parents and caregivers identify abnormal stool colour and prompt early referral to specialty care (Table 2). These applications have a touch-screen interface, utilize the smartphone camera, and apply specially designed colour analyzer software to assess the infant's stool colour. Abnormal stool colour triggers a message to the user to seek consultation with their health care provider.

PoopMD®, developed at John Hopkins University in the United States and released in 2014, was the first stool colour application for iOS and Android devices [55]. The colour recognition software was based on the Taiwan stool colour card images converted to a 16-base colour pallet using RGB digital photo hexcodes. The interface targeted adolescent and young adult parents having an eighth-grade reading proficiency level. The accuracy of the mobile app was determined by seven expert pediatricians based on 34 photographs of infant stool. The application correctly identified all acholic stool photos without any false-negatives. While 11% of the photos were classified as indeterminate, none of the normal stools were identified as acholic (Table 2).

Table 2. Mobile device screening application (Angelico et al. [43], © 2017 reprinted by the permission of Sage Publications).

Characteristics	PoopMD	Baby Poop	PopòApp
Year	2015	2017	2020
Country	USA	Japan	Italy
Reference	[14]	[16]	Current study
Programming language	Java		Java
Operating system	iOS/Android	iOS	iOS/Android
Source of pictures	Previously validated and recorded	Pre-existing images	Newly acquired images taken with the Pop6App
Establishment of the gold standard for stool color	ISCC	Pre-existing BA and non-BA stool images	ISCC
Color analyzer system	RGB parameters	RGB and HSV parameters + machine learning process	RGB system + machine learning process
Clinical assessment of the App	Agreement between 6 doctors who revisited the pictures	Performance tested with pre-classified images	Real-time assessment by 4 doctors who took the images (agreement between 4 doctors)
Classification of stool color	Acholic, cholic, indeterminate	Acholic, cholic	Acholic, cholic, uncertain, indeterminate
Number of pictures for Accuracy test of the App	34	40	160
– Acholic	7	5	60
– Normal	24	35	63
– Uncertain			16
– Indeterminate	3		21
Sensitivity (95% CI)	100%	100% (48–100%)	100% (93.9–100.0%)
Specificity (95% CI)	89%	100% (90–100%)	99% (94.6–99.9%)

BA: biliary atresia; CI: confidence intervals; HSV: hue-saturation-value; ISCC: infant stool color card; RGB: red-green-blue.

Baby Poop® is an iOS-based application developed in Japan and released in 2016 [56]. A total of 54 BA and 100 non-BA stool images were collected to develop the colour detection algorithm. Both RGB and HSV (hue, saturation, and value) attributes were used in the stool colour analysis (Table 2). HSV was demonstrated to be an important component in the accurate identification of abnormal stool colour. The application, in Japanese only, had 100% sensitivity and specificity for the detection of BA based on a test sample of 40 stool pictures including five BA stools. A similar application is being developed in Shanghai [57].

Popòapp®, designed by an Italian team, is another mobile device application for both iOS and Android devices [43]. The colour analyzer algorithm is based on the Japanese seven-stool colour photo panel using an RGB digital colour system. After completing a baseline questionnaire, the user takes a picture of the stool. Results are categorized as "normal", "abnormal", or "uncertain". Any stool colour that cannot be classified by the app is defined as "indeterminate". The application was validated by four pediatric subspecialists using 160 stool samples from infants ≤6 months of age who had been admitted to an inpatient hepatobiliary service. The application performed well without any false-negative results (Table 2).

4.4. BA Screening Using Conjugated or Direct (Fractionated) Bilirubin

The first study to apply a fractionated bilirubin test for newborn BA screening was conducted in the UK in 1998 [44]. The investigators measured conjugated bilirubin levels in infants 4–28 days old using extra plasma collected from routine newborn screening. At the time, in Birmingham and other parts of the UK, routine newborn screening was based on liquid capillary blood specimens. In a follow-up prospective study of 23,214 patients using defined bilirubin cut-offs, testing had a sensitivity of 100%, specificity of 99.6%, and positive predictive value of 10.3% for the detection of BA [45]. Testing also identified other diseases, including Alagille Syndrome, alpha-1-antitrypsin deficiency, and panhypopituitarism. As mentioned previously, the dried "Guthrie" blood spots for newborn screening could not be used to test for fractionated bilirubin measurements.

In the United States, recent studies explored bilirubin testing in the first 24–48 h of life based on the observation that newborns with BA have elevated direct or conjugated bilirubin levels starting at birth [58]. The screening algorithm involves blood procurement for testing all infants before discharge from the newborn nursery. Infants with high levels of fractionated bilirubin were later tested as outpatients at the routine two-week well-child visit, and those with persistently high levels were referred for further evaluation. This screening algorithm for BA was tested in a pilot study of 11,636 infants and a larger follow-up study of 123,279 infants (Table 1, [59]). Screening resulted in significant improvements in the timing of the KPE. Screening also identified other diseases, including Alagille Syndrome, alpha-1-antitrypsin deficiency, progressive intrahepatic cholestasis, and choledochal cyst. Screening newborns for BA with fractionated bilirubin measurements is now also taking place in other US locations, including San Antonio, Salt Lake City and surrounding areas, and New Orleans [60].

5. BA Screening and Public Health Policy: The Challenge of Influencing Policymakers and Considerations for Program Implementation

Advocacy and the realization of a BA screening program requires a strong leadership team to champion the proposal and bring it to fruition. Meticulous and well-coordinated planning with local governmental authorities, newborn screening advisory committees (or similar groups if they exist), and other local experts in the field is an absolute necessity. It is recommended to have strong engagement among patients and their families to help garner support for the program by governmental representatives. Careful consideration of country-specific health care resources and capacities, particularly in the context of the program development plan is key. The choice of screening methodology that is most appropriate to the respective region, the required infrastructure for the operation of the program, and the optimal process for case follow-up are necessary first steps to consider before embarking on the implementation of the program.

There are now several publications to justify the need for a BA screening program that demonstrates the feasibility, efficacy, and cost-effectiveness of screening [27,42,47,61]. It is helpful to have pilot program study data from the respective region to inform stakeholders of the local BA outcome and infant age of KPE in the context of published reports from elsewhere in the world. Every country needs a "homegrown" approach to show that BA screening is needed, and a reliable, easy-to-apply, and suitable screening program for their own population can be proposed.

Despite the scientific evidence of the benefit of early diagnosis and management of BA patients, the creation of a SCC screening program is challenging. In Taiwan, the Department of Health Director became very supportive of the BA screening program after an enthusiastic explanation of the plan by Professor Mei Hwei Chang with the support of the community, care providers, and the local press (personal communication). Universal BA screening in Taiwan was approved following a pilot project that expanded from small regional sites to a national study. In Switzerland, the Swiss reference center for BA patients initiated a national feasibility screening program using the SCC in 2009. It took 10 years before SCC screening for BA was introduced into the Swiss national health booklet (www.paediatrieschweiz.ch, accessed on 24 December 2021) (personal communication). In Germany, the initiative for BA SCC screening was launched in 2016 by the Hannover group [54]. The physicians cooperated with a major German health insurance company and with the local Medical Association in their region in Lower Saxony to establish the screening project. This local initiative opened its doors at the German Federal Joint Committee, and the group was authorized to make binding regulations in the country. Negotiations are still underway for a SCC to be enclosed nationally in German children's health booklets.

In Canada, health care is a federal charter, but newborn screening programs are provincially mandated and directed. A pilot study for the SCC program was first completed in British Columbia before it was supported by the provincial perinatal services and BC Ministry of Health. In France, a private parent organization, the Association Maladies Foie Enfants (AMFE), is promoting the screening of "yellow babies" using stool colour, and has launched many national information campaigns to encourage the screening mode called *"alerte jaune"* ("yellow alert"), including spots on national TV stations and annual national sensitization events (alertjaune.com, accessed on 29 December 2021). In the US, the choice of the diseases to be included in newborn screening involves coordination between federal and state policy makers [62]. At the federal level, the Secretary of the Department of Health and Human Services makes recommendations as to which diseases belong on the Recommended Uniform Screening Panel, or RUSP, based on expert opinions from the Advisory Committee on Heritable Disorders in Newborns and Children. However, individual states are not required to follow the RUSP. The state policy-makers are the ones who decide which diseases will be screened for in their state [2].

Each screening modality requires its own infrastructure and evidence-based data to support its adoption and successful implementation. BA screening using a SCC is simple and inexpensive, whereas the cost-effectiveness of fractionated bilirubin testing is still under investigation in the US. In developing countries, screening using an SCC may be a preferred methodology because of its low cost. For smartphone applications to be effective for BA screening in any given region, comprehensive and widespread distribution and the use of mobile phone technology is necessary, and the quality of the screen needs to meet the standards. Screening applications require further validation studies before they should be adopted. In the US, a SCC screening program may be more difficult to implement universally, given the decentralized structure of the health care system.

For SSC-based screening programs, Taiwanese, Japanese, Canadian and Swiss program leaders have emphasized the importance of having comprehensive educational seminars about the screening program before the program launch. These should be directed towards maternity nurses, other health care professionals on the maternity wards, midwives, and community newborn care providers. The use of webinars, virtual teaching sessions, or scripted educational sheets to uniformly explain the screening process to families is an essential requirement for a program's success. Considerations must be given to families' first language and socioeconomic status to ensure the instructions are clearly understood. Recent input from developing countries support the concept that this screening process is simple and easily understood even in lower socioeconomic groups and those with illiteracy [51].

The SCC requires validated stool colour photos. The Japanese have emphasized the need for reproducible digital photographic images with CYMK-based metafiles to ensure the quality of the stool colours and reproducibility of card-printing [36]. The colour and hue of stool photos on a computer or a smartphone will depend on the resolution of the colour screen, while printouts of the SCC depend on the quality of the colour printer and paper. Caution is advised against using home printers for card distribution. Instead, professionally printed cards on quality paper or stool photos incorporated into a professionally printed health booklet is recommended. In the case of smartphones, the use of applications having valid and real-life proven software colour analytics is necessary.

There are other nuances with the current SCC screening programs. Japan and Taiwan have differing screening processes. The former includes check points at infant age 2 weeks, one month and 1–4 months, while the latter only includes a 30-day follow-up. In Japan, the screening program is under the jurisdiction of each local government and the screening program policies differ regionally. Additionally, the SCC is contained within the Maternal and Child Health handbook, which is distributed to pregnant women in the antenatal period during pregnancy and prior to delivery. In British Columbia and Switzerland, the SCC is distributed at the time of discharge from maternity. Families are instructed at that time to monitor the stool for the first 30 days of life. In British Columbia as in Switzerland there is no formal check-point time with the screening centre or other health care professional. In the US, given the ease of fractionated bilirubin testing newborns in the first 24–48 h of life before hospital discharge, implementation of this BA screening program is now being considered in various US centers.

6. Limitations of the Current BA Screening Programs

Each of the existing SCC screening programs have been hampered by delayed follow-up of patients screening positive for stool colour. This is a major concern and efforts need to be made to ensure prompt recognition and referral of these patients. There are no universally accepted BA diagnostic algorithms, and several of the potential laboratory or imaging studies to diagnose BA take a long time to perform and interpret. Cases identified through a BA screening program need the corresponding infrastructure to facilitate prompt referral to a centre with expertise in BA assessment and management instead of leaving the workup to community care providers.

Two important challenges to the implementation of fractionated bilirubin screening are variations in normal values for fractionated bilirubin assays between laboratories and the process for communicating abnormal results in a timely manner [60]. Assay variations arise because hospital laboratories use either direct or conjugated bilirubin methodology. While conjugated bilirubin methodology is consistent across sites, direct bilirubin methodology can differ slightly from site to site, depending on the reaction conditions used. As a result, providers must interpret direct bilirubin levels using site-specific reference intervals rather than a universal standard that can be used at all sites. Communication challenges arise because the screening algorithm requires outpatient providers to know when an abnormal result occurs in the newborn nursery. In the US, medical care is decentralized and there is no universally shared medical record. As a result, primary care providers may not have access to complete information about the initial newborn hospitalization, including the results of the first direct or conjugated bilirubin measurement. The outpatient providers may not be aware of which infants tested positive and who requires timely follow-up.

Finally, as in other screening programs, there is a risk that BA screening will unnecessarily increase parental anxiety with false-positive cases [63]. Strategies to reduce anxiety focus on improving ways to communicate information to parents. A recent study used a parental questionnaire to investigate parental anxiety with the SCC [49]. The study showed that of the respondents ($n = 109$), most did not experience negative feelings when using the SCC or discussing liver diseases with their physician in the context of SCC use.

7. Conclusions

BA affects infants around the world, with birth prevalence showing regional and, in some cases, seasonal variation. Despite its unknown etiology, the importance of early treatment with the KPE in delaying or avoiding liver transplant is well-established. Newborn screening of BA represents a powerful way to ensure prompt diagnosis of affected infants. Multiple screening modalities have been examined, with the SCC and direct or conjugated bilirubin screening being implemented on the largest scales and also being the most promising. The SCC has been incorporated into national screening strategies and adapted to smartphone apps, whereas fractionated bilirubin screening is still under investigation. Future studies are needed to determine how best to implement screening strategies more widely, taking into account region-specific resources and variations in the process of policy decisions that are needed to ensure broader adoption. Future studies to establish the diagnostic algorithms for BA are required to ensure that screen-positive infants are evaluated efficiently and receive the KPE in a timely manner, ideally before 30 days of life.

Author Contributions: Conceptualization, R.A.S. and S.H.; Formal analysis, S.H.; Writing—original draft, R.A.S., S.H., J.B.F.H. and B.E.W.; Writing—review & editing, R.A.S., S.H., J.B.F.H. and B.E.W. All authors have read and agreed to the published version of the manuscript.

Funding: S.H. is supported by NIH NIDDK K23 DK109207 and R03 DK128535.

Institutional Review Board Statement: Not applicable.

Informed Consent Statement: Not applicable.

Data Availability Statement: Not applicable.

Conflicts of Interest: S.H. serves on the DSMB for a therapeutic trial for biliary atresia (DSMB coordinated by Syneos Health).

References

1. Hartley, J.L.; Davenport, M.; Kelly, D.A. Biliary atresia. *Lancet* **2009**, *37*, 1704–1713. [CrossRef]
2. Sanchez-Valle, A.; Kassira, N.; Varela, V.C.; Radu, S.C.; Paidas, C.; Kirby, R.S. Biliary atresia: Epidemiology, genetics, clinical update and public health perspective. *Adv. Pediatr.* **2017**, *64*, 285–305. [CrossRef] [PubMed]
3. Jimenez-Rivera, C.; Jolin-Dahel, K.S.; Fortinsky, K.J.; Gozdyra, P.; Benchimol, E.I. International incidence and outcomes of biliary atresia. *J. Pediatr. Gastroenterol. Nutr.* **2013**, *56*, 344–354. [CrossRef] [PubMed]
4. Chung, P.H.Y.; Zheng, S.; Tam, P.K.H. Biliary atresia: East versus west. *Semin. Pediatr. Surg.* **2020**, *29*, 150950. [CrossRef] [PubMed]
5. Xu, Y.; Yu, J.; Zhang, R.; Yin, Y.; Ye, J.; Tan, L.; Xia, H. The perinatal infection of cytomegalovirus is an important etiology for biliary atresia in China. *Clin. Pediatr.* **2012**, *51*, 109–113. [CrossRef]
6. Lakshminarayan, B.; Davenport, M. Biliary atresia: A comprehensive review. *J. Autoimmun.* **2016**, *73*, 1–9. [CrossRef]
7. Schreiber, R.A.; Kleinman, R.E. Genetics, immunology and biliary atresia: An opening or a diversion. *J. Pediatr. Gastroenterol. Nutr.* **1993**, *16*, 111–113. [CrossRef]
8. Feldman, A.; Mack, C.L. Biliary atresia: Cellular dynamics and immune dysregulation. *Semin. Pediatr. Surg.* **2012**, *21*, 192–200. [CrossRef]
9. Bezerra, J.A.; Wells, R.G.; Mack, C.L.; Karpen, S.J.; Hoofnagle, J.H.; Doo, E.; Sokol, R.J. Biliary atresia: Clinical and research challenges for the twenty first century. *Hepatology* **2018**, *68*, 1163–1173. [CrossRef]
10. Strickland, A.D.; Shannon, K. Studies in the etiology of extrahepatic biliary atresia: Time-space clustering. *J. Pediatr.* **1982**, *100*, 749–753. [CrossRef]
11. Yoon, P.W.; Bresee, J.S.; Olney, R.S.; James, L.M.; Khoury, M.J. Epidemiology of biliary atresia: A population-based study. *Pediatrics* **1997**, *99*, 376–382. [CrossRef] [PubMed]
12. Lee, K.J.; Kim, J.W.; Moon, J.S.; Ko, J.S. Epidemiology of biliary atresia in Korea. *J. Korean Med. Sci.* **2017**, *32*, 656–660. [CrossRef] [PubMed]
13. Nomden, M.; van Wessel, D.B.; Ioannou, S.; Verkade, H.J.; de Kleine, R.H.; Alizadeh, B.Z.; Bruggink, J.L.; Hulscher, J.B. A higher incidence of isolated biliary atresia in rural area: Results from an epidemiologic study in the Netherlands. *J. Pediatr. Gastroenterol. Nutr.* **2021**, *72*, 202–209. [CrossRef] [PubMed]
14. Livesey, E.; Borja, M.C.; Sharif, K.; Alizai, N.; McClean, P.; Kelly, D.; Hadzic, N.; Davenport, M. Epidemiology of biliary atresia in England and Wales (1999–2006). *Arch. Dis. Child. Fetal Neonatal Ed.* **2009**, *94*, F451–F455. [CrossRef] [PubMed]
15. Fischler, B.; Haglund, B.; Hjern, A. A population-based study on the incidence and possible pre- and perinatal etiologic risk factors of biliary atresia. *J. Pediatr.* **2002**, *141*, 217–222. [CrossRef]
16. Caton, A.R.; Druschel, C.M.; McNutt, L.A. The epidemiology of extrahepatic biliary atresia in New York State, 1983–1998. *Pediatr. Perinat. Epidemiol.* **2004**, *18*, 97–105. [CrossRef]
17. Nomden, M.; de Kleine, R.H.; Bruggink, J.L.; Verkade, H.J.; Burgerhof, J.G.; Hulscher, J.B. Unusual long absence of isolated biliary atresia in COVID lockdown: Coïncidence or association? *J. Pediatr. Gastroenterol. Nutr.* **2021**, *74*, e17–e18. [CrossRef]
18. Kasai, M.; Suzuki, S. A new operation for, 'non-correctable' biliary atresia: Hepatic porto-enterostomy. *Shuiyutsu* **1959**, *13*, 733–739.
19. Lilly, J.R.; Altman, R.P. Hepatic portoenterostomy (the Kasai operation) for biliary atresia. *Surgery* **1975**, *78*, 76–86.
20. Shneider, B.L.; Magee, J.C.; Karpen, S.J.; Rand, E.B.; Narkewicz, M.R.; Bass, L.M.; Schwarz, K.; Whitington, P.F.; Bezerra, J.A.; Kerkar, N.; et al. Total serum bilirubin within 3 months of hepatopoetoenterostomy predicts native liver survival in biliary atresia. *J. Pediatr.* **2016**, *170*, 211–217. [CrossRef]
21. Huang, C.Y.; Chang, M.H.; Chen, H.L.; Ni, Y.H.; Hsu, H.Y.; Wu, J.F. Bilirubin level 1 week after hepatoportoenterostomy predicts native liver survival in biliary atresia. *Pediatr. Res.* **2020**, *87*, 730–734. [CrossRef] [PubMed]
22. Nio, M.; Sasaki, H.; Wada, M.; Kazama, T.; Nishi, K.; Tanaka, H. Impact of age of Kasai operation on short- and long- term outcomes of type III biliary atresia at a single institution. *J. Pediatr. Surg.* **2010**, *45*, 2361–2363. [CrossRef] [PubMed]
23. Pakarinen, M.P.; Johansen, L.S.; Svensson, J.F.; Bjørnland, K.; Gatzinsky, V.; Stenström, P.; Koivusalo, A.; Kvist, N.; Almström, M.; Emblem, R.; et al. Outcomes of biliary atresia in the nordic countries- a mulitcenter study of 158 patients during 2005–2016. *J. Pediatr. Surg.* **2018**, *53*, 1509–1515. [CrossRef] [PubMed]
24. De Vries, W.; de Langen, Z.J.; Groen, H.; Scheenstra, R.; Peeters, P.M.; Hulscher, J.B.; Verkade, H.J. Biliary atresia in the Netherlands: Outcome of patients diagnosed between 1987 and 2008. *J. Pediatr.* **2012**, *160*, 638–644. [CrossRef]
25. Fanna, M.; Masson, G.; Capito, C.; Girard, M.; Guerin, F.; Hermeziu, B.; Lachaux, A.; Roquelaure, B.; Gottrand, F.; Broue, P.; et al. Management of biliary atresia in France 1986–2015: Long-term results. *J. Pediatr. Gastroenterol. Nutr.* **2019**, *69*, 416–424. [CrossRef]
26. Schreiber, R.A.; Barker, C.C.; Roberts, E.A.; Martin, S.R.; Alvarez, F.; Smith, L.; Butzner, J.D.; Wrobel, I.; Mack, D.; Moroz, S.; et al. Biliary atresia: The Canadian experience. *J. Pediatr.* **2007**, *151*, 659–665. [CrossRef]

27. Serinet, M.O.; Wildhaber, B.E.; Broue, P.; Lachaux, A.; Sarles, J.; Jacquemin, E.; Gauthier, F.; Chardot, C. Impact of age at Kasai operation on its results in late childhood and adolescence: A rational basis for biliary atresia screening. *Pediatrics* **2009**, *123*, 1280–1286. [CrossRef]
28. Davenport, M.; Puricelli, V.; Farrant, P.; Hadzic, N.; Mieli-Vergani, G.; Portmann, B.; Howard, E.R. The outcome of the older (≥100 days) infant with biliary atresia. *J. Pediatr. Surg.* **2004**, *39*, 575–581. [CrossRef]
29. Chardot, C.; Carton, M.; Spire-Bendelac, N.; Le Pommelet, C.; Golmard, J.L.; Reding, R.; Auvert, B. Is the Kasai operation still indicated in children older than 3 months diagnosed with biliary atresia. *J. Pediatr.* **2001**, *138*, 224–228. [CrossRef]
30. Volpert, D.; White, F.; Finegold, M.J.; Molleston, J.; DeBaun, M.; Perlmutter, D.H. Outcome of early hepatic portoenterostomy for biliary atresia. *J. Pediatr. Gastroenterol. Nutr.* **2001**, *32*, 265–269. [CrossRef]
31. Calinescu, A.M.; Wilde, J.C.; Korff, S.; McLin, V.A.; Wildhaber, B.E. Perioperative complications after Kasai hepatoportoenterostomy: Data from the Swiss national biliary atresia registry. *Eur. J. Pediatr. Surg.* **2020**, *30*, 364–370. [CrossRef]
32. Kelley-Quon, L.I.; Shue, E.; Burke, R.V.; Smith, C.; Kling, K.; Mahdi, E.; Ourshalimian, S.; Fenlon, M.; Dellinger, M.; Shew, S.B.; et al. The need for early Kasai portoenterostomy; a western pediatric surgery research consortium study. *Pediatr. Surg. Int.* **2021**, *38*, 193–199. [CrossRef]
33. McKieran, P.J. Prompt diagnosis of biliary atresia education has not succeeded, time to move to universal screening. *Arch. Dis. Child.* **2020**, *105*, 709–710. [CrossRef] [PubMed]
34. Zhou, K.; Lin, N.; Xiao, Y.; Wang, Y.; Wen, J.; Zou, G.M.; Gu, X.; Cai, W. Elevated bile acids in newborns with biliary atresia. *PLoS ONE* **2012**, *7*, 49270. [CrossRef] [PubMed]
35. Mowat, A.P.; Davidson, L.L.; Dick, M.C. Earilier identification of biliary atresia and hepatobiliary disease; selective screening in the third week of life. *Arch. Dis. Child.* **1995**, *72*, 90–92. [CrossRef] [PubMed]
36. Matsui, A. Screening for biliary atresia. *Pediatr. Surg. Int.* **2017**, *33*, 1305–1313. [CrossRef] [PubMed]
37. Gu, Y.H.; Yokoyama, K.; Mizuta, K.; Tsuchioka, T.; Kudo, T.; Sasaki, H.; Nio, M.; Tang, J.; Ohkubo, T.; Matsui, A. Stool card screening for early detection of biliary atresia and long term native liver survival: A 19 year cohort study in Japan. *J. Pediatr.* **2015**, *166*, 897–902. [CrossRef]
38. Chang, M.H. Screening for biliary atresia Chang Gung. *Med. J.* **2006**, *29*, 231–233.
39. Hsiao, C.H.; Chang, M.H.; Chen, H.L.; Lee, H.C.; Wu, T.C.; Lin, C.C.; Yang, Y.J.; Chen, A.C.; Tiao, M.M.; Lau, B.H.; et al. Universal screening for biliary atresia using an infant stool color card in Taiwan. *Hepatology* **2008**, *47*, 1233–1240. [CrossRef]
40. Lien, T.H.; Chang, M.H.; Wu, J.F.; Chen, H.L.; Lee, H.C.; Chen, A.C.; Tiao, M.M.; Wu, T.C.; Yang, Y.J.; Lin, C.C.; et al. Effects of the Infant stool color card screening program on 5 year outcome of biliary atresia in Taiwan. *Hepatology* **2011**, *53*, 202–208. [CrossRef]
41. Kong, Y.Y.; Zhao, J.Q.; Wang, J.; Qui, L.; Yang, H.H.; Diao, M.; Li, L.; Gu, Y.H.; Matsui, A. Modified stool color card with digital images was efficient and feasible for early detection of biliary atresia—A pilot study in Beijing, China. *World J. Pediatr.* **2016**, *12*, 415–420. [CrossRef] [PubMed]
42. Woolfson, J.P.; Schreiber, R.A.; Butler, A.E.; MacFarlane, J.; Kaczorowski, J.; Masucci, L.; Bryan, S.; Collet, J.P. Province-wide biliary atresia home screening program in British Columbia: Evaluation of first 2 years. *J. Pediatr. Gastroenterol. Nutr.* **2018**, *66*, 845–849. [CrossRef] [PubMed]
43. Angelico, R.; Liccardo, D.; Paoletti, M.; Pietrobattista, A.; Basso, M.S.; Mosca, A.; Safarikia, S.; Grimaldi, C.; Saffioti, M.C.; Candusso, M.; et al. A novel mobile phone application for infant sotol color recognition: An easy and effective tool to identify acholic stools in newborns. *J. Med. Screen.* **2021**, *28*, 230–237. [CrossRef] [PubMed]
44. Keffler, S.; Kelly, D.A.; Powell, J.E.; Green, A. Population screening for newborn liver disease: A feasibility study. *J. Pediatr. Gastroenterol. Nutr.* **1998**, *27*, 306–311. [CrossRef]
45. Powell, J.E.; Keffler, S.; Kelly, D.A.; Green, A. Population screening for neonatal liver disease. *J. Med. Screen.* **2003**, *10*, 112–116. [CrossRef]
46. Gu, Y.H.; Zhao, J.Q.; Kong, Y.Y.; Yang, H.H.; Diao, M.; Li, L.; Nomachi, S.; Tezuka, M.; Hanai, J.; Matsui, A. Repeatability and reliability of home based stool color card screening for biliary atresia based on results in China and Japan Tohoku. *Exp. Med.* **2020**, *252*, 365–372. [CrossRef]
47. Schreiber, R.A.; Masucci, L.; Kaczorowski, J.; Collet, J.P.; Lutley, P.; Espinosa, V.; Bryan, S. Home based screening for biliary atresia usinf infant stool colour cards: A large scale prospective cohort study and cost effectiveness analysis. *J. Med. Screen.* **2014**, *21*, 126–132. [CrossRef]
48. Morinville, V.; Ahmed, N.; Ibberson, C.; Kovacs, L.; Kaczorowski, J.; Bryan, S.; Collet, J.P.; Schreiber, R. Home based screening for biliary atresia using infant stool colour cards in Canada: Quebec feasibility study. *J. Pediatr. Gastroenterol. Nutr.* **2016**, *62*, 536–541. [CrossRef]
49. Borgeat, M.; Korff, S.; Wildhaber, B. Newborn biliary atresia screening with the stool colour card. *BMJ Paediatr. Open* **2018**, *2*, e000269. [CrossRef]
50. Bezerra, J.A. Biliary atresia in Brazil. *J. Pediatr.* **2010**, *86*, 445–447. [CrossRef]
51. El-Shaabrawi, M.H.; Baroudy, S.R.; Hassanin, F.S.; Farag, A.E. A pilot study of a stool color card as a diagnostic tool for extrahepatic biliary atresia at a single tertiary referral center n a low/middle income country. *Arab J. Gasterol.* **2021**, *22*, 61–65. [CrossRef]
52. Zheng, J.; Ye, Y.; Wang, B.; Zhang, L. Biliary atresia screening in Shenzhen: Implementation and achievements. *Arch. Dis. Child.* **2020**, *105*, 720–723. [CrossRef] [PubMed]

53. Ashworth, J.; Tavares, M.; Silva, E.S.; Lopes, A.I. The stool color card as a screening tool for biliary atresia in the digital version of the Portuguese child and youth health booklet. *Acta Med. Port.* **2021**, *34*, 630–645. [CrossRef] [PubMed]
54. Madadi-Sanjani, O.; Blaser, J.; Voigt, G.; Kuebler, J.F.; Petersen, C. Home based color card screening for biliary atresia: The first steps for implementation of a nationwide newborn screening in Germany. *Pediatr. Surg. Int.* **2019**, *35*, 1217–1222. [CrossRef] [PubMed]
55. Franciscovich, A.; Vaidya, D.; Doyle, J.; Bolinger, J.; Capdevila, M.; Rice, M.; Hancock, L.; Mahr, T.; Mogul, D.B. PoopMD, a mobile health application accurately identifies infant acholic stools. *PLoS ONE* **2015**, *10*, e0132270. [CrossRef] [PubMed]
56. Hoshino, E.; Hayashi, K.; Suzuki, M.; Obatake, M.; Urayama, K.Y.; Nakano, S.; Taura, Y.; Nio, M.; Takahashi, O. An iphone application using a novel stool color detection algorithm for biliary atresia screening. *Pediatr. Surg. Int.* **2017**, *33*, 1115–1121. [CrossRef]
57. Shen, Z.; Zheng, S.; Dong, R.; Chen, G. Saturation of stool colour in HSV color model is a promising objective parameter for screening biliary atresia. *J. Pediatr. Surg.* **2016**, *51*, 2091–2094. [CrossRef]
58. Harpavat, S.; Garcia-Prats, J.A.; Shneider, B.L. Newborn screening for biliary atresia. *NEJM* **2016**, *375*, 605–606. [CrossRef]
59. Harpavat, S.; Garcia-Prats, J.A.; Anaya, C.; Brandt, M.L.; Lupo, P.J.; Finegold, M.J.; Obuobi, A.; ElHennawy, A.A.; Jarriel, W.S.; Shneider, B.L. Diagnostic yield of newborn screening for biliary atresia using direct or conjugated bilirubin measurements. *JAMA* **2020**, *323*, 1141–1150. [CrossRef]
60. Rabbani, T.; Guthery, S.L.; Himes, R.; Shneider, B.L.; Harpavat, S. Newborn screening for biliary atresia: A review of current methods. *Curr. Gastroenterol. Rep.* **2021**, *23*, 28. [CrossRef]
61. Mogul, D.; Zhou, M.; Intihar, P.; Schwarz, K.; Frick, K. Cost-effectiveness analysis of screening for biliary atresia with the stool color card. *J. Pediatr. Gastroenterol. Nutr.* **2015**, *60*, 91–98. [CrossRef] [PubMed]
62. Kemper, A.R.; Green, N.S.; Calonge, N.; Lam, W.K.; Comeau, A.M.; Goldenberg, A.J.; Ojodu, J.; Prosser, L.A.; Tanksley, S.; Bocchini, J.A., Jr. Decision-making process for conditions nominated to the recommended uniform screening panel: Statement of the US department of health and human services secretary's advisory committee on heritable disorders in newborns and children. *Genet. Med.* **2014**, *16*, 183–187. [CrossRef] [PubMed]
63. Hewlett, J.; Waisbren, S.E. A review of the psychosocial effects of false-positive results on parents and current communication practices in newborn screening. *J. Inherit. Metab. Dis.* **2006**, *29*, 677–682. [CrossRef] [PubMed]

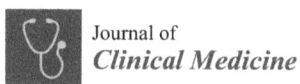 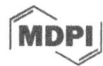

Article

Features of Nodules in Explants of Children Undergoing Liver Transplantation for Biliary Atresia

Ana M. Calinescu [1,2,*], Anne-Laure Rougemont [1,3], Mehrak Anooshiravani [1,4], Nathalie M. Rock [1,5], Valerie A. McLin [1,5,†] and Barbara E. Wildhaber [1,2,†]

1. Swiss Pediatric Liver Center, Geneva University Hospitals, 1205 Geneva, Switzerland; anne-laure.rougemont@hcuge.ch (A.-L.R.); mehrak.dumont@hcuge.ch (M.A.); nathalie.rock@hcuge.ch (N.M.R.); valerie.mclin@hcuge.ch (V.A.M.); barbara.wildhaber@hcuge.ch (B.E.W.)
2. Division of Child and Adolescent Surgery, Department of Pediatrics, Gynecology, and Obstetrics, Geneva University Hospitals, University of Geneva, 1205 Geneva, Switzerland
3. Division of Clinical Pathology, Diagnostic Department, Geneva University Hospitals, University of Geneva, 1205 Geneva, Switzerland
4. Unit of Pediatric Radiology, Diagnostic Department, Geneva University Hospitals, University of Geneva, 1205 Geneva, Switzerland
5. Gastroenterology, Hepatology and Nutrition Unit, Division of Pediatric Specialties, Department of Pediatrics, Gynecology, and Obstetrics, Geneva University Hospitals, University of Geneva, 1205 Geneva, Switzerland
* Correspondence: ana-maria.calinescu@hcuge.ch; Tel.: +41-22-372-4662
† These authors contributed equally.

Abstract: (1) Background: In patients with biliary atresia (BA) liver nodules can be identified either by pre-transplant imaging or on the explant. This study aimed to (i) analyze the histopathology of liver nodules, and (ii) to correlate histopathology with pretransplant radiological features. (2) Methods: Retrospective analysis of liver nodules in explants of BA patients transplanted in our center (2000–2021). Correlations with pretransplant radiological characteristics, patient age at liver transplantation (LT), time from Kasai hepatoportoenterostomy (KPE) to LT, age at KPE and draining KPE. (3) Results: Of the 63 BA-patients included in the analysis, 27/63 (43%) had nodules on explants. A majority were benign macroregenerative nodules. Premalignant (low-grade and high-grade dysplastic) and malignant (hepatocellular carcinoma) nodules were identified in 6/63 and 2/63 patients, respectively. On pretransplant imaging, only 13/63 (21%) patients had liver nodules, none meeting radiological criteria for malignancy. The occurrence of liver nodules correlated with patient age at LT ($p < 0.001$), time KPE-LT ($p < 0.001$) and draining KPE ($p = 0.006$). (4) Conclusion: In BA patients, pretransplant imaging did not correlate with the presence of liver nodules in explants. Liver nodules were frequent in explanted livers, whereby 25% of explants harboured malignant/pre-malignant nodules, emphasizing the need for careful surveillance in BA children whose clinical course may require LT.

Keywords: biliary atresia; liver nodules; hepatocellular carcinoma; regenerative nodules; focal nodular hyperplasia

1. Introduction

Biliary atresia (BA) is the main indication for liver transplantation (LT) in children [1,2]. Every BA patient, after Kasai hepatoportoenterostomy (KPE) or in the absence of it, will eventually develop some degree of liver fibrosis or cirrhosis. As biliary cirrhosis is associated with malignant transformation, children with BA warrant careful monitoring [3]. The usual modalities for the follow up of BA patients are ultrasound (US) and/or computed tomography (CT) and/or magnetic resonance imaging (MRI). If liver nodules identified on imaging exhibit malignant characteristics, biopsy is warranted [4]. The detection of malignant or premalignant nodules is clinically important, as it accelerates the need for LT [5]. It is known that explants of patients undergoing LT for BA can harbor various benign (regenerative nodules, focal nodular hyperplasia (FNH), adenomas), premalignant (low-grade and high-grade dysplastic nodules), or malignant (hepatocellular carcinoma (HCC), hepatoblastoma, and cholangiocarcinoma) nodules, yet the detection of these nodules through conventional imaging remains a challenge [3,4].

We aimed to analyze the histopathology of nodules identified on liver explants of patients undergoing LT for BA and to correlate histological findings with pre-LT radiological features. We hypothesized that there would be limited correlation between pre-LT radiological and post-LT pathological findings.

2. Materials and Methods

2.1. Patients

We conducted a retrospective study of all children diagnosed with BA and having undergone LT between 2000–2021 in our national referral center. Patient inclusion criteria were: primary diagnosis of BA and LT. Patient exclusion criteria were patients who did not have a primary diagnosis of BA, or BA patients who were not transplanted yet.

The following data were collected from the national BA database: demographics, age at KPE, cholangitis episodes (defined as i) fever associated with discolored stool and/or jaundice, or ii) fever associated with inflammatory parameters and/or cholestasis and/or increased transaminases and/or positive blood cultures), draining KPE (defined as conjugated bilirubin < 20 µmol/L at 6 months after KPE), pre-LT laboratory values (aspartate aminotransferase (AST), alanine aminotransferase (ALT), γ-glutamyl transferase (GGT), total and conjugated bilirubin, alpha-fetoprotein (AFP)), presence or not of pre-LT portal hypertension (defined as both splenomegaly + 2SD and thrombocytopenia (platelet count less than 100,000 G/L) or history of a complication of portal hypertension such as varices, ascites, etc.), age at LT, imaging (US performed at 6 weeks, 6 months, 1 year, 2 years pre-LT and/or CT performed prior to LT, see Section 2.2) and pathology results (see Section 2.3). The study was approved by the local ethics committee (CE 06-050).

2.2. Imaging Analysis

The routine imaging work-up consisted of color Doppler US and contrast enhanced CT scans that were performed by pediatric radiologists (3–25 years of experiece). The US machines were Acuson Sequoia 512 and Acuson S3000 (Siemens Healthineers, Erlangen, Germany) with curved-array 6 MHz and linear-array 9 MHz probes.

All CTs were obtained by using multi-detector machines: GE Lightspeed 16, GE Lightspeed VCT 64 (GE Medical Systems, WI, USA) and Somatom Definition Edge machine (Siemens Healthcare Systems, Erlangen, Germany). We used a low-dose technique based on patient weight and automatic exposure control. Parameters were: KV 80–120, 50–150 mA (care-dose modulation) and 2–5 mm slice thickness. Arterial and portal venous phase images were obtained after injecting Iohexol 300 (2 mL/kg). Imaging studies were reviewed by one author (MA) (25 years experience), first blindly, i.e., before knowing the results of the pathology report, and secondly after having received the results, to check for possibly missed nodules. For each nodule, the location (liver segments) and size (largest diameter), echogenicity on US and vascular uptake pattern on CT were reported.

2.3. Morphological and Histological Evaluation

Liver explants were submitted for gross and histological analysis. Specimens were handled according to guidelines, weighed and measured in all three dimensions, and serially cut along the transverse plane. For cirrhosis, the uniformity or variability of the nodules was recorded. After adequate fixation in 10% neutral buffered formalin, representative sections of the hilum, and of the right and left liver lobes were taken. Nodules standing out from the background liver because of size, differences in color or texture, or with a more pronounced bulging surface, were recorded and submitted for histological analysis.

Hematoxylin and Eosin stains were performed on 3 µm thick sections of the paraffin-embedded tissue. Special stains were routinely performed on selected paraffin blocks: Masson's trichrome for collagen, reticulin for architecture evaluation, Perl's Prussian blue for iron deposition, and PAS-diastase for hyaline globules. A reticulin stain and a Masson's trichrome stain were performed on the nodules when required.

2.4. Statistical Analysis

Categorical variables were compared using the chi-square and Fisher exact test, accordingly. Continuous data were expressed as median and interquartile range. Continuous variables were compared using the Student t-test. Hazard ratios were estimated with the univariate Cox proportional hazards model. Survival curves were compared using the log-rank test. Differences were considered statistically significant if $p < 0.05$.

3. Results

During the study period, 168 patients had a LT. Sixty-three patients (33 females) were included in the study with a median age at LT of 12 (9–24.5) months. Sixty (60/63) of the patients underwent KPE. Median age at KPE was 58 (45–74) days. At 6 months, 27/60 (45%) patients had a draining KPE. Thirty-nine 39/60 (65%) patients after KPE experienced one or more cholangitis episodes and were treated with two to three weeks of IV antibiotics. Portal hypertension was present in 55/63 (87%) patients at LT. The median time from KPE to LT was 11 (6–73.5) months. Thirteen 13/63 (21%) patients had nodules on pretransplant imaging, while 27/63 (43%) had nodules on explants.

3.1. Nodules on Imaging

Thirteen 13/63 (21%) patients were radiologically diagnosed with 25 liver nodules prior to LT, none with features clearly in favor of malignancy (Table 1).

Table 1. Clinical, biological and imaging characteristics of patients with nodules on pretransplant imaging. LT, liver transplantation; US, ultrasound; CT, computed tomography; KPE, Kasai hepatoportoenterostomy; F, female; M, male; m, months; NA, not acquired.

Patient	Age at LT (m)	Time KPE-LT (m)	Sex	Size (mm)	Location	US	CT Arterial/Portal Phases	AFP (µg/L)	Pathology
1	6	4	F	17 25	IV	Hypoechoic Hypoechoic with central scar	Isodense/hypodense Isodense/hypodense with central scar	363	Macroregenerative nodule Focal nodular hyperplasia
2	10	8	F	5	V	No nodule	Hyperdense/hyperdense	3255	No nodule
3	10	8	M	6	VI	No	NA/Hyperdense	12.9	No nodule
4	13	11	M	7	IV	4 Hyperechoic hilar nodules	Hypodense/hypodense segment IV Hypodense/hypodense segment III	26.6	Regenerative steatotic nodule
5	15	14	M	11	VI	Hyperechoic nodule	Isodense/hypodense	7	Regenerative steatotic nodule
6	25	23	F	12	Left lobe	2 isoechoic nodules	No nodule	1.6	No nodule
7	47	6	M	60	III	Heterogeneous isoechoic	Isodense/isodense with a small central componenet hyperdense/hyperdense	32.7	Macroregenerative nodule
8	66	65	F	30	V	Isoechoic	NA	NA	Macroregenerative nodule

Table 1. Cont.

Patient	Age at LT (m)	Time KPE-LT (m)	Sex	Size (mm)	Location	US	CT Arterial/Portal Phases	AFP (µg/l)	Pathology
9	84	83	F	30 60	I V	No nodule	Isodense/isodense Isodense/hyperdense	2.1	Macroregenerative nodule
10	133	132	F	30	IV, VII, VIII	No nodule	Isodense/hypodense	1	Low-grade dysplastic nodule Regenerative cholestatic nodule
11	174	173	M	80	Diffuse	Isoechoic	Isodense/isodense	2.6	Macroregenerative nodules
12	201	200	F	27	III	No nodule	Isodense/isodense	2.3	High-grade dysplastic nodule
13	203	201	M	16	III	Hypoechoic nodule	No nodule	2.2	No nodule

Radiological findings in 7/13 (54%) patients correlated with the final histological diagnosis: one patient with FNH and 6 with regenerative nodules (Figure 1).

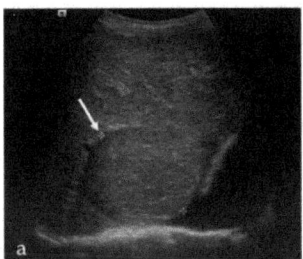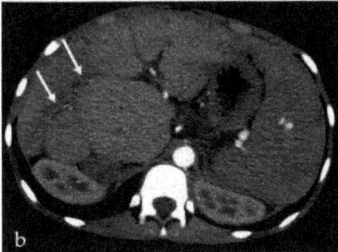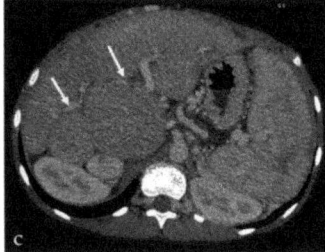

Figure 1. Macroregenerative nodules in a 14-years old boy with biliary atresia. US (**a**) with large isoechoic nodules with no vascularization on Doppler. CT with arterial (**b**) and venous (**c**) acquisition: multiple diffuse isodense iso-enhancing nodules.

3.2. Nodules in Liver Explants

Histological examination of liver explants revealed 55 nodules in 26 patients, 1 patient had 3 types of nodules and 4 other patients had 2 types of nodules. The liver of the 27th patient displayed nodules too-numerous-to-count (Figure 2). Half of the liver explants (14/27) presented with more than one nodule. Figures 1, 3 and 4 show representative imaging, gross and histological findings, in selected patients.

Most nodules were benign, with the majority being regenerative nodules (38) and the multiple nodules observed in the 27th liver explant, whereby 9 regenerative nodules displayed more pronounced cholestasis and/or steatosis than the background liver (Figure 3a). Identified in the majority of the patients presenting nodules (22/27), macroregenerative nodules were mainly seen in a central location, in segments IV, V and VIII (Table 2). Benign lesions also comprised 2 FNH, both located in segment IV (Figures 3b and 4a), and one biliary infarct.

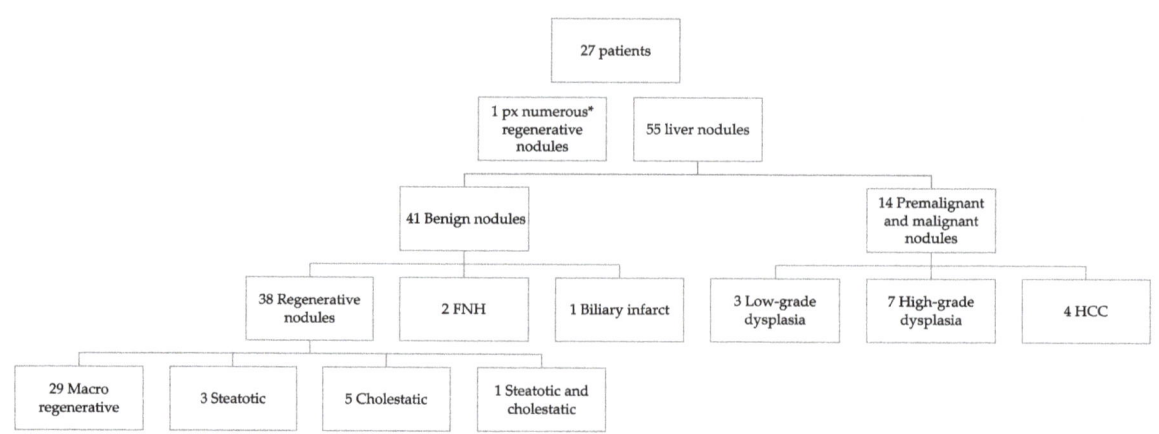

Figure 2. *Nodule types* on liver explants of biliary atresia patients (FNH, focal nodular hyperplasia; HCC, hepatocellular carcinoma; px, patient; * too-numerous-to-count).

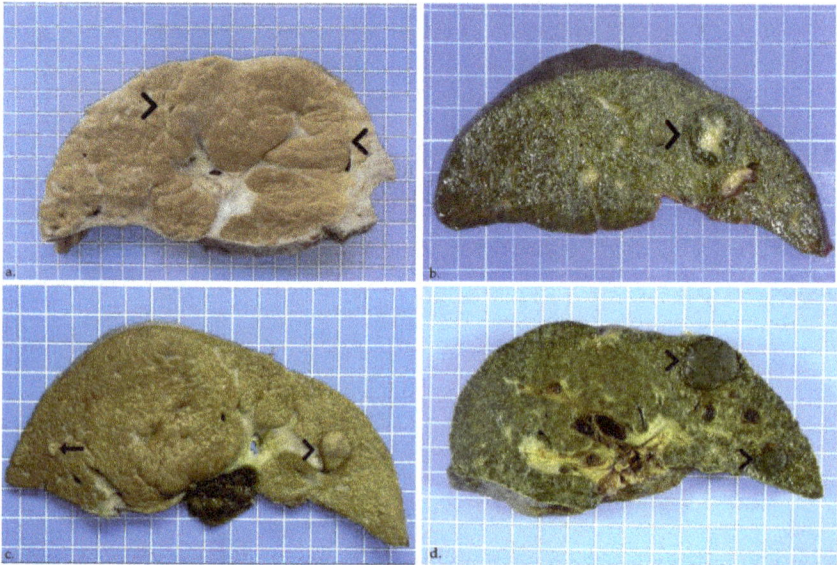

Figure 3. (**a**) Regenerative nodule in a male patient 7-years-old at liver transplantation. On cut section, a rather ill-defined 8-cm large regenerative macronodule involves segments IV, V and VIII (delineated by arrowheads). (**b**) Focal nodular hyperplasia in a 13-month-old girl. On cut section, a 2.5-cm lobulated and well-defined though unencapsulated cholestatic lesion with a central scar is seen in segment IV (arrowhead). (**c**) High-grade dysplastic nodule in a female patient aged 3 years and 5 months at transplantation. Macroscopy shows a 1.5-cm bulging brown nodule in liver segment III (arrowhead), and a further 0.4-cm nodule in segment VI (arrow). (**d**) Well-differentiated hepatocellular carcinoma. Two large cholestatic nodules in segments II and III, measuring 2.3 and 1.1 cm in greatest diameters, bulge out from the cut section (arrowheads).

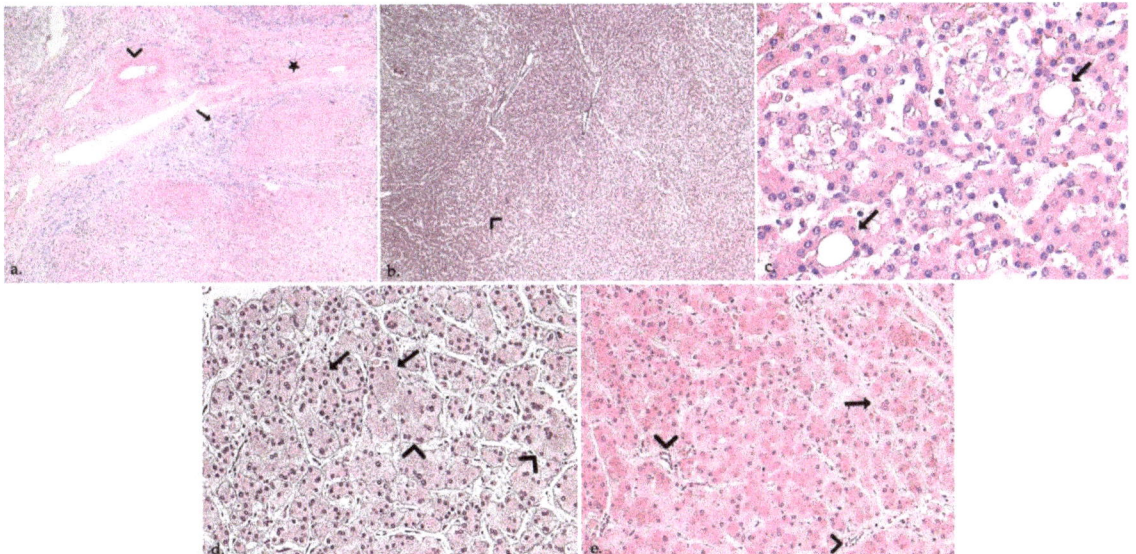

Figure 4. (**a**) Focal nodular hyperplasia in a 13-month-old girl. Histology shows benign hepatocellular nodules separated by thick fibrous septa (star) radiating from the central scar, containing thick-walled abnormal-appearing arteries (arrowhead) and a ductular reaction (arrow) (Hematoxylin & Eosin, H&E, original magnification ×40). (**b**,**c**) High-grade dysplastic nodule in a female patient aged 3 years and 5 months at transplantation, reticulin stain (5b, ×40) highlights a vaguely "nodular within nodule" growth (arrowhead), and increased cell density, while H&E stain (5c, ×400) shows small cell changes (arrowhead) and pseudoglands (arrows). (**d**,**e**) Well-differentiated hepatocellular carcinoma in a 1-year-old girl. Plate thickening (arrowheads) and focal loss of reticulin staining (arrows) is seen, together with variation in tumor cell size, multinucleation (arrow) and several unpaired arteries (arrowheads) (5d, reticulin stain, 5e, H&E, ×400).

Table 2. Histo-pathological characteristics of nodules identified in liver explants. * One nodule can overlap multiple liver segments. ** Largest diameter for every nodule, median (range) diameter for every *nodule type*. KPE, Kasai hepatoportoenterostomy; LT, liver transplantation.

Nodules	Nodule Type	Number of Nodules	Location * (Segments)	Size ** (mm)
Benign nodules	Macro regenerative nodules	29/55 (53%)	3xI/1xII/1xIII/8xIV/6xV/2xVI/5xVII/7xVIII	9 (3–80)
	Regenerative cholestatic nodules	5/55 (9%)	1xII/2xIII/1xVI/1xVII	12 (6–60)
	Regenerative steatotic nodules	3/55 (5%)	1xIII/1xIV	8.5 (5–12)
	Regenerative cholestatic and steatotic nodules	1/55 (2%)	1xVIII	7
	Focal nodular hyperplasia	2/55 (4%)	2xIV	20 (15–25)
	Biliary infarction nodules	1/55 (2%)	III	17
Premalignant and malignant nodules	Low-grade dysplasia nodules	3/55 (5%)	2xIV/1xV	7 (7–15)
	High-grade dysplasia nodules	7/55 (13%)	1xII 2xIII/1xIV/2xV/1xVI	7 (3–32)
	Hepatocellular carcinoma	4/55 (7%)	1xII/2xIII/1xV	14.5 (7–23)

Ten premalignant and four malignant tumors were seen in 7 patients (7/27, 26%). Premalignant lesions were composed of 3 low-grade dysplastic nodules, and of 7 high-grade dysplastic nodules, measuring between 0.3 and 3.2 cm in the largest diameter (Figures 3c and 4b,c).

Malignant tumors were 4 well-differentiated HCCs, seen in 2 patients (2/27), measuring between 0.7 and 2.3 cm in the largest diameter (Table 2) (Figures 3d and 4d,e). In the first patient, premalignant and malignant tumors co-existed: the liver explant of this female patient, aged 15 years at LT, showed co-occurrence of 2 well-differentiated HCCs, 2 high-grade dysplastic nodules and 3 macroregenerative nodules. The liver of the second 1-year-old patient with 2 well-differentiated HCCs, also showed a cholestatic 0.7 cm regenerative nodule.

3.3. Correlation between Imaging and Histopathology

Even after reviewing the US and CT scans, none of the malignant and premalignant nodules were detected on the pre-LT imaging. No further benign nodules were identified neither.

3.4. Patient Characteristics of Groups with and without Nodules in Liver Explants

Patients with histologically detected nodules on their liver explant were significantly older both at KPE ($p = 0.05$) and LT ($p < 0.001$) than patients without nodules. When LT was performed beyond the first year of life, significantly more explants presented *with* nodules, compared with patients receiving their LT in the first year of life: HR 1.6 [0.9–2.9] ($p = 0.08$); when LT was performed after the second year of life almost all liver explants displayed nodules (Figure 5). In the group *with* nodules, more patients had a draining KPE at 6 months, when compared with the group *without* liver nodules ($p = 0.006$). Significantly more patients had normal bilirubin values in their second year of life in the group *with* nodules when compared to the group *without* liver nodules ($p = 0.003$). No difference was identified between the two groups regarding the incidence of cholangitis ($p = 0.63$) or portal hypertension ($p = 0.67$) (Table 3). AFP was increased only in one of the two HCC patients.

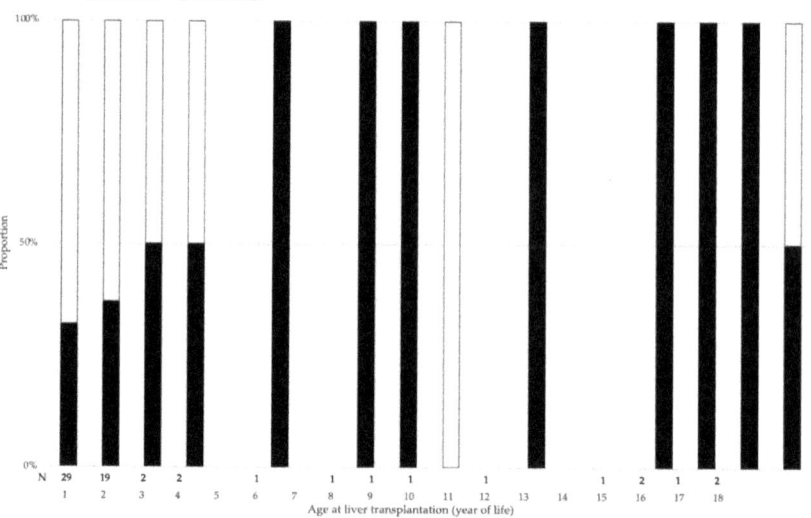

Figure 5. Percentage of patients *with* histologically detected nodules on their liver explant according to age.

Table 3. Characteristics of biliary atresia patients *with* and *without* nodules on liver explant. KPE, Kasai hepatoportoenterostomy; LT, liver transplantation.

Characteristics	With Nodules (n = 27)	Without Nodules (n = 36)	p-Value
Age at LT (months)	15 (5–207)	11 (3–203)	<0.001
KPE before LT	26/27 (96.2%)	34/36 (94.4%)	0.78
Age at Kasai (days)	53 (18–87)	64 (25–126)	0.05
Draining KPE at 6 months post KPE	17/26 (65.3%)	10/34 (29.4%)	0.006
Cholangitis episode(s) before LT	16/26 (61.5%)	23/34 (67.6%)	0.63
Portal hypertension	23/27 (85.1%)	32/36 (88.8%)	0.67
Direct bilirubin before LT (µmol/L)	34 (13–169.5)	163 (40–271.5)	0.39
Time period KPE to LT (months)	17 (3–1412)	8 (1–1338)	<0.001

Overall patient survival was not different in the group *with* nodules when compared with the group *without* liver nodules ($p = 0.79$). Likewise, there was no difference in survival between patients with premalignant or malignant nodules ($p = 0.41$). None of the patients had died or had been treated with chemotherapy at the end of follow-up (101 (48.5–156.5) months). No patient with malignant or premalignant nodules on liver explants presented with a recurrence.

4. Discussion

Nearly 50% of patients in this representative series of patients having undergone LT for BA displayed liver nodules upon histological examination of the explant, with one in four patients harboring malignant or premalignant lesions, most of which were not detected by pre-transplant imaging or serum AFP levels. Time from KPE to LT was associated with the occurrence of nodules, with more patients having identified nodules when LT was performed beyond the first year of life. The prevalence of liver nodules, their histopathological features, and the lack of correlation with imaging are all findings which differ somewhat from previous reports and warrant discussion.

4.1. Half of Explants with Nodules

The prevalence of liver nodules in this series reached nearly 50%. This is clearly higher than in previous series that report 11% of "liver nodules" on BA liver explants or [6] "benign and malignant" hepatic tumors in 8% of BA patients [3]. We hypothesized that the actual incidence of nodules in BA patients is underestimated due to underreporting.

There are several hypotheses concerning the physiopathology leading to these liver nodules. Vascular changes are frequently noted in the setting of chronic hepatic disease and also for BA patients we often observe an enlarged hepatic artery and a hypoplastic portal vein. These hemodynamic changes may induce the development of nodules such as FNH and regenerative nodules. Besides smoother bile drainage after KPE, Ijiri et al. formulate the hypothesis of a better blood supply of the porta hepatis, partially explaining the formation of hilar nodules [7]. Concerning the more peripheral nodules, Itai et al. formulate the hypothesis that the portal blood supply might not be able to reach the liver capsule in cases of diminished portal perfusion and thus contribute to the development of more peripheral nodules [7,8]. The link between KPE and nodules has been postulated by Hussein et al. in a comparative study of unoperated and post-KPE BA patients undergoing LT, no regenerative nodules were documented in the liver explants with diffuse biliary cirrhosis of the 6 patients without prior KPE. The authors therefore conclude that regenerative nodules are not purely a consequence of BA, and instead represent a consequence of KPE [9]. The highly regenerative modifications in the hilum might be a trigger for dysplasia and later HCC [9–11]. Further, the contact of the biliary epithelium with enteric contents has been reported as another accepted trigger for the development of bile duct malignancies [11,12]. Cholangitis might be another potential explanation to the appearance of liver nodules in BA patients. In our study, cholangitis occurrence was not statistically different between patients with and without nodules. Last, but not least, fibrosis grade at the time of KPE could play a role in the development of nodules. It has already been shown by Salzedas-Neto et al., that there is a negative correlation between the fibrosis grade on liver biopsy at KPE and a draining KPE [13]. As patients with a draining KPE exhibited more nodules in our series, we can speculate that there is a negative correlation between fibrosis grade and nodule occurrence.

4.2. Features of Benign Nodules

4.2.1. Focal Nodular Hyperplasia

In our series, there were two FNHs, one detected by imaging. Both were centrally located, in segment IV. FNH, a benign hepatic lesion commonly seen in vascular liver disease rather than biliary cirrhosis, was found to be the most common lesion in a recent imaging series (6/13) [3]. There is one report of an FNH increasing in size after treatment of varices, congruent with the theory of hemodynamic changes [14]. Even if in 65% of the previously reported cases FNH are radiologically diagnosed, 3/17 were not detected on pre-LT imaging and other 3/17 were potentially diagnosed as HCC or hepatoblastoma [3,6,14–17]. In the present series, both of the FNH nodules were associated with other nodule types: a low-grade dysplastic nodule in a first patient and a macroregenerative nodule in a second one. The speculation that the hemodynamic changes encountered in the evolution of BA patients ultimately lead to the development of nodules needs further research [7].

4.2.2. Regenerative Nodules

In this series, 24% of explanted livers displayed at least one regenerative nodule. Yet, the prevalence of regenerative nodules on explants of BA patients is described to be as low as 3.3% [4,7,18]. We assume that the discrepancy with previous reports may be due to underreporting. Indeed, only 22 cases of regenerative nodules are described in literature, versus 32 HCC [4,7,18], a ratio which seems very unlikely. Given that the malignant potential of macroregenerative nodules is still debated, close follow up of these patients is probably indicated [18,19].

For both FNH and regenerative nodules, the time elapsed from KPE to nodule detection is controversial: while it was found to be one per year in a cohort of 55 patients, other studies suggest a five to nine year-period until their first diagnosis [6]. Overall, in our series, patients with liver nodules had a longer time period from KPE to LT than those without nodules, suggesting that the longer the patient lives with his native liver, the higher the risk for developing nodules. That said, in our cohort clearly more patients develop nodules after the first year of life, underlining the need for screening already beyond the age of one year.

4.2.3. Other Benign Nodules

Other benign nodules described in association with BA include mesenchymal hamartoma and adenomas, none of which were observed in our series [3,6,20]. Mesenchymal hamartoma and adenoma have both been presented as case reports in patients with BA. The pathophysiological relationship with BA is difficult to explain in both cases, raising the question of incidental findings [6,20].

4.3. Features of Malignant Nodules

The striking feature of the present series is the lack of correlation between pre-LT imaging and histopathological findings. None of the HCC nodules reported here were detectable on imaging, even on a post-hoc analysis, despite their detectable size (Table 2).

4.3.1. Hepatocellular Carcinoma

The discrepancy between imaging and histopathology in the setting of BA has been reported in 32 pediatric cases [2,3,10,21–33]. The prevalence of HCC in explants of 544 children transplanted for BA was reported to be 1.2% [3,10,26]. Half of HCC seem to be missed during pre-LT imaging, and 41% of BA patients with HCC have a normal AFP [3]. The calculated sensitivity for the radiological diagnosis of HCC within the available literature of BA is 62.5% [2,3,10,21–27,29–33]. AFP was also of very limited use in our series, since it was only increased in one of the two patients with HCC. Indeed, AFP monitoring in BA patients and imaging has a low sensitivity of detecting small HCC. Nevertheless, increasing AFP in a BA patient should clearly encourage further imaging such as MRI with a hepatobiliary phase to rule out malignancy. The sensitivity of MRI to detect nodules is higher than both US and CT, and affords the opportunity to distinguish between regenerative nodules and malignancy using diffusion sequences and hepatospecific contrast agents. Small and borderline nodules (dysplastic and early HCC) may still be challenging to diagnose by MRI. Contrast-enhanced ultrasound, a non ionizing technique, is increasingly used in children for detecting and characterizing focal liver lesions and may be helpful in the follow-up of BA patients. As for other techniques, the difficulty lies in the analysis of nodules within a cirrhotic liver with global parenchymal changes [34]. Thus, in case of increased AFP and detected nodules, targeted biopsies should help to plan the appropriate management [28].

4.3.2. Dysplastic Nodules

Dysplastic nodules are considered to be preoplastic conditions [21]. Even if radiological investigations were negative for malignancy, a 3.3% incidence of HCC was reported in a series of dysplastic nodules [35]. The mean diameter of dysplastic nodules in our series correlated with the degree of dysplasia: the size increased from low grade dysplasia, to high grade dysplasia, to HCC, supporting the hypothesis of progression through the stages of carcinogenesis with the increasing diameter [5]. Given that half of the dysplastic nodules in the present series were located in the hilar area, especially segment IV, and the hilar region being known for having particular regenerative properties in BA patients, it is tempting to speculate about the role of the hilar hepatic regeneration in the development of dysplastic nodules and later HCC [9,10].

4.3.3. Other Malignant Tumors

Other malignant tumors such as cholangiocarcinoma and hepatoblastoma have been reported to be found in liver explants of BA patients [2,36,37]. None of these tumors were found on liver explants in our series.

4.4. Limitations of This Study

The findings of this study have to be seen in the light of several limitations. First, there is a certain selection bias. This study started with a design in which we only investigated patients who finally underwent LT. KPE-succeeded BA patients spend a longer period of life with cirrhotic liver than KPE-failed patients. Therefore, KPE-succeeded BA patients might have more chances for the development of hepatic nodules. Associating successful KPE with the frequent occurrence of hepatic nodules after collecting LT candidates thus corresponds to a selection bias. However, this selection bias is inherent to the design and aim of our study that sought the correlations between pre-LT radiology and pathology of nodules of the explant.

Second, there is a literature gap regarding the pathophysiology of the development of nodules in BA patients. Our study incites for further research to clarify this aspect.

Third, the small sample size might limit the generalization of our results. Nevertheless, our data is representative as our center is the national referral center for BA patients and all patients are centralized.

5. Conclusions

Liver nodules were more frequently encountered in explanted livers after KPE than previously reported. A high proportion of liver nodules was not detected radiologically. One quarter of the lesions was malignant or pre-malignant, emphasizing the need for careful surveillance of BA patients and meticulous explant analysis. Older age at KPE, a draining KPE, and thus a longer time interval from KPE to LT, were associated with the presence of nodules on explants. How to improve detection of these nodules and whether patients require tailored follow-up are questions for future research.

Author Contributions: Conceptualization, A.M.C. and B.E.W.; methodology, A.M.C. and B.E.W.; software, A.M.C.; validation, B.E.W., A.-L.R., N.M.R., V.A.M. and M.A.; formal analysis, A.M.C., V.A.M. and B.E.W.; investigation, A.M.C., A.-L.R. and M.A.; resources, A.M.C.; data curation, A.M.C.; writing—original draft preparation, A.M.C., A.-L.R., V.A.M. and B.E.W.; writing—review and editing, B.E.W., A.M.C., A.-L.R., N.M.R., M.A. and V.A.M.; visualization, B.E.W., A.M.C., A.-L.R., N.M.R., V.A.M. and M.A.; supervision, B.E.W.; project administration, A.M.C.; funding acquisition, none. All authors have read and agreed to the published version of the manuscript.

Funding: This research received no external funding.

Institutional Review Board Statement: The study was conducted according to the guidelines of the Declaration of Helsinki, and approved by the Ethics Committee (CE 06-050), approval date 29 March 2021.

Informed Consent Statement: Informed consent was obtained from all subjects involved in the study.

Data Availability Statement: The data presented in this study are available on request from the corresponding author. The data are not publicly available due to ethical and legal reasons.

Acknowledgments: The authors would like to thank Hélène Ara-Somohano, Luigi Cataldi and Simona Korff for their help with the samples and data management.

Conflicts of Interest: The authors declare no conflict of interest.

References

1. Arnon, R.; Annunziato, R.A.; D'Amelio, G.; Chu, J.; Shneider, B.L. Liver Transplantation for Biliary Atresia: Is There a Difference in Outcome for Infants? *J. Pediatr. Gastroenterol. Nutr.* **2016**, *62*, 220–225. [CrossRef] [PubMed]
2. Tatekawa, Y.; Asonuma, K.; Uemoto, S.; Inomata, Y.; Tanaka, K. Liver transplantation for biliary atresia associated with malignant hepatic tumors. *J. Pediatr. Surg.* **2001**, *36*, 436–439. [CrossRef] [PubMed]
3. Yoon, H.J.; Jeon, T.Y.; Yoo, S.Y.; Kim, J.H.; Eo, H.; Lee, S.K.; Kim, J.S. Hepatic tumours in children with biliary atresia: Single-centre experience in 13 cases and review of the literature. *Clin. Radiol.* **2014**, *69*, e113–e119. [CrossRef] [PubMed]
4. Liu, Y.W.; Concejero, A.M.; Chen, C.L.; Cheng, Y.F.; Eng, H.L.; Huang, T.L.; Chen, T.Y.; Wang, C.C.; Wang, S.H.; Lin, C.C.; et al. Hepatic pseudotumor in long-standing biliary atresia patients undergoing liver transplantation. *Liver Transplant.* **2007**, *13*, 1545–1551. [CrossRef] [PubMed]
5. Libbrecht, L.; Bielen, D.; Verslype, C.; Vanbeckevoort, D.; Pirenne, J.; Nevens, F.; Desmet, V.; Roskams, T. Focal lesions in cirrhotic explant livers: Pathological evaluation and accuracy of pretransplantation imaging examinations. *Liver Transplant.* **2002**, *8*, 749–761. [CrossRef] [PubMed]
6. Song, H.J.; Suh, Y. Newly formed hepatic masses in children with biliary atresia after Kasai Hepatic Portoenterostomy. *Korean J. Pathol.* **2011**, *45*, 160–169. [CrossRef]
7. Ijiri, R.; Tanaka, Y.; Kato, K.; Misugi, K.; Ohama, Y.Y.; Shinkai, M.; Nishi, T.; Aida, N.; Kondo, F. Clinicopathological study of a hilar nodule in the livers of long-term survivors with biliary atresia. *Pathol. Int.* **2001**, *51*, 16–19. [CrossRef] [PubMed]
8. Itai, Y.; Matsui, O. Blood flow and liver imaging. *Radiology* **1997**, *202*, 306–314. [CrossRef]
9. Hussein, A.; Wyatt, J.; Guthrie, A.; Stringer, M.D. Kasai portoenterostomy–new insights from hepatic morphology. *J. Pediatr. Surg.* **2005**, *40*, 322–326. [CrossRef]
10. Hadzic, N.; Quaglia, A.; Portmann, B.; Paramalingam, S.; Heaton, N.D.; Rela, M.; Mieli-Vergani, G.; Davenport, M. Hepatocellular carcinoma in biliary atresia: King's College Hospital experience. *J. Pediatr.* **2011**, *159*, 617–622.e1. [CrossRef]
11. Tocchi, A.; Mazzoni, G.; Liotta, G.; Lepre, L.; Cassini, D.; Miccini, M. Late development of bile duct cancer in patients who had biliary-enteric drainage for benign disease: A follow-up study of more than 1,000 patients. *Ann. Surg.* **2001**, *234*, 210–214. [CrossRef] [PubMed]
12. Chakhunashvili, K.; Pavlenishvili, I.; Kakabadze, M.; Kordzaia, D.; Chakhunashvili, D.; Kakabadze, Z. Biliary Atresia: Current Concepts and Future Prospects (Review). *Georgian Med. News* **2016**, 104–111.
13. Salzedas-Netto, A.A.; Chinen, E.; de Oliveira, D.F.; Pasquetti, A.F.; Azevedo, R.A.; da Silva Patricio, F.F.; Cury, E.K.; Gonzalez, A.M.; Vicentine, F.P.; Martins, J.L. Grade IV fibrosis interferes in biliary drainage after Kasai procedure. *Transplant. Proc.* **2014**, *46*, 1781–1783. [CrossRef] [PubMed]
14. Sato, A.; Rai, T.; Takahashi, A.; Saito, H.; Takagi, T.; Shibukawa, G.; Wakatsuk, T.; Takahashi, Y.; Irisawa, A.; Ise, K.; et al. A case of rapidly expanding and increasing focal nodular hyperplasia. *Fukushima J. Med. Sci* **2006**, *52*, 149–155. [CrossRef] [PubMed]

15. Ohtomo, K.; Itai, Y.; Hasizume, K.; Kosaka, N.; Iio, M. CT and MR appearance of focal nodular hyperplasia of the liver in children with biliary atresia. *Clin. Radiol.* **1991**, *43*, 88–90. [CrossRef]
16. Cha, D.I.; Yoo, S.Y.; Kim, J.H.; Jeon, T.Y.; Eo, H. Clinical and imaging features of focal nodular hyperplasia in children. *AJR Am. J. Roentgenol.* **2014**, *202*, 960–965. [CrossRef] [PubMed]
17. Okugawa, Y.; Uchida, K.; Inoue, M.; Kawamoto, A.; Ohtake, K.; Sakurai, H.; Uchida, K.; Isaji, S.; Miki, C.; Kusunoki, M. Focal nodular hyperplasia in biliary atresia patient after Kasai hepatic portoenterostomy. *Pediatr. Surg. Int.* **2008**, *24*, 609–612. [CrossRef] [PubMed]
18. Liang, J.L.; Cheng, Y.F.; Concejero, A.M.; Huang, T.L.; Chen, T.Y.; Tsang, L.L.; Ou, H.Y. Macro-regenerative nodules in biliary atresia: CT/MRI findings and their pathological relations. *World J. Gastroenterol.* **2008**, *14*, 4529–4534. [CrossRef] [PubMed]
19. Rougemont, A.L.; McLin, V.A. Central Liver Nodules in Alagille Syndrome and Biliary Atresia After Kasai Portoenterostomy. *J. Pediatr. Gastroenterol. Nutr.* **2016**, *63*, e41–e42. [CrossRef] [PubMed]
20. Lack, E.E. Mesenchymal hamartoma of the liver. A clinical and pathologic study of nine cases. *Am. J. Pediatr. Hematol. Oncol.* **1986**, *8*, 91–98. [PubMed]
21. Esquivel, C.O.; Gutierrez, C.; Cox, K.L.; Garcia-Kennedy, R.; Berquist, W.; Concepcion, W. Hepatocellular carcinoma and liver cell dysplasia in children with chronic liver disease. *J. Pediatr. Surg.* **1994**, *29*, 1465–1469. [CrossRef]
22. Van Wyk, J.; Halgrimson, C.G.; Giles, G.; Lilly, J.; Martineau, G.; Starzl, T.E. Liver transplantation in biliary atresia with concomitant hepatoma. *S. Afr. Med. J.* **1972**, *46*, 885–889. [PubMed]
23. Okuyama, K. Primary Liver Cell Carcinoma Associated with Biliary Cirrhosis Due to Congenital Bile Duct Atresia. *J. Pediatr.* **1965**, *67*, 89–93. [CrossRef]
24. Kohno, M.; Kitatani, H.; Wada, H.; Kajimoto, T.; Matuno, H.; Tanino, M.; Nakagawa, T.; Takarada, A. Hepatocellular carcinoma complicating biliary cirrhosis caused by biliary atresia: Report of a case. *J. Pediatr. Surg.* **1995**, *30*, 1713–1716. [CrossRef]
25. Superina, R.; Bilik, R. Results of liver transplantation in children with unresectable liver tumors. *J. Pediatr. Surg.* **1996**, *31*, 835–839. [CrossRef]
26. Hol, L.; van den Bos, I.C.; Hussain, S.M.; Zondervan, P.E.; de Man, R.A. Hepatocellular carcinoma complicating biliary atresia after Kasai portoenterostomy. *Eur. J. Gastroenterol. Hepatol.* **2008**, *20*, 227–231. [CrossRef] [PubMed]
27. Brunati, A.; Feruzi, Z.; Sokal, E.; Smets, F.; Fervaille, C.; Gosseye, S.; Clapuyt, P.; de Ville de Goyet, J.; Reding, R. Early occurrence of hepatocellular carcinoma in biliary atresia treated by liver transplantation. *Pediatr. Transplant.* **2007**, *11*, 117–119. [CrossRef] [PubMed]
28. Iida, T.; Zendejas, I.R.; Kayler, L.K.; Magliocca, J.F.; Kim, R.D.; Hemming, A.W.; Gonzalez-Peralta, R.P.; Fujita, S. Hepatocellular carcinoma in a 10-month-old biliary atresia child. *Pediatr. Transplant.* **2009**, *13*, 1048–1049. [CrossRef] [PubMed]
29. Romano, F.; Stroppa, P.; Bravi, M.; Casotti, V.; Lucianetti, A.; Guizzetti, M.; Sonzogni, A.; Colledan, M.; D'Antiga, L. Favorable outcome of primary liver transplantation in children with cirrhosis and hepatocellular carcinoma. *Pediatr. Transplant.* **2011**, *15*, 573–579. [CrossRef] [PubMed]
30. Zen, Y.; Srinivasan, P.; Kitagawa, M.; Suzuki, K.; Heneghan, M.; Prachalias, A. De novo perihilar cholangiocarcinoma arising in the allograft liver 15 years post-transplantation for biliary atresia. *Pathol. Int.* **2020**, *70*, 563–567. [CrossRef]
31. Hirzel, A.C.; Madrazo, B.; Rojas, C.P. Two Rare Cases of Hepatocellular Carcinoma after Kasai Procedure for Biliary Atresia: A Recommendation for Close Follow-Up. *Case Rep. Pathol.* **2015**, *2015*, 982679. [CrossRef] [PubMed]
32. Kim, J.M.; Lee, S.K.; Kwon, C.H.; Joh, J.W.; Choe, Y.H.; Park, C.K. Hepatocellular carcinoma in an infant with biliary atresia younger than 1 year. *J. Pediatr. Surg.* **2012**, *47*, 819–821. [CrossRef] [PubMed]
33. Squires, J.H.; Bill, A.; Thieret, J.; Squires, J.E. Identification of Suspected Hepatocellular Carcinoma with Contrast-Enhanced Ultrasound. *J. Pediatr.* **2017**, *182*, 398–398.e1. [CrossRef] [PubMed]
34. Fang, C.; Anupindi, S.A.; Back, S.J.; Franke, D.; Green, T.G.; Harkanyi, Z.; Jungert, J.; Kwon, J.K.; Paltiel, H.J.; Squires, J.H.; et al. Contrast-enhanced ultrasound of benign and malignant liver lesions in children. *Pediatr. Radiol.* **2021**, *51*, 2181–2197. [CrossRef] [PubMed]
35. Kobayashi, M.; Ikeda, K.; Hosaka, T.; Sezaki, H.; Someya, T.; Akuta, N.; Suzuki, F.; Suzuki, Y.; Saitoh, S.; Arase, Y.; et al. Dysplastic nodules frequently develop into hepatocellular carcinoma in patients with chronic viral hepatitis and cirrhosis. *Cancer* **2006**, *106*, 636–647. [CrossRef] [PubMed]
36. Amir, A.Z.; Sharma, A.; Cutz, E.; Avitzur, Y.; Shaikh, F.; Kamath, B.M.; Ling, S.C.; Ghanekar, A.; Ng, V.L. Hepatoblastoma in Explanted Livers of Patients with Biliary Atresia. *J. Pediatr. Gastroenterol. Nutr.* **2016**, *63*, 188–194. [CrossRef] [PubMed]
37. Taat, F.; Bosman, D.K.; Aronson, D.C. Hepatoblastoma in a girl with biliary atresia: Coincidence or co-incidence. *Pediatr. Blood Cancer* **2004**, *43*, 603–605. [CrossRef] [PubMed]

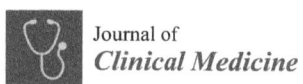 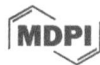

Article

Variability of Care and Access to Transplantation for Children with Biliary Atresia Who Need a Liver Replacement

Jean de Ville de Goyet [1,*], Toni Illhardt [2], Christophe Chardot [3], Peace N. Dike [4], Ulrich Baumann [5], Katherine Brandt [6], Barbara E. Wildhaber [7], Mikko Pakarinen [8], Fabrizio di Francesco [1], Ekkehard Sturm [2], Marianna Cornet [3], Caroline Lemoine [6], Eva Doreen Pfister [5], Ana M. Calinescu [7], Maria Hukkinen [8], Sanjiv Harpavat [4], Fabio Tuzzolino [9] and Riccardo Superina [6]

1. Department of Pediatrics, IRCCS-ISMETT (Institute for Scientific-Based Care and Research—Mediterranean Institute for Transplantation and Advanced Specialized Therapies), 90127 Palermo, Italy; fdifrancesco@ismett.edu
2. Department of General, Visceral and Transplant Surgery, University Hospital Tübingen, 72076 Tübingen, Germany; toni.illhardt@med.uni-tuebingen.de (T.I.); ekkehard.sturm@med.uni-tuebingen.de (E.S.)
3. Division of Pediatric Surgery, Necker Enfants Malades Hospital, 75015 Paris, France; christophe.chardot@nck.aphp.fr (C.C.); marianna.cornet@aphp.fr (M.C.)
4. Division of Pediatric Gastroenterology, Hepatology and Nutrition, Department of Pediatrics, Baylor College of Medicine, Texas Children's Hospital, Houston, TX 77030, USA; peace.dike@bcm.edu (P.N.D.); harpavat@bcm.edu (S.H.)
5. Division of Pediatric Gastroenterology and Hepatology, Department of Pediatric Kidney, Liver and Metabolic Diseases, Hannover Medical School, 30625 Hannover, Germany; baumann.u@mh-hannover.de (U.B.); pfister.eva-doreen@mh-hannover.de (E.D.P.)
6. Division of Transplant Surgery, Ann & Robert H. Lurie Children's Hospital of Chicago, Chicago, IL 60611, USA; kabrandt@luriechildrens.org (K.B.); clemoine@luriechildrens.org (C.L.); rsuperina@luriechildrens.org (R.S.)
7. Swiss Pediatric Liver Center, Child and Adolescent Surgery Division, Geneva University Hospitals (HUG), 1205 Geneva, Switzerland; barbara.wildhaber@hcuge.ch (B.E.W.); ana-maria.calinescu@hcuge.ch (A.M.C.)
8. Children's Hospital, University of Helsinki, 00029 Helsinki, Finland; mikko.pakarinen@hus.fi (M.P.); maria.hukkinen@hus.fi (M.H.)
9. Research Department, IRCCS-ISMETT (Institute for Scientific-Based Care and Research—Mediterranean Institute for Transplantation and Advanced Specialized Therapies), 90127 Palermo, Italy; ftuzzolino@ismett.edu
* Correspondence: jdeville@ismett.edu

Abstract: Background & Aims: Biliary atresia (BA) is the commonest single etiology indication for liver replacement in children. As timely access to liver transplantation (LT) remains challenging for small BA children (with prolonged waiting time being associated with clinical deterioration leading to both preventable pre- and post-transplant morbidity and mortality), the care pathway of BA children in need of LT was analyzed—from diagnosis to LT—with particular attention to referral patterns, timing of referral, waiting list dynamics and need for medical assistance before LT. Methods: International multicentric retrospective study. Intent-to-transplant study analyzing BA children who had indication for LT early in life (aged < 3 years at the time of assessment), over the last 5 years (2016–2020). Clinical and laboratory data of 219 BA children were collected from 8 transplant centers (6 in Europe and 2 in USA). Results: 39 patients underwent primary transplants. Children who underwent Kasai in a specialist -but not transplant- center were older at time of referral and at transplant. At assessment for LT, the vast majority of children already were experiencing complication of cirrhosis, and the majority of children needed medical assistance (nutritional support, hospitalization, transfusion of albumin or blood) while waiting for transplantation. Severe worsening of the clinical condition led to the need for requesting a priority status (i.e., Peld Score exception or similar) for timely graft allocation for 76 children, overall (35%). Conclusions: As LT currently results in BA patient survival exceeding 95% in many expert LT centers, the paradigm for BA management optimization and survival have currently shifted to the pre-LT management. The creation of networks dedicated to the timely referral to a pediatric transplant center and possibly centralization of care

Citation: de Ville de Goyet, J.; Illhardt, T.; Chardot, C.; Dike, P.N.; Baumann, U.; Brandt, K.; Wildhaber, B.E.; Pakarinen, M.; di Francesco, F.; Sturm, E.; et al. Variability of Care and Access to Transplantation for Children with Biliary Atresia Who Need a Liver Replacement. *J. Clin. Med.* **2022**, *11*, 2142. https://doi.org/10.3390/jcm11082142

Academic Editors: Claus Petersen and Hidekazu Suzuki

Received: 29 January 2022
Accepted: 9 March 2022
Published: 12 April 2022

Publisher's Note: MDPI stays neutral with regard to jurisdictional claims in published maps and institutional affiliations.

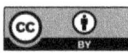

Copyright: © 2022 by the authors. Licensee MDPI, Basel, Switzerland. This article is an open access article distributed under the terms and conditions of the Creative Commons Attribution (CC BY) license (https:// creativecommons.org/licenses/by/ 4.0/).

should be considered, in combination with implementing all different graft type surgeries in specialist centers (including split and living donor LTs) to achieve timely LT in this vulnerable population.

Keywords: biliary atresia; Kasai portoenterostomy; transplant waiting list; pediatric liver transplantation; referral practice; outcome

1. Introduction

Biliary atresia (BA) is the most common single indication for liver replacement and transplantation (LT) in children. It is the most common cause of death from liver disease in that age group, and was the indication for 39% of all LT in Europe between 1968 and 2017 [1]. LT is currently proposed as a cure for all children with BA in need of a liver replacement. In the absence of severe comorbidities or contraindications, the risk of these children dying from biliary cirrhosis depends in fact directly on the possibility of obtaining a LT as a timely cure [2–6].

The predictable, progressive and irreversible worsening of their clinical condition during the wait for LT contributes directly to added morbidity and a risk of death in both pre- and post-LT periods [7–11]. Although it is clear and self-evident that a late referral to transplant centers (LTC) and prolonged waiting time for LT are associated with worse outcomes, there are only a few studies analyzing the dynamics of these children's referrals and of their pathway to LT.

For this study, attention was paid to analyzing the clinical evolution of small children diagnosed with BA and needing LT early in life (<3 years of age), from their diagnosis until LT, and to bring evidence of possible determinants for a successful path to LT (intent-to-transplant analysis).

One hypothesis was that children who are referred secondarily to LTC may experience some delay of assessment and LT (and possible increased morbidity). The analysis aimed at comparing patterns of referral and, in particular, comparing patients who were managed outside an LTC initially, with those who were immediately referred at diagnosis and managed in the center that eventually offered LT. Particular attention was paid to the timing of referral, waiting list dynamics and the need for medical assistance before LT.

2. Methods

This study was an international multicentric retrospective analysis. The study concept was generated spontaneously during brainstorming for future research projects on the BA theme, within the BARD association (BA-Related Disorders—http://www.bard-online.com, accessed on 10 March 2022). Eight centers (six in Europe and two in the USA) collaborated for the study.

2.1. Study Design and Analysis Plan

Since medical care, transplant medicine and surgery have evolved rapidly, and because liver graft availability/use has varied significantly in the last decades, only the recent and limited period of time (recent five consecutive years) was analyzed. This allowed for analysis of the very current health pathways and ability to further propose methods for improvement in the near future.

Since the reason for liver replacement in BA patients varies with the age, with rapidly progressive liver dysfunction being seen mostly in the younger ones and indications in older ones are mostly related to chronic cirrhosis and portal hypertension or its collateral effects, it was decided to concentrate only on the younger ones, i.e., less than 3 years old, at assessment/registration on the transplant list.

In view of the liver graft allocation policies and graft type, as a consequence, waiting list dynamics substantially differ between Europe and the USA [12,13]. For this reason, separate analyses were run in these two world areas, in order to both compare the two health systems and provide specific conclusions/recommendations for future care.

As all contributing centers were experts in managing children with liver disease and as the time period covered only the recent years, it was considered that clinical approaches and management protocols were sufficiently homogenous enough over the whole period of the study to exclude analyzing/comparing the quality and type of care proposed in these centers (both for pre- and post-LT care, including immunosuppression protocol and surgical techniques).

2.2. Study Population: Inclusion and Exclusion Criteria

All consecutive children with BA managed in the respective centers were enrolled if they fulfilled the following criteria: (i) <3 years of age at assessment for LT, and (ii) assessed and transplanted within the contributing centers between 1 January 2016 and 31 December 2020. For those who had been transplanted, only those with a minimum of 3 months follow-up after LT were included at the time of selection and data gathering.

As the study was an "intent-to-LT" analysis, the endpoints were "transplant" or "death (while waiting for LT)". Patients who were still waiting on the list at the study closure date were excluded, as well as those who were removed from the list during the study period because of being "too-well" or clinically improving to the point that LT was not recommended. On the contrary, those who died while waiting, and those who were removed from the list because they were considered too sick (i.e., a contraindication to LT), were included in the study group. Lastly, patients who had been assessed in one of the contributing centers but were later transferred to another center were excluded from the analysis performed by the former center.

2.3. Data for Analysis

All data were retrospective and retrieved from the patients' medical and operational records. This was performed once and only for the purpose of the analyses by one of the co-authors of the caring center.

Data and information were collected about: (1) The history of prematurity, comorbidities and associated malformations, poly-malformative atresia or not. (2) The type of initial surgery for BA (no-surgery, laparotomy or Kasai procedure) and the type of center for Kasai ((a) non-liver-expert center (i.e., no multidisciplinary pediatric liver service), (b) liver-expert center (i.e., multidisciplinary pediatric liver service available but no transplant service) and (c) pediatric LT center (LTC including multidisciplinary pediatric liver services). (3) Age at initial operation, age at assessment and age at registration on the transplant list. (4) Clinical condition (weight, ascites or not, nutritional support or not and type, Pediatric End-Stage Liver score (PELD)) at the time of assessment and registration on the list. (5) Waiting time on the list before LT, and clinical evolution while waiting (ascites, albumin or blood transfusions, need for hospitalization). (6) Age, weight, PELD and clinical condition (home, hospital- or intensive care unit (ICU)-bound) at LT. (7) Type of donor (deceased or living donor (LD)) and liver graft type (full-size, reduced, split or living donor). (8) Cause of death before LT, cause of death or graft loss after LT and age at last clinical check.

2.4. Data Management and Statistical Analyses

Data were initially analyzed as a whole with comparisons between subgroups, and secondly as follows:

1. To analyze referral pathways and their dynamic, subgroups were defined as per the type of initial BA surgery: (A) no-surgery, (B) explorative laparotomy only (no-Kasai), (C) Kasai procedure performed in non-expert liver center, (D) Kasai procedure performed in expert liver center other than the LTC and (E) Kasai procedure performed in the LTC where the transplant was performed later.

2. As access to LT and waiting time for LT are very different when a candidate for LT is proposed to LD-LT, a second analysis was performed with the same subgrouping method, and comparing all patients who had living donor LT versus all others.

For studying correlations, at the level of the centers: between regional allocation rules, waiting list dynamics, LD-LT use and the proportion of LT using PELD exception (or similar priority) request, one center was excluded because regional allocation was not PELD/MELD-based, but center-driven in an otherwise unique national set-up. For this specific study, all mean values were rounded to the nearest integer.

For the statistical analysis, continuous variables were expressed as mean and standard deviations, or as median and range where appropriate. They were compared with the T-Test, Wilcoxon rank sum test or the Mann–Whitney test, and the ANOVA test, together with Levene's Test, for assessing the homogeneity of variance between the groups. The categorical variables were compared by using Fisher's exact test or the Chi-square test when appropriate. All the data were analyzed by using SAS 9.4 Software.

$p < 0.05$ was considered statistically significant.

3. Results

General demographics and results of the analysis are detailed in Tables 1–3.

3.1. Europe

During the study period, 165 patients were assessed for LT in 6 LTC. Of the 165 children, 11 had a history of prematurity, 25 had malformative polysplenia syndrome and 27 had other comorbidities (Table 1). Of the 165 patients, 136 underwent Kasai porto-enterostomy after the diagnosis of BA (82%) (mean age at Kasai ± SD, 60.3 ± 25.0 days). A detailed analysis is provided in Tables 1 and 3.

During their waiting time for a LT, the clinical condition of 150/165 children worsened with any (or a combination) of the following problems: increasing ascites (73%), the need for albumin infusion (59%) or blood transfusions (29%), the need for enteral (40%) or parenteral nutrition (PN) support (22%), the need for short (<5 days) or long (>5 days) hospitalizations (25% and 61%, respectively), or the need for recovery in the ICU (13%).

No deaths occurred during their LT waiting time and all the children were finally transplanted.

Of all LT, 120 (72.7%) were performed in children aged less than 1 year at the time of transplant. At the time of the LT, 88 children were at home, while 63 cases were hospital-bound, and another 14 children were in the ICU. LT were performed with full-size livers ($n = 20$), reduced livers ($n = 5$), split liver grafts ($n = 60$) and grafts procured from LD ($n = 80$). Of all 165 children transplanted over a period of 5 years, death occurred after LT in 5 cases (overall patient survival = 97%). Death occurred within the first post-operative trimester in 4/5 cases (graft primary non-function in 2 cases, sepsis in 1 case and pulmonary hypertension in 1 case), or during the second year in another case (cardiac complication).

Comparison of subgroups A to E (as per type of initial surgery at BA diagnosis) evidenced statistical differences between the subgroups for age at assessment, weight at assessment and initial PELD score (Table 1). The children who had primary transplants and those who had the Kasai operation performed within the center where they received the transplant were younger, weighed less and had lower PELD scores at any time of their management course (from assessment to LT) compared to the other groups.

A comparison of those who benefited from LD versus others showed that children in the former group were similar for age but lower in weight, though they were significantly more likely to develop ascites and the management of the ascites required more albumin infusion and was associated with significantly more hospitalization (including in the ICU). Although their waiting time for LT was significantly shorter, those receiving a LD-LT had worsening PELD scores while waiting and had significantly higher PELD scores at LT compared to the latter group. Interestingly, the duration of respiratory assistance after LT, and the length of stay both in the ICU and in hospital overall, were all significantly shorter in the LD group (Table 3).

3.2. USA

General demographics and results of the analysis are detailed in Tables 2 and 3.

In the American phase of the study, 55 patients in 2 LT centers were included. Only 5 (9%) babies were born prematurely. Of the 55, 9 (16.4%) had polysplenia, 45/55 babies underwent a Kasai portoenterostomy, while 10 (18.2%) either underwent no surgery or just an exploration. The mean age at Kasai operation for the American cohort was 60.0 ± 27.2 days.

During the waiting period, many of the children suffered from a deterioration in their condition: 31/55 (56.4%) experienced worsening ascites and 32/55 (58.2%) required albumin infusions during the waiting period. Though at referral for assessment, 28/55 (51%) had enteral support and only 10/55 (18%) had PN, the latter ratio increased to 27/55 (49.1%) during the waiting time (Table 2). Additionally, 27/55 (49.1%) required at least one blood transfusion, and 40/55 (72.7%) required at least one hospital admission of greater than 5 days as well as at least one admission shorter than 5 days (26/55, 47.2%).

One child died before LT: though he was waiting in ICU and had a PELD exception priority, his condition deteriorated to the point where a LT would be contraindicated and he was removed from the list.

Slightly more than half of the 54 transplanted patients (28/54, 52%) received a transplant while waiting at home, and more than a third (19/54, 35.2%) were in hospital but not in the ICU, with 7 (12.7%) being in the ICU at the time of the transplant.

Of the children undergoing a transplant, 36/54 (67%) were less than a year of age. The average age at transplant was 9.8 months (7.6–13 interquartile range).

The distribution of organ types in the American cohort was 30 (56%) whole livers, 16 (30%) split livers, 2 (4%) reduced size and 6 (11%) living donor left lobes or segment II–III grafts.

Most patients (5/6, 83.3%) who received a LD-LT were in hospital, and 1/6 was in the ICU. Only 1 patient (1/6, 16.7%) was at home at the time of the LD transplant, in contrast to the European live donor patients, most of whom (47/80, 58.7%) were at home at the time of the transplant.

Overall survival in the 5-year period was 51/54 (94.4%), including 6/6 surviving in the live donor group and 45/48 (94%) in the deceased donor group.

A comparison between the five groups (A–E) according to where and if they had a Kasai operation demonstrated that the infants who had either no surgery or an exploration alone (groups A and B) were significantly younger at assessment, listing and transplant than all the other groups. This was followed by the patients who had a Kasai operation and the transplant at the same center (group E) compared to those who had a Kasai at a liver-expert center different from the transplant center (group D). The average age at listing was significantly different among groups, including 5.9 ± 1.1 months for group A, 7.2 ± 4.4 months for Group C, 12.4 ± 7.3 months for Group D and 7.3 ± 2.7 for Group E ($p = 0.026$). Similarly, the age at transplantation was younger for groups A and E (8.1 ± 1.8 and 10.9 ± 4.2 months, respectively) compared to groups C and D (13.0 ± 7.2 and 16.2 ± 10.1 months, respectively). Group B was only 4 patients and did not permit statistical comparison.

Differences in the PELD scores at either listing or transplantation did not differ significantly in the five groups, although PELD score at the time of the transplant tended to be higher in groups A and E, but the difference was not significant (Table 1). The waiting time on the list was shorter in groups A and E but the difference was not significant among the five groups. Group C patients had a higher rate of whole liver transplantations than all other groups, but this was a function of the different donor characteristics and referral patterns between the two American centers rather than because of any differences in the patients themselves.

Table 1. Europe group: analysis of subgroups as per initial surgery for biliary atresia.

			A	B	C	D	E	p
			NO Surgery	Explorative Laparotomy	KASAI in Non-Liver-Expert Centre	KASAI in Liver-Expert Other Centre	KASAI and Transplant in Same Center	
		N (%)	25 (15%)	4 (2%)	44 (27%)	12 (7%)	80 (49%)	
Polysplenia Syndrome		N (%)	5 (20%)	1 (25%)	6 (14%)	2 (17%)	11 (14%)	0.9126
Age at Kasai (if kasai)	(Days)	Mean ± SD	-	-	62.0 ± 25	69.0 ± 18.7	58.2 ± 26.0	0.4499
At assessment	Age (months)	Mean ± SD	5.8 ± 3.1	6.0 ± 1.4	10.5 ± 7.2	9.0 ± 5.0	5.8 ± 3.9	0.0068
	Weight (Kgs)	Mean ± SD	6.6 ± 1.55	6.8 ± 1.2	7.6 ± 2.3	8.0 ± 2.0	6.34 ± 1.9	0.0058
	PELD score	score	19.4 ± 7.2	24.5 ± 7.55	16.2 ± 8.9	17.5 ± 7.8	11 ± 7.8	0.0009
	Presence of ascites	N (%)	20 (80%)	3 (75%)	27 (61%)	8 (67%)	47 (59%)	0.3943
	Enteral nutrition support	N (%)	7 (28%)	1 (25%)	17 (39%)	2 (17%)	35 (44%)	0.3079
	Parenteral nutrition support	N (%)	-	-	5 (11%)	3 (25%)	12 (15%)	0.1639
At registration on list	Age (months)	Mean ± SD	6.6 ± 3.3	8.25 ± 2.2	12.2 ± 7.5	11.7 ± 5.7	6.5 ± 4.2	0.0012
	Weight (Kgs)	Mean ± SD	6.8 ± 1.6	7.2 ± 0.7	8.1 ± 2.2	8.4 ± 2.8	6.6 ± 1.9	0.0005
	PELD score	score	17.8 ± 6.9	20.7 ± 6.8	15.4 ± 8.2	17.9 ± 8.7	11.5 ± 7.8	0.0005
Delta Peld score 1	assessment to registration on list	delta	1.6 ± 4.4	3.7 ± 2.4	0.8 ± 3.4	0.9 ± 3.2	1.4 ± 3.8	0.5916
While waiting for LT	Worsening ascites	N (%)	20 (80%)	3 (75%)	28 (64%)	10 (83%)	59 (74%)	0.5196
	Albumin infusion(s)	N (%)	15 (60%)	2 (50%)	26 (59%)	10 (83%)	45 (57%)	0.5254
	Blood transfusion(s)	N (%)	4 (15%)	1 (25%)	13 (30%)	7 (58%)	23 (29%)	0.1311
	Enteral nutrition support	N (%)	11 (44%)	1 (25%)	18 (41%)	6 (50%)	30 (38%)	0.8922
	parenteral nutrition support	N (%)	3 (12%)	-	13 (30%)	5 (42%)	16 (20%)	0.1504
	1 Hospital admission < 5 days	N (%)	3 (12%)	1 (25%)	6 (14%)	-	10 (12%)	0.6655
	>1 Hospital admission < 5 days	N (%)	5 (20%)	-	4 (9%)	5 (42%)	8 (10%)	**0.0227**
	1 Hospital admission > 5 days	N (%)	14 (56%)	1 (25%)	19 (43%)	8 (67%)	43 (54%)	0.4318
	>1 Hospital admission > 5 days	N (%)	3 (12%)	-	2 (5%)	-	10 (12%)	0.3952
	Recovery in ICU	N (%)	1 (4%)	-	1 (2%)	4 (33%)	16 (20%)	0.0062
At Liver transplant	Age (months)	Mean ± SD	9.1 ± 6.05	18 ± 21.4	14.6 ± 8.5	13.4 ± 7.1	8.9 ± 6.1	0.0012
	Weight (Kgs)	Mean ± SD	7.5 ± 2.1	8.8 ± 2.9	9.0 ± 2.4	8.9 ± 3.2	7.6 ± 2.1	0.0072
	PELD score	score	21.6 ± 6.5	24.0 ± 12.1	17.7 ± 10.5	18.7 ± 10.0	14.9 ± 9.7	0.0184
Clinical condition at LT	Elective-Home	N (%)	11 (44%)	3 (75%)	29 (66%)	5 (42%)	40 (50%)	0.1300
	Hospital-bound	N (%)	13 (52%)	1 (25%)	15 (34%)	5 (42%)	29 (36%)	
	ICU-bound	N (%)	1 (4%)	-	-	2 (16%)	11 (14%)	
Waiting time	Assessment to LT (Days)	Median (p25–p75)	40 (25–72)	34 (26–695)	77 (45–149)	80 (22–157)	71 (34–121)	0.3530
Delta PELD score 2	Assessment to LT	Mean ± SD	3.8 ± 9.0	3.2 ± 5.25	2.4 ± 5.4	0.7 ± 7.4	3.4 ± 6.4	0.6658
Graft type	Full-size	N (%)	5 (20%)	-	3 (7%)	-	12 (15%)	0.6108
	Split liver graft	N (%)	7 (28%)	1 (25%)	16 (36%)	5 (42%)	31 (39%)	
	Reduced liver	N (%)	-	-	1 (2%)	-	4 (5%)	
	Living donor left lobe	N (%)	13 (52%)	3 (75%)	24 (54%)	7 (58%)	33 (41%)	
post-LT recovery	Respiratory assistance (time—days)	Median (p25–p75)	1 (1–5)	0 (0–2)	1 (0–2)	1 (0–7)	2 (0–6)	0.1415
	Enteral nutrition support need	N (%)	17 (68%)	-	26 (59%)	8 (67%)	71 (89%)	**<0.0001**
	Parenteral nutrition need	N (%)	19 (76%)	2 (50%)	29 (66%)	8 (67%)	65 (81%)	0.2565
	ITU stay (days)	Median (p25–p75)	7 (2–11)	2 (2–2.5)	4.5 (2–15.5)	4.5 (2–20)	6 (3–12)	0.3665

Table 1. Cont.

			A	B	C	D	E	
			NO Surgery	Explorative Laparotomy	KASAI in Non-Liver-Expert Centre	KASAI in Liver-Expert Other Centre	KASAI and Transplant in Same Center	p
	Hospital stay (days)	Median (p25–p75)	27 (22–35)	24.5 (16.5–32.5)	24 (17–34)	30 (20–44.5)	26 (21–35)	0.5731
Outcome	Death while waiting	N (%)	-	-	-	-	-	
	Death after LT	N (%)	-	-	1 (2%)	-	4 (5%)	0.6584
	Alive and well	N (%)	25 (100%)	4 (100%)	43 (98%)	12 (100%)	76 (95%)	
	Current age of survivors (months)	Mean ± SD	47.5 ± 21.3	46.7 ± 5.3	48.4 ± 18.2	50.3 ± 15.7	38.3 ± 17.7	*0.0157*

Italic and bold: significant values of *p*.

Table 2. USA group: analysis of subgroups as per initial surgery for biliary atresia.

			A	B	C	D	E	
			NO Surgery	Explorative Laparotomy	KASAI in Non-Liver-Expert Centre	KASAI in Liver-Expert Other Centre	KASAI and Transplant in Same Center	p
		N	6 (11%)	4 (7%)	18 (33%)	5 (9%)	22 (40%)	
Polysplenia Syndrome		N	1 (17%)	-	2 (11%)	-	6 (27%)	0.4409
Age at Kasai (if kasai)	(Days)	Mean ± SD	-	-	66.8 ± 28.9	53.0 ± 17.3	55.2 ± 27.0	0.157
At assessment	Age (months)	Mean ± SD	5.9 ± 1.4	4.2 ± 0.5	6.5 ± 4.1	12.2 ± 6.9	6.7 ± 2.7	*0.0032*
	Weight (Kgs)	Mean ± SD	7.2 ± 1.0	6.7 ± 0.7	6.1 ± 1.8	8.7 ± 3.7	6.6 ± 1.4	0.0821
	PELD score	score	20.7 ± 7.6	12.8 ± 7.7	12.9 ± 7.7	12.6 ± 14.3	13.5 ± 7.0	0.329
	Presence of ascites	N (%)	4 (67%)	2 (50%)	12 (67%)	3 (60%)	13 (59%)	0.9682
	Enteral nutrition support	N (%)	3 (50%)	-	10 (56%)	2 (40%)	13 (59%)	0.2739
	Parenteral nutrition support	N (%)	2 (33%)	-	6 (33%)	-	2 (9%)	0.1399
At registration on list	Age (months)	Mean ± SD	5.9 ± 1.1	4.9 ± 0.8	7.2 ± 4.4	12.4 ± 7.3	7.3 ± 2.7	*0.0264*
	Weight (Kgs)	Mean ± SD	7.2 ± 1.0	6.9 ± 0.5	6.4 ± 1.8	8.5 ± 3.9	6.6 ± 1.1	0.181
	PELD score	score	20.8 ± 8.5	13.5 ± 7.5	12.9 ± 7.7	14.4 ± 17.2	14.1 ± 7.6	0.459
Delta Peld score 1	assessment to registration on list	delta	0.2 ± 1.3	0.8 +/1 1.5	0.1 ± 0.2	1.8 ± 4.0	0.6 ± 4.3	0.618
While waiting for LT	Worsening ascites	N (%)	5 (83%)	2 (50%)	8 (44%)	2 (40%)	14 (64%)	0.4201
	Albumin infusion(s)	N (%)	5 (83%)	2 (50%)	7 (39%)	2 (40%)	16 (73%)	0.135
	Blood transfusion(s)	N (%)	4 (67%)	2 (50%)	8 (44%)	1 (20%)	12 (55%)	0.5826
	Enteral nutrition support	N (%)	3 (50%)	4 (100%)	5 (28%)	2 (40%)	9 (41%)	0.1255
	parenteral nutrition support	N (%)	4 (67%)	2 (50%)	9 (50%)	-	12 (55%)	0.212
	1 Hospital admission < 5 days	N (%)	1 (17%)	1 (25%)	5 (28%)	3 (60%)	5 (23%)	0.5118
	>1 Hospital admission < 5 days	N (%)	1 (17%)	2 (50%)	4 (22%)	1 (20%)	3 (14%)	0.574
	1 Hospital admission > 5 days	N (%)	5 (83%)	1 (25%)	7 (39%)	1 (20%)	10 (46%)	0.2195
	>1 Hospital admission > 5 days	N (%)	1 (17%)	2 (50%)	5 (28%)	-	8 (36%)	0.4159
	Recovery in ICU	N (%)	4 (67%)	1 (25%)	7 (39%)	-	6 (27%)	0.1787
At Liver transplant	Age (months)	Mean ± SD	8.1 ± 1.8	8.9 ± 0.7	13.0 ± 7.2	16.2 ± 10.1	10.9 ± 4.2	0.0511
	Weight (Kgs)	Mean ± SD	8.9 ± 1.6	8.2 ± 0.8	9.3 ± 2.6	8.5 ± 5.2	7.9 ± 1.7	0.559
	PELD score	score	22.0 ± 10.3	23.3 ± 8.3	12.8 ± 11.7	16.2 ± 16.0	21.5 ± 10.7	0.139
Clinical condition at LT	Elective-Home	N (%)	2 (33%)	2 (50%)	11 (65%)	4 (80%)	9 (41%)	0.4352
	Hospital-bound	N (%)	2 (33%)	1 (25%)	4 (24%)	1 (20%)	11 (50%)	
	ICU-bound	N (%)	2 (33%)	1 (25%)	2 (12%) *	-	2 (9%)	

Table 2. Cont.

			A	B	C	D	E	p
			NO Surgery	Explorative Laparotomy	KASAI in Non-Liver-Expert Centre	KASAI in Liver-Expert Other Centre	KASAI and Transplant in Same Center	
Waiting time	Assessment to LT (Days)	Median (p25–p75)	43 (36.8–62)	135 (103.5–151.5)	112 (74–303)	117 (49–146)	82.5 (52.3–133.3)	0.1688
Delta PELD score 2	Assessment to LT	Mean ± SD	1.6 ± 11.4	10.5 ± 5.5	0.2 ± 11.7	3.6 ± 5.5	8.0 ± 10.8	0.163
Graft type	Full-size	N (%)	2 (33%)	3 (75%)	16 (94%)	3 (60%)	6 (27%)	
	Split liver graft	N (%)	2 (33%)	1 (25%)	-	2 (40%)	11 (50%)	**0.0202**
	Reduced liver	N (%)	-	-	-	-	2 (9%)	
	Living donor left lobe	N (%)	2 (33%)	-	1 (6%)	-	3 (14%)	
post-LT recovery	Respiratory assistance (time - days)	Median (p25–p75)	22.5 (9.3–46.3)	16.5 (10.8–44.3)	17 (5–30)	2 (1–7)	9 (5–20.3)	0.2132
	Enteral nutrition support need	N (%)	6 (100%)	4 (100%)	14 (82%)	3 (60%)	19 (91%)	0.268
	Parenteral nutrition need	N (%)	6 (100%)	3 (75%)	11 (65%)	1 (20%)	13 (59%)	0.0953
	ITU stay (days)	Median (p25–p75)	24.5 (10.5–40)	19.5 (12–46.8)	17 (8–38)	3 (3–8)	10 (6.3–19.8)	0.0802
	Hospital stay (days)	Median (p25–p75)	33 (19–54.5)	27 (24.5–70.5)	28 (19–81)	10 (9–11)	19.5 (11.3–33.3)	0.0621
Outcome	Death while waiting	N (%)	-	-	1 (6%)	-	-	0.8969
	Death after LT	N (%)	-	-	1 (6%)	-	2 (9%)	
	Alive and well	N (%)	6 (100%)	4 (100%)	16 (89%)	5 (100%)	20 (91%)	
	Current age of survivors (months)	Mean ± SD	41.6 ± 9.5	45.6 ± 17.6	37.3 ± 15.9	47.8 ± 21.1	39.8 ± 21.6	0.804

* One other child, not transplanted, was waiting in ICU and having a PELD exception score; he was removed from list because of being too sick, and died. Bold: significant values of *p*.

Table 3. Demographics, data and outcomes of transplanted patients according to type of donor.

			EUROPE				USA			
			ALL	Living Donor LT	Deceased Donor LT	p	ALL	Living Donor LT	Deceased Donor LT	p
N		N (%)	165	80 (48.5%)	85 (51.5%)		54	6 (11.1%)	48 (88.9%)	
Prematurity		N (%)	11 (6.7%)	7 (63.6%)	4 (36.4%)	0.2008	5 (9.3%)	-	5 (10.4%)	0.9339
Co-morbidity	Cardiac	N (%)	9 (5.5%)	6 (42.9%)	3 (23.1%)	0.4810	1 (1.9%)	-	1 (2.1%)	0.3916
	Digestive	N (%)	10 (6.1%)	5 (35.7%)	5 38.5%)		2 (3.7%)	-	2 (4.2%)	
	Other	N (%)	8 (4.8%)	3 (21.4%)	5 (38.5%)		2 (3.7%)	1 (16.7%)	1 (2.1%)	
Polysplenia Syndrome		N (%)	25 (15.2%)	11 (16.5%)	14 (16.5%)	0.6262	8 (14.8%)	-	8 (16.7%)	0.2786
Type of initial surgery for BA	NONE	N (%)	25 (15.2%)	13 (16.2%)	12 (14.2%)	0.5065	6 (11.1%)	2 (33.3%)	4 (8.3%)	0.1587
	Explorative laparotomy	N (%)	4 (2.4%)	3 (3.7%)	1 (1.2%)		4 (7.4%)	-	4 (8.3%)	
	Kasai	N (%)	136 (82.4%)	64 (80.0%)	72 (84.7%)		44 (81.5%)	4 (66.7%)	40 (83.3%)	
Kasai Centre	Non-liver expert	N (%)	44 (26.7%)	24 (37.5%)	20 (27.8%)	0.2611	17 (38.6%)	1 (25.0%)	16 (40.0%)	0.5321
	Liver-expert other	N (%)	12 (7.3%)	7 (10.9%)	5 (6.9%)		5 (11.4%)	-	5 (12.5%)	
	Same as LT centre	N (%)	80 (48.5%)	33 (51.6%)	47 (65.3%)		22 (50.0%)	3 (75.0%)	19 (47.5%)	
Age at Kasai (if kasai)	(months)	Mean ± SD	60.3 ± 25.0	62.2 ± 24.0	58.5 ± 25.7	0.3826	60.0 ± 27.2	50.0 ± 30.3	60.8 ± 27.4	0.4594
At assessment	Age (months)	Median (p25–p75)	6 (4–8)	6 (4–10)	5 (4–7)	0.0508	6.2 (4.1–7.7)	6.3 (6.2–6.5)	5.5 (4.0–7.9)	0.6095
	Weight (Kgs)	Mean ± SD	6.8 ± 2.1	6.59 ± 2.0	7.1 ± 2.0	0.1438	6.7 ± 1.8	6.9 ± 1.2	6.7 ± 1.9	0.8159
	PELD score	Mean ± SD	14.2 ± 8.3	14.7 ± 8.6	13.7 ± 8.0	0.3990	13.9 ± 8.1	18.3 ± 6.7	13.1 ± 8.3	0.1595
	Presence of ascites	N (%)	85 (51.5%)	57 (71.2%)	48 (56.5%)	**0.0486**	34 (63.0%)	5 (83.3%)	29 (60.4%)	0.2731

Table 3. Cont.

				EUROPE				USA			
			ALL	Living Donor LT	Deceased Donor LT	p	ALL	Living Donor LT	Deceased Donor LT	p
N		N (%)	165	80 (48.5%)	85 (51.5%)		54	6 (11.1%)	48 (88.9%)	
	Enteral nutrition support	N (%)	62 (37.6%)	25 (31.2%)	37 (43.5%)	0.1036	28 (51.9%)	3 (50.0%)	25 (52.1%)	0.9232
	Parenteral nutrition support	N (%)	20 (12.1%)	9 (11.2%)	11 (12.9%)	0.7394	10 (18.5)	-	10 (20.8)	0.2155
At registration on list	Age (months)	Median (p25–p75)	7 ± (4–10)	6 (4–8)	8 (4–11)	0.0543	6.4 (5.0–8.0)	6.8 (6.6–7.4)	6.0 (5.0–8.4)	0.448
	Weight (Kgs)	Mean ± SD	7.2 ± 2.1	6.8 ± 2.0	7.5 ± 2.2	0.0283	6.8 ± 1.8	6.9 ± 1.2	6.8 ± 1.8	0.9755
While waiting for LT	Worsening ascites	N (%)	120 (72.7%)	69 (86.2%)	51 (60.0%)	0.0002	30 (55.6%)	6 (100.0%)	24 (50.0%)	**0.0201**
	Enteral nutrition support	N (%)	66 (40%)	36 36.1%)	30 (45.0%)	0.2496	22 (40.7%)	2 (33.3%)	20 (47.7%)	0.6953
	Parenteral nutrition support	N (%)	37 (22.4%)	17 (21.2%)	20 (23.8%)	0.6951	26 (48.1%)	2 (33.3%)	24 (50.0%)	0.4411
	Albumin infusion(s)	N (%)	98 (59.4%)	56 (70.0%)	42 (50.0%)	0.0090	31 (57.4%)	6 (100.0%)	25 (52.1%)	**0.0252**
	Blood transfusion(s)	N (%)	48 (29.1%)	26 (32.5%)	22 (25.9%)	0.3496	26 (48.1%)	3 (50.0%)	23 (47.9%)	0.9233
	1 Hospital admission < 5 days	N (%)	20 (12.1%)	9 (11.2%)	11 (12.9%)	0.7394	15 (27.8%)	1 (16.7%)	14 (29.2%)	*0.5192*
	> 1 Hospital admission < 5 days	N (%)	21 (12.7%)	7 (8.7%)	15 (17.6%)	0.0929	10 (18.5%)	1 (16.7%)	9 (18.8%)	0.9014
	1 Hospital admission > 5 days	N (%)	85 (51.5%)	35 (43.7%)	50 (58.8%)	0.0528	24 (44.4%)	5 (83.3%)	19 (39.6%)	**0.042**
	> 1 Hospital admission > 5 days	N (%)	15 (9.1%)	8 (10.0%)	7 (8.2%)	0.6935	15 (27.8%)	1 (16.7%)	14 (29.2%)	*0.5192*
	Recovery in ICU	N (%)	22 (13.3%)	6 (7.5%)	16 (18.8%)	0.0325	17 (31.5%)	3 (50.0%)	14 (29.2%)	0.3002
At Liver transplant	Age (months)	Median (p25–p75)	8 (6–13)	8 (6–10)	10 (6–18)	0.0294	9.8 (7.6–13)	9.3 (8.3–10.5)	10.0 (7.3–14.3)	0.6297
	Weight (Kgs)	Med ± SD	8.1 ± 2.3	7.4 ± 2.0	8.7 ± 2.5	0.0007	8.5 ± 2.4	8.4 ± 1.7	8.6 ± 2.5	0.8853
	PELD score	Med ± SD	17.2 ± 9.8	18.8 ± 9.8	15.6 ± 9.6	0.0395	18.5 ± 11.8	18.2 ± 12.7	18.5 ± 11.8	0.9421
Clinical condition at LT	Elective-Home	N (%)	88 (53.3%)	47 (58.7%)	41 (48.2%)	0.1990	28 (51.9%)	1 (16.7%)	27 (56.2%)	0.1666
	Hospital-bound	N (%)	63 (38.2%)	29 (36.2%)	34 (40.0%)		19 (35.2%)	4 (66.7%)	15 (31.2%)	
	ICU-bound	N (%)	14 (8.5%)	4 (5.0%)	10 (11.8%)		7 (13.0%)	1 (16.7%)	6 (12.5%)	
Waiting time	Assessment to LT (Days)	Median (p25–p75)	63 (33–124)	55 (33–98)	82 (32–180)	0.0717	90 (49.3–148.8)	95.5 (56.3–128.8)	90.5 (49.8–152.3)	0.7726
Delta PELD score	Assessment to LT	Med ± SD	3.0 ± 6.6	4.0 ± 6.0	2.0 ± 7.0	0.0470	4.6 ± 10.9	-0.2 ± 15.3	5.2 ± 10.3	0.2575
Graft type	Full-size	N (%)	20 (12.1%)	-	20 (23.5%)		30 (55.6%)	-	30 (62.5%)	
	Split liver graft	N (%)	60 (36.4%)	-	60 (70.6%)		16 (29.6%)	-	16 (33.3%)	
	Reduced liver	N (%)	5 (3%)	-	5 (5.9%)		2 (3.7%)	-	2 (4.2%)	
	Living donor left lobe	N (%)	80 (48.5%)	80 (100%)	-		6 (11.1%)	6 (100.0%)	-	
LT recovery	Respiratory assistance (time - days)	Median (p25–p75)	1.0 (0–5)	0.0 (0.0–3.5)	3.0 (1.0–6.0)	<0.0001	10 (5–24.5)	9 (6.5–16.8)	10.5 (4.3–25.8)	0.7726
	Enteral nutrition support need	N (%)	122 (74%)	49 (61.2%)	73 (85.9%)	0.0003	46 (86.8%)	6 (100.0%)	40 (85.1%)	0.3103
	Parenteral nutrition need	N (%)	123 (74%)	61 (76.2%)	62 (72.9%)	0.6258	34 (63.0%)	5 (83.3%)	29 (60.4%)	0.2731
	ITU stay (days)	Median (p25–p75)	6 (2–12)	3.5 (2–8.5)	8.0 (4–15)	0.0002	12 (6.3–27.0)	10.5 (7.5–18)	12.5 (7.5–18.0)	0.9341
	Hospital stay (days)	Median (p25–p75)	26 (21–35)	24.5 (17–31.5)	27 (21–38)	0.0312	23 (11.3–38)	28.5 (20.5–33.5)	22.0 (11.0–39.8)	0.6794
	Death after LT	N (%)	5 (3%)	2 (2.5%)	3 (3.5%)	0.6999	3 (5.6%)	-	3 (6.3%)	0.529
	Alive and well	N (%)	160 (97.0%)	78 (97.5%)	82 (96.5%)		51 (94.4%)	6 (100.0%)	45 (93.8%)	

Italic and bold: significant values of p.

3.3. Center's Waiting List Dynamics in Relation to Regional Allocation Rules

Overall, per the allocation system, the lowest use of the exception status was observed in the Eurotransplant area (centers C5 and C6—Figures 1 and 2). At the center level, there was a straight correlation—proportionally to the total activity in a given center (i.e., between a high proportion of LD-LT and a very low proportion of priority requests—in that center), or the opposite, between a high proportion of whole liver grafts and a very high number of priority requests (Figure 3).

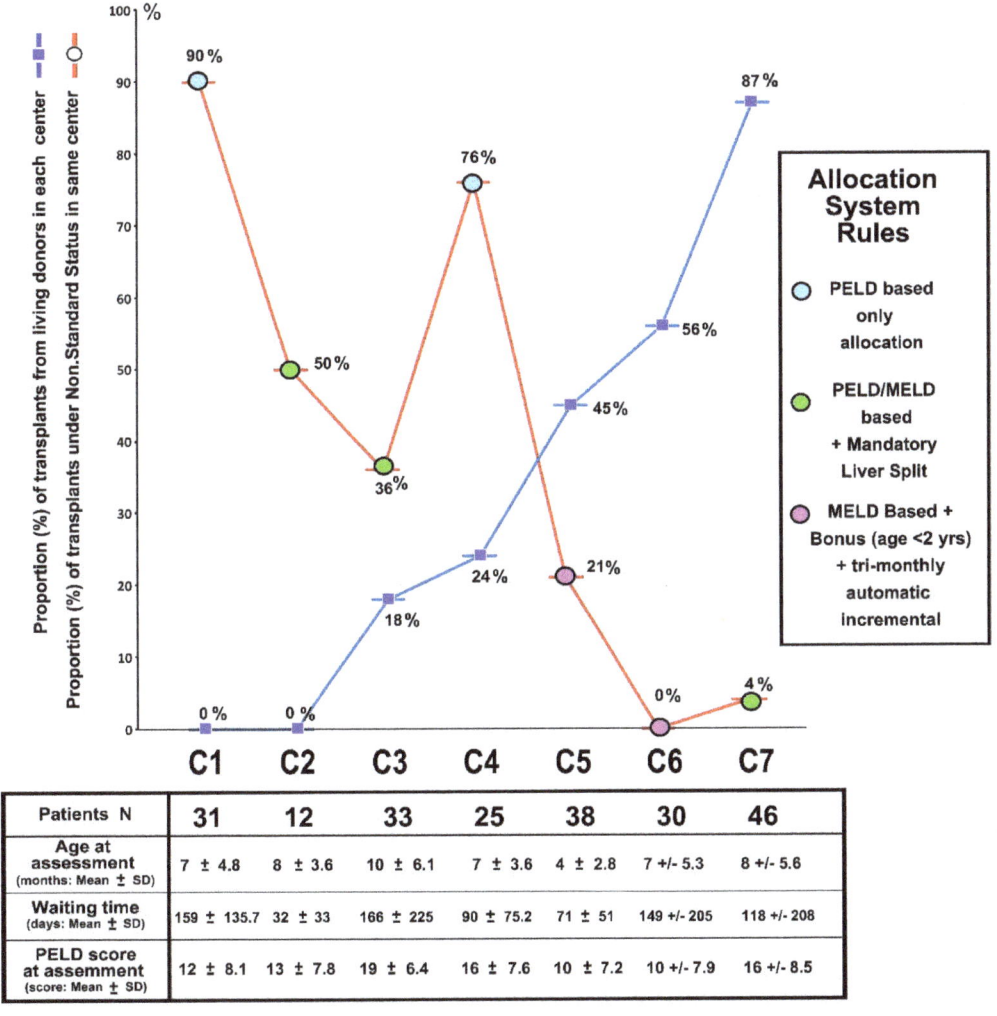

Figure 1. Waiting list dynamics in 7 centers participating in organ sharing/allocation system and use of PELD exception or priority status for timely transplants. Specific waiting list data from 7 separate centers (C1 to C7). 1—Age, weight and PELD score at the time of patient assessment for liver transplantation (bottom table: values given as mean ± SD) (all mean values were rounded to the nearest integer), and 2—proportion (%) of transplants performed in each center using a living related donation (blue line and dark blue spot ■) and a request for a PELD exception or similar priority score (red line) (values in % of all transplants in each center). Center organ sharing/allocation system type (see legend on the right side) are referred to as per the color spot in the figure (blue, green and purple).

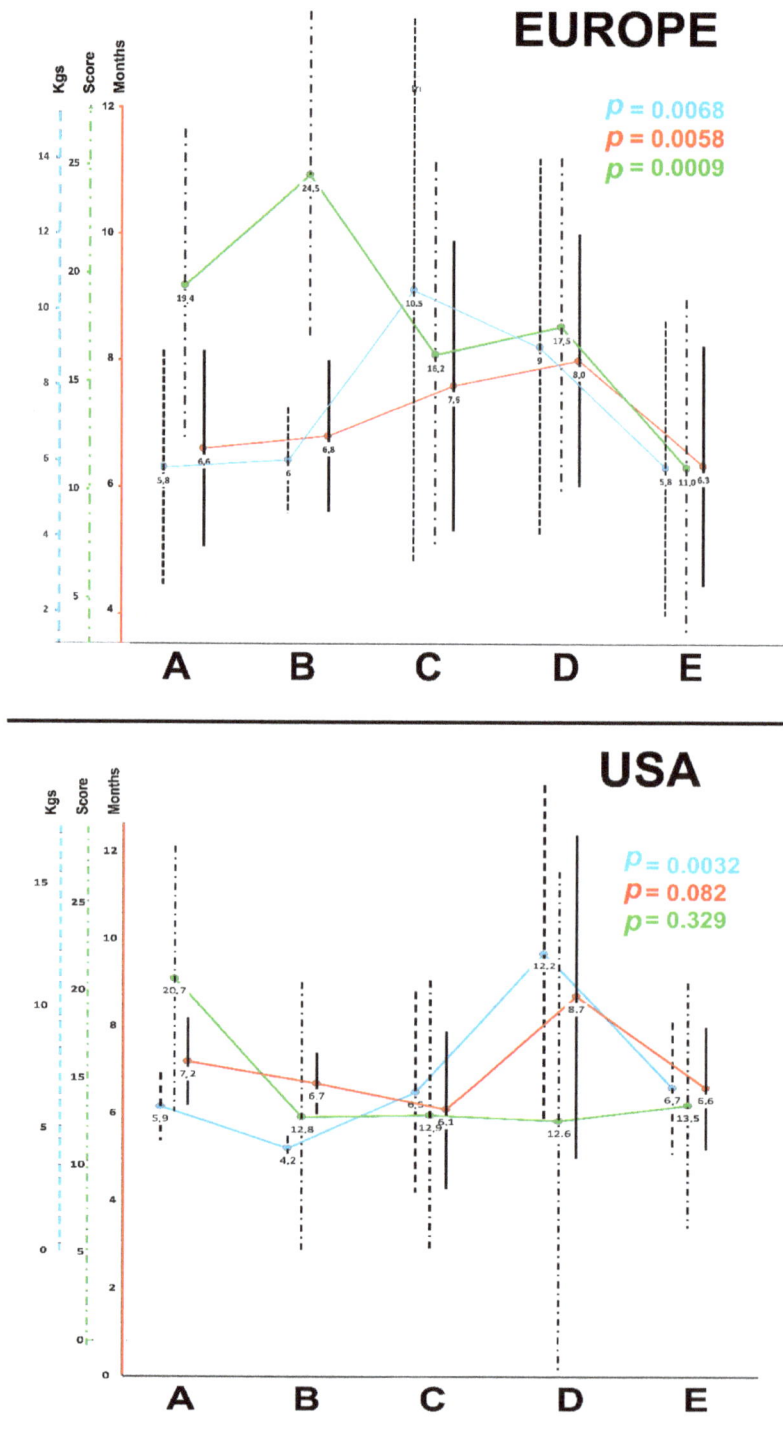

Figure 2. Patient characteristics at assessment for liver transplantation, as per initial management of biliary atresia. Age, weight and PELD score at assessment for liver transplantation (the dots represent

the median value, with the black vertical bars representing SD): distribution per subgroups according to initial management of biliary atresia (subgroups as follow: A—no intervention and primary transplant, B—explorative laparotomy only, C—Kasai portoenterostomy in a non-specialist center, D—Kasai portoenterostomy in a specialist, but not transplant, center, and E—Kasai portoenterostomy in the transplant center).

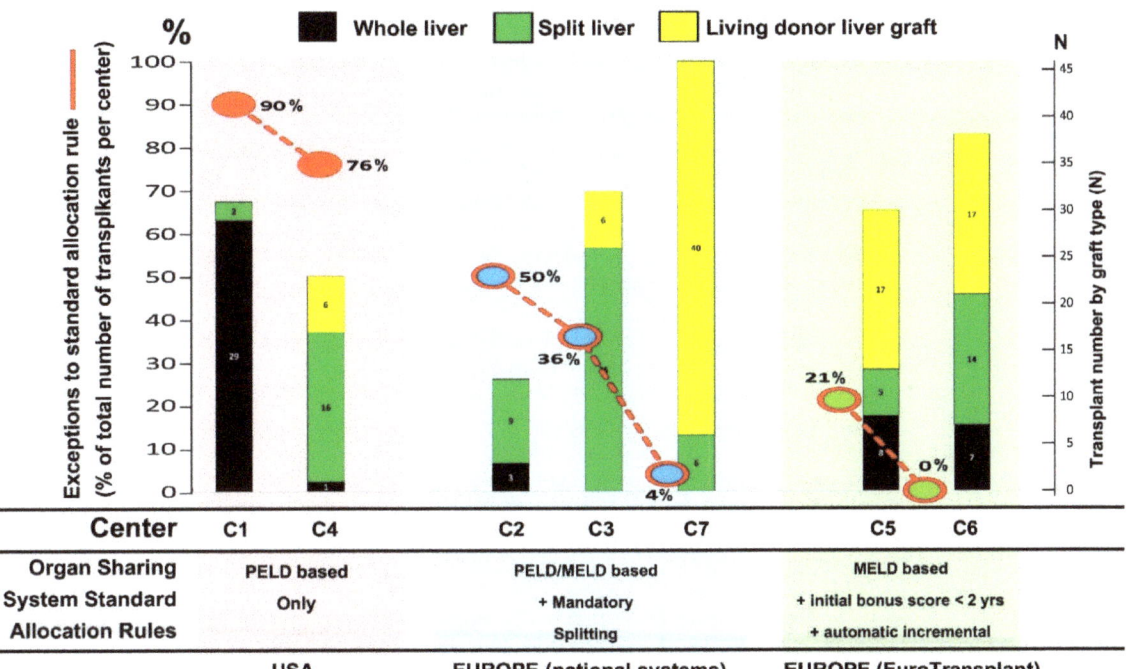

Figure 3. Use of PELD exception or priority status for biliary atresia patients registered on the waiting list before age 3 years, according to the type of allocation rules and types of organ used. Transplant data from 7 centers. 1—Proportion of transplants performed under PELD exception or priority status (red line) (values in % in each transplant), and 2—number of transplants and graft types used: whole livers (black), split livers (green) and living donor grafts (yellow). Centers (defined as in Figure 1) are aligned left to right according to their affiliation to one of 3 allocation systems that differ about allocation rules for small children (see legend on the bottom).

In seven centers, LT activity relied on a large national or multi-national organ exchange and allocation system that was PELD/MELD-based; although similar, rules for allocation were slightly different and three major systems were identified. All three systems had in common: (1) an emergency status for critical cases (fulminant hepatitis, urgent re-LT), (2) few priority status for special indications where PELD scores do not well-represent the condition and (3) the possibility of submitting special requests for priority status based on the critical condition of the patients as a PELD exception or similar. Differences were, however, observed between the three systems in that one also had a mandatory split approach in standard donors, and one used a variant PELD (Pediatric MELD—Eurotransplant area (https://www.eurotransplant.org, accessed on 15 March 2022)), and for children registered at age < 2 years, a bonus score at the start with an automatic score increment, every 90 days (Figures 1 and 3).

Requesting some sort of priority for graft allocation because of severe clinical deterioration or complications was possible in all allocation systems—though the type of priority varied from system to system, according to the rules of the respective regional allocation system (PELD exception, bonus score points, or emergency status). In Europe, a priority status had been obtained for 29 cases (27.6%), while in the USA, a PELD exception score or an emergency status had been obtained for 47/56 cases (84%).

4. Discussion

A recent survey of pediatric LT in Europe over the last five decades [1] has evidenced that the outcome has steadily improved overall with time, with current results being better than ever for children in need of a LT, although the progress in the last decade is modest compared to the previous one. The former study, however, also confirmed that the youngest patients (<1 year of age at LT) continued having worse outcomes compared to the older ones, which is also suggested in previous studies [3,5,7–11,14–17].

Moreover, aside from the lower survival after LT, the literature provides strong evidence that those aged less than 1 year when waiting for a LT have a lower chance of benefiting from LT in time, and waiting list mortality peaks up to around 10% in this youngest group [5,6,8,11,14–17]. Prolonged waiting time is also associated with clinical deterioration, hospital boundness and/or LT under urgent conditions—all conditions associated with increased (although preventable) peri-transplant morbidity and mortality.

4.1. Advanced Liver Disease at Registration on Waiting List

The current study brings deeper insights into the morbidity related to the waiting period, in particular when the study evidenced that 14.1% of all patients had primary transplants (31/220 cases), and that mean age at Kasai operation was almost identical (American and European patients: 60.3 ± 25.0 days and 60.0 ± 27.2 days, respectively) (Tables 1 and 2). This suggests that enough time was available to manage BA patients who had no chance with Kasai, or no Kasai, and planning the best timing for LT. The data demonstrate that children in both Europe and the United States were assessed for LT with already a relatively advanced stage of their liver disease, with mean (±SD) calculated PELD, at assessment, being 14.2 (±8.3) in Europe and 13.9 (±8.1) in the United States.

The proportion of children with complications at the time of their assessment was also high, including (A) the presence of clinical ascites (a marker of serious condition and poor prognosis for those awaiting LT [18,19]) in 105/165 children (63.6%) in Europe, and 31/55 cases (56%) in the United States, and (B) the need for nutrition enteral support (62/165 (37.6%) in Europe, 28/55 (51%) in the United States) or needing PN (20/165 (12%) in Europe, 10/55 (18%) in the United States). In the American patients, unlike the European ones, there were fewer differences between the live donor and deceased donor groups, except for worse ascites, greater need for albumin infusions and more hospital admissions in the live donor group (Table 3).

4.2. Variability of Timing in Registration on Waiting List

As the progression of biliary cirrhosis (hence of hepatic dysfunction and associated portal hypertension) is predictable when bile flow is not established, one would expect a timely referral to an LTC. The large variation in the timing for assessment (based on age at assessment in the study) is a surprising observation, with the following findings:

(1) In Europe, children who had no surgery at diagnosis were not brought to assessment at an earlier age compared to other groups. This might, however, be due to the fact that no surgery had been proposed because their diagnosis was late in life—too late for proposing a Kasai operation. In contrast, in the USA cohort, the no surgery group were listed significantly earlier than infants in the other groups. One possible reason for the delay in the surgery group is the practice of waiting three months or more to determine if bile drainage would occur in the Kasai group.

(2) There was a large variation in terms of timing of the referral for LT assessment for those who had undergone Kasai, depending on where the Kasai had been performed, particularly in the European arm of the study. Children in the European centers were younger ($p = 0.00012$) and in a better condition (as per PELD score, $p = 0.0009$) when

they had been followed from diagnosis to LT within the same center (Table 1, Figure 1). In the American series, although a similar observation was found for age at assessment ($p = 0.0032$), weight and PELD score at assessment were similar in all subgroups (Table 2, Figure 1).

(3) In the 4 European patients who only had an explorative laparotomy at BA diagnosis, the mean PELD at assessment was 24.5 (SD: ±7.55), which suggests that they were referred very late, although they had no chance of cure without a LT. In contrast, the 4 US patients who only had exploratory laparotomy had a mean PELD score at assessment of 13.5 ± 7.5. These patients were evaluated for LT the earliest of all US patients (4.9 ± 0.8 months), although the numbers were too small for meaningful statistical comparisons. Interestingly, of all patients who had no Kasai (39/220, 17.7% of the cohort), all eventually did get a LT and all survived, while the actual survival of those who had the Kasai operation was 172/181 (95%) (97% and 94% actual survival after LD-LT or deceased donor LT, respectively).

(4) Overall, 31 children had primary transplants. The 2 groups (25 in Europe and 6 in USA—15% and 11% of LT, respectively) were very similar for age, weight and PELD score at assessment, and this shows that this category of patients is probably the worst as they are young, have a low weight and have the highest PELD scores in the whole series.

Overall, the trend for a variability of timing for referral was less striking in the USA cohort, suggesting that timely referral for transplant in the US is taking place from centers that do not run their own transplant programs. Nevertheless, findings in this cohort suggest that from a healthcare delivery point of view, the current situation is far from optimal, generally speaking, and is a problem to address in the future. Kohaut et al. [20], Karakoyun et al. [21] and Lampela et al. [22] had made similar observations in single-center series, showing that, in their experience, children referred for LT after Kasai performed in a different center had a poorer clinical condition and/or higher peri-transplant morbidity.

4.3. Burden of Care While Waiting for LT

Independently of patient death secondary to prolonged waiting time and inevitable clinical deterioration, there is a very high price to pay for those who ultimately succeed to LT and survive. This can be seen in the many aspects of child health, such as malnutrition, worsening growth retardation, recurrent infections and need for hospitalization, secondary multi-resistant bacterial colonization, neurocognitive developmental or psychomotor delay, hepatic osteodystrophy and fractures and significant psychosocial stress on both the child and the family [23–27].

More worrisome is the fact that not all these problems are easily or rapidly reversed after LT (i.e., bone demineralization and scoliosis, neurocognitive definitive retardation and social or scholarly integration). This data strongly suggests that reducing the waiting time and the associated clinical deterioration is a vital objective [28–30]. In this series, these aspects were not analyzed specifically, and only approached by looking at the need for medical support while waiting (management of worsening ascites, need for albumin or blood transfusion, hospitalizations and worsening of PELD; Tables 1 and 2); as an example, though PN support was necessary—at referral—in 12% and 18% of cases, respectively, in European and American cohorts, these ratios increased during waiting time, to 22% and 49% of patients, respectively. Although there was also no cost assessment, another limitation of this study, it is obvious that this all translated into higher costs for the pre-transplant care, and very likely was associated with a higher cost of LT itself, as a worse condition at the time of LT is associated with longer ICU and hospital stays, respiratory assistance and need for nutritional support after LT. It is a limitation of this study, and a call for further dedicated studies [16].

Overall, this analysis and the results are a plea for earlier referral to a TC, but also a call to TC for shortening the waiting time by all means. In fact, providing all options for LT and developing more aggressive strategies for allocating liver grafts to these patients, such as splitting more livers and expanding the use of living donation, which are options that can be and should be developed further and are precisely meeting the needs for the youngest children who are most in need [31–37]. In the European series, the use of living donation has been important (48.5% of the series) and likely contributed to both shortening the waiting time and the excellent general outcome (97.5% actual survival over 5 years). Although the children who were proposed for living donor LT (LD-LT) were significantly younger, smaller and in a worse (PELD) condition at transplantation, they had shorter respiratory assistance and ICU/hospital stays. It confirms the important role that LD-LT can play in improving the care planning of BA children in the future, particularly in countries where the availability of deceased donor organs is limited, and LT cannot be offered in a timely manner. In countries where only a single donor option is available—LD or deceased donation—mortality on the waiting list remains high for the infants [3,5,7,8,14,38].

4.4. Steadily Increasing Prioritization Requests

In order to meet the needs of children who often compete with adults for organs in an environment of deceased donor shortage, one solution has been to request—and obtain—priority on the waiting list by either giving pediatric priority to organs from pediatric donors (under age 18 years), and/or by obtaining priority by bonus points or exceptions to the PELD score. The latter strategy was used in both Europe and in the USA—mostly for small infants waiting for livers whose PELD score may not accurately reflect the risk of mortality. In this study cohort, exception points were used on a surprisingly large scale, being 35% of LT, overall. Although it well-reflects that listed BA infants often rapidly deteriorate, it also suggests that graft allocation is still not adequate to this group of fragile and urgent patients.

Two very recent analyses (by SPLIT and OPTN) [39,40] confirmed that prioritization has become a necessary strategy to get infants transplanted in time. Both showed that more than half of pediatric LT in the USA are currently performed in children who received an exception score. Though the prioritization system was associated with excellent outcomes, the OPTN report showed that the proportion of PELD exception LT has steadily increased during the last decade. This strategy rapidly expanded—from 40% exception LT in 2008, to 79% in 2019—although it is not a real solution to the problem of organ shortage. Worse still, the priority allocated to one patient leaves another case a step backwards on the waiting list. This system functions as a vicious loop and the number of requests will eventually increase to become the new standard if true solutions are not implemented.

The comparison of waiting list dynamics in different allocation systems (Figures 1 and 3) has evidenced that implementing a bonus score at registration for the youngest patients (<2 years of age at registration) and adding an automatic score increment every three months (Eurotransplant system) was possibly the most efficient timely allocation with the lowest number of requests for priority status. Although this strategy is an efficient redistribution of organs based on the "sickest first" concept, and also helps to increase the number of available grafts (most of the allocated donor livers would be split in this age group), it is not helpful in solving the donor shortage at the end. Surprisingly, this analysis did not evidence a major contribution of the "mandatory split" strategy, as of the three centers who benefited from that rule, two had a high proportion of priority requests (50% and 36% in centers C2 and C3, respectively—Figures 1 and 3). Lastly and more interestingly, there was a good inverse correlation between a low number of special requests and a higher use of LD in a given center—with the latter observation being even clearer when comparing centers within a same allocation system (Figure 3). Altogether, this evidence calls for consideration of implementing specific allocation rules for small children at the level of the organ sharing system, and considering implementation of LD on a larger scale at the level of transplantation centers.

Many pediatric programs, both in Europe and in the USA, are still reluctant to offer split LTs on a large scale, and even more so to offer LD-LT. This situation is probably more extreme in the USA, where in 2019, whole livers were still used in around 2/3 of pediatric LT, while split and LD represented only 20.3% and 14.3%, respectively [40,41]. In Europe, whole livers, LD and splits represented approximatively one third each for pediatric LT in the last decade [1]. As split and LD are now both associated with excellent results [11,34,42–46], offering all the possible surgical solutions available can help to ensure timely access of children to organs and prevent the deterioration of their clinical condition or even death while on the waiting list [12]. It has been shown that the children with the highest mortality on the waiting list are those under the age of 1 year.

4.5. Paradigm Shift in Caring for BA and Roadmap for Future Management

In December 2021, the EASL–Lancet Liver Commission (an expert panel of health professionals from various medical disciplines, nurses and patients) called for a paradigm shift in the liver disease response in Europe (Published Online on 2 December 2021 https://doi.org/10.1016/S0140-6736(21)01701-3, accessed on 15 March 2022). After a three-year analysis, they concluded that the future health of Europeans relies on "a necessary shift in the way in which liver disease needs to be prevented, diagnosed and treated". Their analysis confirmed that centralization of rare disease cases in multidisciplinary specialist service centers was associated with higher caseloads and, in turn, with enhanced quality of care to patients with rare diseases, such as those with primary sclerosing cholangitis and biliary atresia. The EASL–Lancet Liver Commission commented that "Early diagnosis and cost-saving therapies can be achieved by establishing effective case-finding procedures, standardized treatment protocols, and centralization of patients to high-volume pediatric liver units".

In line with optimization of BA care, some have opted for care-centralization as the United Kingdom did in the mid-nineties. Three pediatric centers were designated for delivering a national comprehensive service for diagnosis, management and surgery of BA, including transplant services. The centralization of services and the subsequent effect on outcome was followed with attention and reported by Davenport et al. in 2004 [2], and further in 2011 [47]. Davenport et al. concluded that *"National outcome measures in BA appear better than those from previously published series from comparable countries and may be attributed to centralization of surgical and medical resources"*. In 2008, Stringer also insisted on the fact that, independently of the service type, the improvement of the general outcome is mostly dependent on timely access to transplantation [48]. More recently, centralization of BA management in Finland led to a major change and a significant increase of overall survival—from 64% to 92% [22]. Lastly, in a recent review of BA registries and outcomes, Verkade et al. [49] mentioned that the United Kingdom and Switzerland (both centralized services) had the best overall patient survival (89% and 90% at 5 years, respectively) [38,47].

Centralization of BA care is more controversial in the United States and Canada. This is perhaps in part due to the large sizes of the respective countries in contrast to European nations, but also due to the nature of pediatric surgery in America where sub-specialization among pediatric surgeons is not embraced except in very few centers. In both European and American areas, the children in Group D (who had their Kasai at one transplant center but then ultimately were transplanted at another center) were the group who were evaluated, listed and transplanted at the latest time point. Although there was no significant difference in the American series (because of the small number of patients in group D (5/55 cases)), there were significant differences in Europe for the PELD score (both at assessment and at LT), for the need for short hospitalization, or for recovery in the ICU during the waiting time. This suggests that LTs in children should be concentrated in liver-specialized pediatric units who can seamlessly take care of an infant from diagnosis of BA to the performance of LT.

As an alternative to centralization, improving integration and collaboration between non-LTC and LTC could be a solution and optimization of the current situation. It would imply a set of innovative strategies or optimizations. Focusing on substantially earlier recognition of Kasai failure, earlier contacts to the LTC for sharing information and optimizing timing for referral, sharing post-Kasai and LT protocols may improve delayed adequate healthcare delivery and lead to earlier referral and listing. These proposals have already been made by various authors but have not been implemented: they could be the cornerstone of a roadmap for improving the management of BA children in the future [50–56]. Additionally, as the data evidence that children who did not undergo the Kasai were referred and transplanted earlier in both European and American cohorts, part of the solution could be to define parameters (other than presentation at age > 120 days or significant portal hypertension) that allow predicting success, or not, with the Kasai operation. Schneider et al., for example, suggested that failure to normalize serum bilirubin within three months after Kasai should elicit prompt evaluation for LT as extended native liver survival is exceptional among these patients [50]. Moreover, though a "Kasai success predicting score" remains far from reality, other groups support more research in that direction as part of BA management—a strategy that would allow early primary transplantation [47,54,57–61].

4.6. More than Ever, Room for Technical Solutions

The zero mortality in Europe during the waiting time is remarkable and may reflect the larger use of LD and split liver grafts in Europe (48.5%). Pre-transplant mortality in America is also low, possibly more a reflection of the greater access to pediatric organs (54% of LT were with full-size livers in the American cohort, versus 12% of cases in Europe)— even though the latter access is not present in all geographic American areas [48]. Though the very low waiting list mortality in this cohort could suggest that allocation systems are efficient and sufficient, the frequent need for an exception status (especially in America) and the high demand for medical support before LT evidence that access to LT can and must be improved worldwide. The best approach for an expert pediatric LTC is to combine offering all possible transplant modalities, i.e., implementing split as a standard procedure in every optimal multi-organ donor and considering a living donor program [11,12,34,43–46,62–64]. Since deceased donor organs are a limited resource, and because not all recipients can benefit from a LD for their LT, the combination of both approaches is in fact synergistic and strategic—the most highly probable manner for a single LTC to meet the needs of all their patients in a timely fashion [1,6,11,21,31,35,42,47].

Major differences between the European and the American cohorts are the use of living donors and split LTs. The European study reports an almost 50–50 division in the use of living and deceased donor transplants. In the deceased donor group, 70% of grafts are split LTs, and only 20 of 165 transplants are whole livers. In contrast, the American group had only 11% (6/54) utilization of live donors and only 16/54 (30%) of the rest were split livers. A surprising 30 of 54 LTs utilized whole organs. This difference in utilization of graft types and donor types is more a function of the disparity between the two American centers than it is between Europe and America; while not analyzed here, the vast majority of the whole LTs came from one center, and the majority of the live donors and split LTs from the other center [46,64,65]. This highlights not only different practices between Europe and North America, but between regions in the United States. European centers also differed, as two main allocation rule types were identified; interestingly, it was associated with differences in terms of transplant practice and the need for requesting exceptional status (Figure 3). This deserves further studies.

4.7. Study Limits and Strengths

The observations and results in this study are subject to some limitations. First, the study was retrospective. Due to its observational-only character, it was not adjusted for other elements that may have played a role in a timely referral of patients to the transplant center (i.e., socio-familial issues, intercurrent infections), nor in the timing of LT (i.e., local policies for LD, graft allocation rules). Second, the study was a joint venture between centers who were members of the BARD association and partners in the European reference network on pediatric hepatological diseases (The study is part of a European reference network for the pediatric hepatological diseases (ERN RARE-LIVER) initiative, and was promoted by the BARD association (www.bard-online.com, accessed on 15 March 2022). All European center authors are partners of the ERN RARE-LIVER). Due to their special interest in managing BA children, and their expertise, the results may be not representative of those of the main transplant network.

Despite the limitations, the analysis also has several strengths. Firstly, despite important differences between Europe and the USA, in terms of both organization of the health system and allocation of liver grafts to children, very similar findings were evidenced. Secondly, the study was limited to only the last five years of managing BA children, thus reflecting the current medical practice very well, and the cohort was large (220 BA patients) enough to eventually represent the management of BA children in both Europe and the USA.

5. Conclusions

Developing improved healthcare solutions not only imposes an obligation for scrupulous and frequent analysis of clinical practice and standards, but also relies on auditing clinical outcomes—a systemic reflective practice. However, if this reflection does not result in bringing new skills and improving the knowledge of the practitioners, nor in convincing health providers and healthcare administrators to implement changes that will result in new practices, it is unlikely that patients will benefit and eventually get better care.

In managing BA—a disease that was associated with close to a 100% death rate until five decades ago—both the Kasai portoenterostomy and LT have been instrumental in allowing a continuously growing number of children to survive. As LT currently results in BA patient survival exceeding 95% in many expert LT centers, the paradigm for BA management optimization and survival has now shifted overall to the pre-LT management [6].

Evidence has now accumulated that demonstrates that BA management can only be improved by either the centralization of care (as already performed or proposed for some other rare conditions in a few countries [66–69]), or the creation of networks dedicated to the timely referral to a pediatric transplant center of excellence. As a new way of thinking and because a large proportion of BA will eventually come to LT, post-Kasai care should be aimed at identifying children in need of LT. Standard Kasai follow-up should be a time not only for pediatric hepatologists to monitor the progress of the baby, but also for involving pediatric transplant surgeons more closely than in the past.

Pre-emptive LT assessment, early listing and timely transplant are likely the next necessary steps to further improve the general outcome. In a non-centralized system as seen in the USA, cooperation between expert centers and other tertiary hospitals is also essential to deliver the strategies of caring for BA children who are potential candidates for LT, and ensuring the necessary medical and surgical support to offer a timely transplant.

Lastly, this series suggests that both mandatory liver splitting policy and LD may play an important role in the immediate future to offer LT in a timely manner to all BA candidates in need, and in particular for the younger ones.

Author Contributions: J.d.V.d.G.: concept generation and research design, principal investigator and corresponding author, data analysis and interpretation, writing, editing, reviewing and finalizing the manuscript. R.S. and S.H.: co-investigators for data gathering in the USA and statistical analysis, co-writing and reviewing of the manuscript. All authors, each for his own center: data acquisition and analysis. All authors: participation in reviewing and revising the manuscript, and acceptance of the final draft. F.T.: data analysis, statistical analysis, review of the manuscript. All European center authors are partners in the European reference network on pediatric hepatological diseases (ERN RARE-LIVER) and members of the BARD association (www.bard-online.com, accessed on 15 March 2022). All authors have read and agreed to the published version of the manuscript.

Funding: This research received no external funding.

Institutional Review Board Statement: The ethical committee of the principal investigator's center approved the study during a meeting held on 24 March 2021, under the Study Code number IRRB/03/21. Local institutional review boards and ethical committees were involved as well where appropriate and as per local rules.

Informed Consent Statement: The study concept was approved by the Ethical committee of the center of the principal investigator (first author) (ref: IRRB/03/21). Approval from Institutional Review/Scientific Board and/or Ethical committee, was obtained locally by each participating center; procedures for information and consent followed the rules established in each center by local Institutional Review/Scientific Boards for studies involving humans.

Acknowledgments: The authors acknowledge Claus Petersen for his contribution by promoting this BARD (Biliary Atresia and Related Diseases group) initiative, within the activity of the ERN RARE-LIVER, and for this support in quality of Guest Editor.

Conflicts of Interest: Harpavat Sanjiv is on the Data Safety Monitoring Board for a BA therapeutic study, which is organized by Syneos Health. No other author declares any conflict of interest concerning this manuscript.

Abbreviations

ERN RARE-LIVER	European reference network for pediatric hepatological diseases.
BARD	Biliary Atresia and Related Diseases (multi-purpose online platform for study of biliary atresia and related diseases: http://www.bard-online.com, accessed on 10 March 2022)
BA	Biliary atresia
LT	Liver transplantation
PELD	Pediatric End-Stage Liver score
ICU	Intensive care unit
LD	Living donor
LTC	Pediatric liver transplant center
PN	Parenteral nutrition

References

1. De Ville de Goyet, J.; Baumann, U.; Karam, V.; Adam, R.; Nadalin, S.; Heaton, N.; Reding, R.; Branchereau, S.; Mirza, D.; Klempnauer, J.L.; et al. European Liver Transplant Registry: Donor and transplant surgery aspects of 16,641 liver transplantations in children. *Hepatology* **2022**, *75*, 634–645. [CrossRef] [PubMed]
2. Davenport, M.; Goyet, J.D.V.D.; Stringer, M.; Mieli-Vergani, G.; Kelly, D.; McClean, P.; Spitz, L. Seamless management of biliary atresia in England and Wales (1999–2002). *Lancet* **2004**, *363*, 1354–1357. [CrossRef]
3. Kasahara, M.; Umeshita, K.; Sakamoto, S.; Fukuda, A.; Furukawa, H.; Uemoto, S. Liver transplantation for biliary atresia: A systematic review. *Pediatr. Surg. Int.* **2017**, *33*, 1289–1295. [CrossRef]
4. Chardot, C.; Buet, C.; Serinet, M.-O.; Golmard, J.-L.; Lachaux, A.; Roquelaure, B.; Gottrand, F.; Broué, P.; Dabadie, A.; Gauthier, F.; et al. Improving outcomes of biliary atresia: French national series 1986–2009. *J. Hepatol.* **2013**, *58*, 1209–1217. [CrossRef] [PubMed]
5. Malenicka, S.; Ericzon, B.; Jørgensen, M.H.; Isoniemi, H.; Karlsen, T.H.; Krantz, M.; Naeser, V.; Olausson, M.; Rasmussen, A.; Rönnholm, K.; et al. Impaired intention-to-treat survival after listing for liver transplantation in children with biliary atresia compared to other chronic liver diseases: 20 years' experience from the Nordic countries. *Pediatr. Transplant.* **2017**, *21*, e12851. [CrossRef] [PubMed]
6. De Ville de Goyet, J.; Grimaldi, C.; Tuzzolino, F.; Di Francesco, F. A paradigm shift in the intention-to-transplant children with biliary atresia: Outcomes of 101 cases and a review of the literature. *Pediatr. Transplant.* **2019**, *23*, e13569. [CrossRef] [PubMed]
7. Van der Doef, H.P.J.; van Rheenen, P.F.; van Rosmalen, M.; Rogiers, X.; Verkade, H.J. Wait-list mortality of young patients with Biliary atresia: Competing risk analysis of a eurotransplant regis-try-based cohort. *Liver Transplant.* **2018**, *24*, 810–819. [CrossRef]
8. Leung, D.H.; Narang, A.; Minard, C.G.; Hiremath, G.; Goss, J.A.; Shepherd, R. A 10-Year united network for organ sharing review of mortality and risk factors in young children awaiting liver transplantation. *Liver Transplant.* **2016**, *22*, 1584–1592. [CrossRef]
9. De Vries, W.; de Langen, Z.J.; Aronson, D.C.; Hulscher, J.B.; Peeters, P.M.; Jansen-Kalma, P.; Verkade, H.J. Mortality of biliary atresia in children not undergoing liver transplantation in The Netherlands. *Pediatr. Transplant.* **2011**, *15*, 176–183. [CrossRef]
10. D'Souza, R.; Grammatikopoulos, T.; Pradhan, A.; Sutton, H.; Douiri, A.; Davenport, M.; Verma, A.; Dhawan, A. Acute-on-chronic liver failure in children with biliary atresia awaiting liver transplantation. *Pediatr. Transplant.* **2019**, *23*, e13339. [CrossRef]
11. Tessier, M.E.M.; Harpavat, S.; Shepherd, R.W.; Hiremath, G.S.; Brandt, M.L.; Fisher, A.; Goss, J.A. Beyond the Pediatric end-stage liver disease system: Solutions for infants with biliary atresia requiring liver transplant. *World J. Gastroenterol.* **2014**, *20*, 11062–11068. [CrossRef] [PubMed]
12. Hsu, E.; Mazariegos, G.V. Global lessons in graft type and pediatric liver allocation: A path toward improving outcomes and eliminating wait-list mortality. *Liver Transplant.* **2017**, *23*, 86–95. [CrossRef] [PubMed]
13. Fischler, B.; Baumann, U.; D'Agostino, D.; D'Antiga, L.; Dezsofi, A.; Debray, D.; Durmaz, O.; Evans, H.; Frauca, E.; Hadzic, N.; et al. Similarities and Differences in Allocation Policies for Pediatric Liver Transplantation Across the World. *J. Pediatr. Gastroenterol. Nutr.* **2019**, *68*, 700–705. [CrossRef]

14. Kasahara, M.; Umeshita, K.; Sakamoto, S.; Fukuda, A.; Furukawa, H.; Sakisaka, S.; Kobayashi, E.; Tanaka, E.; Inomata, Y.; Kawasaki, S.; et al. Living donor liver transplantation for biliary atresia: An analysis of 2085 cases in the registry of the Japanese Liver Transplantation Society. *Am. J. Transplant.* **2018**, *18*, 659–668. [CrossRef] [PubMed]
15. Sundaram, S.S.; Mack, C.L.; Feldman, A.G.; Sokol, R.J. Biliary atresia: Indications and timing of liver transplantation and optimization of pretransplant care. *Liver Transplant.* **2017**, *23*, 96–109. [CrossRef]
16. Bondec, A.; Bucuvalas, J. The tip of the iceberg: Outcomes after liver transplantation for very young infants. *Pediatr. Transplant.* **2016**, *20*, 880–881. [CrossRef]
17. Rana, A.; Kueht, M.; Desai, M.; Lam, F.; Miloh, T.; Moffett, J.; Galvan, N.T.N.; Cotton, R.; O'Mahony, C.; Goss, J. No Child Left Behind: Liver Transplantation in Critically Ill Children. *J. Am. Coll. Surg.* **2017**, *224*, 671–677. [CrossRef]
18. Ziogas, I.A.; Ye, F.; Zhao, Z.; Cao, S.; Rauf, M.A.; Izzy, M.; Matsuoka, L.K.; Gillis, L.A.; Alexopoulos, S.P. Mortality Determinants in Children with Biliary Atresia Awaiting Liver Transplantation. *J. Pediatr.* **2021**, *228*, 177–182. [CrossRef]
19. Pugliese, R.; Fonseca, E.A.; Porta, G.; Danesi, V.; Guimaraes, T.; Porta, A.; Miura, I.K.; Borges, C.; Candido, H.; Benavides, M.; et al. Ascites and serum sodium are markers of increased waiting list mortality in children with chronic liver failure. *Hepatology* **2014**, *59*, 1964–1971. [CrossRef]
20. Kohaut, J.; Guérin, F.; Fouquet, V.; Gonzales, E.; de Lambert, G.; Martelli, H.; Jacquemin, E.; Branchereau, S. First liver transplantation for biliary atresia in children: The hidden effects of non-centralization. *Pediatr. Transplant.* **2018**, *22*, e13232. [CrossRef]
21. Karakoyun, M.; Baran, M.; Turan, C.; Kilic, M.; Ergun, O.; Aydogdu, S. Infants with extrahepatic biliary atresia: Effect of follow-up on the survival rate at Ege University Medical School transplantation center. *Turk. J. Gastroenterol.* **2017**, *28*, 298–302. [CrossRef] [PubMed]
22. Lampela, H.; Ritvanen, A.; Kosola, S.; Koivusalo, A.; Rintala, R.; Jalanko, H.; Pakarinen, M. National centralization of biliary atresia care to an assigned multidisciplinary team provides high-quality outcomes. *Scand. J. Gastroenterol.* **2012**, *47*, 99–107. [CrossRef] [PubMed]
23. Tessitore, M.; Sorrentino, E.; Di Cola, G.S.; Colucci, A.; Vajro, P.; Mandato, C. Malnutrition in Pediatric Chronic Cholestatic Disease: An Up-to-Date Overview. *Nutrients* **2021**, *13*, 2785. [CrossRef] [PubMed]
24. Triggs, N.D.; Beer, S.; Mokha, S.; Hosek, K.; Guffey, D.; Minard, C.G.; Munoz, F.M.; Himes, R.W. Central line-associated bloodstream infection among children with biliary atresia listed for liver transplantation. *World J. Hepatol.* **2019**, *11*, 208–216. [CrossRef]
25. Samyn, M.; Davenport, M.; Jain, V.; Hadzic, N.; Joshi, D.; Heneghan, M.; Dhawan, A.; Heaton, N. Young People with Biliary Atresia Requiring Liver Transplantation: A Distinct Population Requiring Specialist Care. *Transplantation* **2019**, *103*, e99–e107. [CrossRef]
26. Mohammad, S.; Alonso, E.M. Approach to Optimizing Growth, Rehabilitation, and Neurodevelopmental Outcomes in Children After Solid-organ Transplantation. *Pediatr. Clin. N. Am.* **2010**, *57*, 539–557. [CrossRef]
27. Ng, V.L.; Mazariegos, G.V.; Kelly, B.; Horslen, S.; McDiarmid, S.V.; Magee, J.C.; Loomes, K.M.; Fischer, R.; Sundaram, S.S.; Lai, J.C.; et al. Barriers to ideal outcomes after pediatric liver transplantation. *Pediatr. Transplant.* **2019**, *23*, e13537. [CrossRef]
28. Sun, Y.; Jia, L.; Yu, H.; Zhu, M.; Sheng, M.; Yu, W. The Effect of Pediatric Living Donor Liver Transplantation on Neurocognitive Outcomes in Children. *Ann. Transplant.* **2019**, *24*, 446–453. [CrossRef]
29. Parmar, A.; VanDriel, S.M.; Ng, V.L. Health-related quality of life after pediatric liver transplantation: A systematic review. *Liver Transplant.* **2017**, *23*, 361–374. [CrossRef]
30. Vimalesvaran, S.; Souza, L.N.; Deheragoda, M.; Samyn, M.; Day, J.; Verma, A.; Vilca-Melendez, H.; Rela, M.; Heaton, N.; Dhawan, A. Outcomes of adults who received liver transplant as young children. *eClinicalMedicine* **2021**, *38*, 100987. [CrossRef]
31. Angelico, R.; Trapani, S.; Spada, M.; Colledan, M.; De Goyet, J.V.; Salizzoni, M.; De Carlis, L.; Andorno, E.; Gruttadauria, S.; Ettorre, G.; et al. A national mandatory-split liver policy: A report from the Italian experience. *Am. J. Transplant.* **2019**, *19*, 2029–2043. [CrossRef]
32. Kitajima, T.; Sakamoto, S.; Sasaki, K.; Narumoto, S.; Kazemi, K.; Hirata, Y.; Fukuda, A.; Imai, R.; Miyazaki, O.; Irie, R.; et al. Impact of graft thickness reduction of left lateral segment on outcomes following pediatric living donor liver transplantation. *Am. J. Transplant.* **2018**, *18*, 2208–2219. [CrossRef] [PubMed]
33. Bourdeaux, C.; Darwish, A.; Jamart, J.; Tri, T.T.; Janssen, M.; Lerut, J.; Otte, J.B.; Sokal, E.; de Ville de Goyet, J.; Reding, R. Living-Related Versus Deceased Donor Pediatric Liver Transplantation: A Multivariate Analysis of Technical and Immunological Complications in 235 Recipients. *Am. J. Transplant.* **2007**, *7*, 440–447. [CrossRef] [PubMed]
34. Montenovo, M.I.; Bambha, K.; Reyes, J.; Dick, A.; Perkins, J.; Healey, P. Living liver donation improves patient and graft survival in the pediatric population. *Pediatr. Transplant.* **2019**, *23*, e13518. [CrossRef] [PubMed]
35. Austin, M.T.; Feurer, I.D.; Chari, R.S.; Gorden, D.L.; Wright, J.K.; Pinson, C.W. Survival after pediatric liver transplantation: Why does living donation offer an advantage? *Arch. Surg.* **2005**, *140*, 465–467. [CrossRef] [PubMed]
36. Kehar, M.; Parekh, R.S.; Stunguris, J.; De Angelis, M.; Van Roestel, K.; Ghanekar, A.; Cattral, M.; Fecteau, A.; Ling, S.; Kamath, B.M.; et al. Superior Outcomes and Reduced Wait Times in Pediatric Recipients of Living Donor Liver Transplantation. *Transplant. Direct* **2019**, *5*, e430. [CrossRef]

37. Barbetta, A.; Butler, C.; Barhouma, S.; Hogen, R.; Rocque, B.; Goldbeck, C.; Schilperoort, H.; Meeberg, G.; Shapiro, J.; Kwon, Y.K.; et al. Living Donor Versus Deceased Donor Pediatric Liver Transplantation: A Systematic Review and Meta-analysis. *Transplant. Direct* **2021**, *7*, e767. [CrossRef]
38. Wildhaber, B.E.; Majno, P.; Mayr, J.; Zachariou, Z.; Hohlfeld, J.; Schwoebel, M.; Kistler, W.; Meuli, M.; Le Coultre, C.; Mentha, G.; et al. Biliary Atresia: Swiss National Study, 1994–2004. *J. Pediatr. Gastroenterol. Nutr.* **2008**, *46*, 299–307. [CrossRef]
39. Elisofon, S.A.; Magee, J.C.; Ng, V.L.; Horslen, S.P.; Fioravanti, V.; Economides, J.; Erinjeri, J.; Anand, R.; Mazariegos, G.V.; Dunn, S.; et al. Society of pediatric liver transplantation: Current registry status 2011–2018. *Pediatr. Transplant.* **2020**, *24*, e13605. [CrossRef]
40. Kwong, A.J.; Kim, W.R.; Lake, J.R.; Smith, J.M.; Schladt, D.P.; Skeans, M.A.; Noreen, S.M.; Foutz, J.; Booker, S.E.; Cafarella, M.; et al. OPTN/SRTR 2019 Annual Data Report: Liver. *Am. J. Transplant.* **2021**, *21* (Suppl. 2), 208–315. [CrossRef]
41. Yoeli, D.; Goss, M.; Galván, N.T.N.; Desai, M.S.; Miloh, T.A.; Rana, A. Trends in pediatric liver transplant donors and deceased donor circumstance of death in the United States, 2002–2015. *Pediatr. Transplant.* **2018**, *22*, e13156. [CrossRef] [PubMed]
42. Saidi, R.F.; Jabbour, N.; Li, Y.; Shah, S.A.; Bozorgzadeh, A. Outcomes in partial liver transplantation: Deceased donor split-liver vs. live donor liver transplantation. *HPB* **2011**, *13*, 797–801. [CrossRef] [PubMed]
43. Cauley, R.P.; Vakili, K.; Potanos, K.; Fullington, N.; Graham, D.A.; Finkelstein, J.A.; Kim, H.B. Deceased donor liver transplantation in infants and small children: Are partial grafts riskier than whole organs? *Liver Transpl.* **2013**, *19*, 721–729. [CrossRef] [PubMed]
44. Mogul, D.B.; Luo, X.; Bowring, M.G.; Chow, E.; Massie, A.B.; Schwarz, K.B.; Cameron, A.M.; Bridges, J.F.; Segev, D.L. Fifteen-Year Trends in Pediatric Liver Transplants: Split, Whole Deceased, and Living Donor Grafts. *J. Pediatr.* **2018**, *196*, 148–153.e2. [CrossRef] [PubMed]
45. Perito, E.R.; Roll, G.; Dodge, J.L.; Rhee, S.; Roberts, J.P. Split Liver Transplantation and Pediatric Waitlist Mortality in the United States: Potential for Improvement. *Transplantation* **2019**, *103*, 552–557. [CrossRef]
46. Valentino, P.L.; Emre, S.; Geliang, G.; Li, L.; Deng, Y.; Mulligan, D.; I Rodriguez-Davalos, M. Frequency of whole-organ in lieu of split-liver transplantation over the last decade: Children experienced increased wait time and death. *Am. J. Transplant.* **2019**, *19*, 3114–3123. [CrossRef]
47. Davenport, M.; Ong, E.; Sharif, K.; Alizai, N.; McClean, P.; Hadzic, N.; Kelly, D.A. Biliary atresia in England and Wales: Results of centralization and new benchmark. *J. Pediatr. Surg.* **2011**, *46*, 1689–1694. [CrossRef]
48. Stringer, M.D. Biliary atresia: Service delivery and outcomes. *Semin. Pediatr. Surg.* **2008**, *17*, 116–122. [CrossRef]
49. Verkade, H.J.; Bezerra, J.A.; Davenport, M.; Schreiber, R.A.; Mieli-Vergani, G.; Hulscher, J.B.; Sokol, R.J.; Kelly, D.A.; Ure, B.; Whitington, P.F.; et al. Biliary atresia and other cholestatic childhood diseases: Advances and future challenges. *J. Hepatol.* **2016**, *65*, 631–642. [CrossRef]
50. Shneider, B.L.; Magee, J.C.; Karpen, S.J.; Rand, E.B.; Narkewicz, M.R.; Bass, L.M.; Schwarz, K.; Whitington, P.F.; Bezerra, J.A.; Kerkar, N.; et al. Total Serum Bilirubin within 3 Months of Hepatoportoenterostomy Predicts Short-Term Outcomes in Biliary Atresia. *J. Pediatr.* **2016**, *170*, 211–217.e2. [CrossRef]
51. Nakajima, H.; Koga, H.; Okawada, M.; Nakamura, H.; Lane, G.J.; Yamataka, A. Does time taken to achieve jaundice-clearance influence survival of the native liver in post-Kasai biliary atresia? *World J. Pediatr.* **2018**, *14*, 191–196. [CrossRef] [PubMed]
52. Nightingale, S.; Stormon, M.O.; O'Loughlin, E.V.; Shun, A.; Thomas, G.; Benchimol, E.I.; Day, A.S.; Adams, S.; Shi, E.; Ooi, C.Y.; et al. Early Posthepatoportoenterostomy Predictors of Native Liver Survival in Biliary Atresia. *J. Pediatr. Gastroenterol. Nutr.* **2017**, *64*, 203–209. [CrossRef] [PubMed]
53. Serinet, M.-O.; Broué, P.; Jacquemin, E.; Lachaux, A.; Sarles, J.; Gottrand, F.; Gauthier, F.; Chardot, C. Management of patients with biliary atresia in France: Results of a decentralized policy 1986–2002. *Hepatology* **2006**, *44*, 75–84. [CrossRef]
54. Hukkinen, M.; Kerola, A.; Lohi, J.; Heikkilä, P.; Merras-Salmio, L.; Jahnukainen, T.; Koivusalo, A.; Jalanko, H.; Pakarinen, M.P. Treatment Policy and Liver Histopathology Predict Biliary Atresia Outcomes: Results after National Centralization and Protocol Biopsies. *J. Am. Coll. Surg.* **2018**, *226*, 46–57. [CrossRef]
55. Wong, Z.H.; Davenport, M. What Happens after Kasai for Biliary Atresia? A European Multicenter Survey. *Eur. J. Pediatr. Surg.* **2019**, *29*, 1–6. [CrossRef] [PubMed]
56. Alexopoulos, S.P.; Merrill, M.; Kin, C.; Matsuoka, L.; Dorey, F.; Concepcion, W.; Esquivel, C.; Bonham, A. The impact of hepatic portoenterostomy on liver transplantation for the treatment of biliary atresia: Early failure adversely affects outcome. *Pediatr. Transplant.* **2012**, *16*, 373–378. [CrossRef]
57. Superina, R. Biliary atresia and liver transplantation: Results and thoughts for primary liver transplantation in select patients. *Pediatr. Surg. Int.* **2017**, *33*, 1297–1304. [CrossRef]
58. Kim, H.B.; Elisofon, S.A. Biliary Atresia: Biliary-Enteric Drainage or Primary Liver Transplant? *Hepatology* **2020**, *71*, 751–752. [CrossRef]
59. Goda, S.S.; Khedr, M.A.; Elshenawy, S.Z.; Ibrahim, T.M.; El-Araby, H.A.; Sira, M.M. Preoperative Serum IL-12p40 Is a Potential Predictor of Kasai Portoenterostomy Outcome in Infants with Biliary Atresia. *Gastroenterol. Res. Pract.* **2017**, *2017*, 9089068. [CrossRef]
60. Yassin, N.; El-Tagy, G.; Abdelhakeem, O.N.; Asem, N.; El-Karaksy, H. Predictors of Short-Term Outcome of Kasai Portoenterostomy for Biliary Atresia in Infants: A Single-Center Study. *Pediatr. Gastroenterol. Hepatol. Nutr.* **2020**, *23*, 266–275. [CrossRef]
61. Caruso, M.; Ricciardi, C.; Paoli, G.D.; Di Dato, F.; Donisi, L.; Romeo, V.; Petretta, M.; Iorio, R.; Cesarelli, G.; Brunetti, A.; et al. Machine Learning Evaluation of Biliary Atresia Patients to Predict Long-Term Outcome after the Kasai Procedure. *Bioengineering* **2021**, *8*, 152. [CrossRef] [PubMed]

62. Ge, J.; Lai, J.C. Split-Liver Allocation: An Underused Opportunity to Expand Access to Liver Transplantation. *Liver Transplant.* **2019**, *25*, 690–691. [CrossRef] [PubMed]
63. Ge, J.; Perito, E.R.; Bucuvalas, J.; Gilroy, R.; Hsu, E.K.; Roberts, J.P.; Lai, J.C. Split liver transplantation is utilized infrequently and concentrated at few transplant centers in the United States. *Am. J. Transplant.* **2020**, *20*, 1116–1124. [CrossRef] [PubMed]
64. Godown, J.; McKane, M.; Wujcik, K.; Mettler, B.A.; Dodd, D.A. Expanding the donor pool: Regional variation in pediatric organ donation rates. *Pediatr. Transplant.* **2016**, *20*, 1093–1097. [CrossRef]
65. Battula, N.R.; Platto, M.; Anbarasan, R.; Perera, M.T.; Ong, E.; Roll, G.R.; Ferraz Neto, B.H.; Mergental, H.; Isaac, J.; Muiesan, P. Intention to split policy: A successful strategy in a combined pediatric and adult liver transplant center. *Ann. Surg.* **2017**, *265*, 1009–1015. [CrossRef]
66. Patroniti, N.; Zangrillo, A.; Pappalardo, F.; Peris, A.; Cianchi, G.; Braschi, A.; Iotti, G.A.; Arcadipane, A.; Panarello, G.; Ranieri, V.M.; et al. The Italian ECMO network experience during the 2009 influenza A(H1N1) pandemic: Preparation for severe respiratory emergency outbreaks. *Intensive Care Med.* **2011**, *37*, 1447–1457. [CrossRef] [PubMed]
67. Benson, C.; Judson, I. Role of expert centres in the management of sarcomas—A UK perspective. *Eur. J. Cancer* **2014**, *50*, 1951–1956. [CrossRef]
68. Congiu, M.E. The Italian National Plan for Rare Diseases. *Blood Transfus.* **2014**, *12*, s614–s616. [CrossRef]
69. Gatta, G.; Botta, L.; Comber, H.; Dimitrova, N.; Leinonen, M.; Pritchard-Jones, K.; Siesling, S.; Trama, A.; Van Eycken, L.; van der Zwan, J.; et al. The European study on centralisation of childhood cancer treatment. *Eur. J. Cancer* **2019**, *115*, 120–127. [CrossRef]

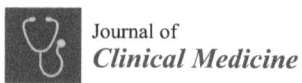

Article

Primary Liver Transplantation vs. Transplant after Kasai Portoenterostomy for Infants with Biliary Atresia

Caroline P. Lemoine, John P. LeShock, Katherine A. Brandt and Riccardo Superina *

Division of Transplant and Advanced Hepatobiliary Surgery, Ann & Robert H. Lurie Children's Hospital of Chicago, Northwestern University Feinberg School of Medicine, 225 E. Chicago Avenue Box 57, Chicago, IL 60611, USA; clemoine@luriechildrens.org (C.P.L.); john.leshock@northwestern.edu (J.P.L.); kabrandt@luriechildrens.org (K.A.B.)
* Correspondence: rsuperina@luriechildrens.org; Tel.: +1-(312)-227-4040; Fax: +1-(312)-227-9387

Abstract: Introduction: Primary liver transplants (pLT) in patients with biliary atresia (BA) are infrequent, since most babies with BA undergo a prior Kasai portoenterostomy (KPE). This study compared transplant outcomes in children with BA with or without a prior KPE. We hypothesized that pLT have less morbidity and better outcomes compared to those done after a failed KPE. Methods: A retrospective review of patients with BA transplanted at our institution was performed. Patients were included if they received a pLT or if they were transplanted less than 2 years from KPE. Outcomes were compared between those groups. Comparisons were also made based on era (early: 1997–2008 vs. modern: 2009–2020). $p < 0.05$ was considered significant. Results: Patients who received a pLT were older at diagnosis (141.5 ± 46.0 vs. KPE 67.1 ± 25.5 days, $p < 0.001$). The time between diagnosis and listing for transplant was shorter in the pLT group (44.5 ± 44.7 vs. KPE 140.8 ± 102.8 days, $p < 0.001$). In the modern era, the calculated PELD score for the pLT was significantly higher (23 ± 8 vs. KPE 16 ± 8, $p = 0.022$). Two waitlist deaths occurred in the KPE group (none in pLT, $p = 0.14$). Both the duration of transplant surgery and transfusion requirements were similar in both groups. There was a significant improvement in graft survival in transplants after KPE between eras (early era 84.3% vs. modern era 97.8%, $p = 0.025$). The 1-year patient and graft survival after pLT was 100%. Conclusions: Patient and graft survival after pLT are comparable to transplants after a failed KPE but pLT avoids a prior intervention. There was no significant difference in pre- or peri-transplant morbidity between groups other than wait list mortality. A multicenter collaboration with more patients may help demonstrate the potential benefits of pLT in patients predicted to have early failure of KPE.

Keywords: biliary atresia; kasai portoenterostomy; primary liver transplantation; outcomes

Citation: Lemoine, C.P.; LeShock, J.P.; Brandt, K.A.; Superina, R. Primary Liver Transplantation vs. Transplant after Kasai Portoenterostomy for Infants with Biliary Atresia. *J. Clin. Med.* 2022, 11, 3012. https://doi.org/10.3390/jcm11113012

Academic Editor: Katsunori Yoshida

Received: 20 February 2022
Accepted: 23 May 2022
Published: 26 May 2022

Publisher's Note: MDPI stays neutral with regard to jurisdictional claims in published maps and institutional affiliations.

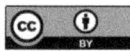

Copyright: © 2022 by the authors. Licensee MDPI, Basel, Switzerland. This article is an open access article distributed under the terms and conditions of the Creative Commons Attribution (CC BY) license (https://creativecommons.org/licenses/by/4.0/).

1. Introduction

Biliary atresia (BA) is a disease characterized by inflammation and obstruction of the biliary tree leading to the development of biliary cirrhosis in infancy if left untreated [1]. It was originally deemed "uncorrectable" until Kasai described a portoenterostomy, allowing bile drainage from the liver [2]. The Kasai portoenterostomy (KPE) remains the conventionally accepted treatment of BA by most pediatric surgeons.

The success of KPE is defined by two indices: clearance of jaundice and transplant free survival. In a recent analysis of North American results among pediatric liver centers of excellence, 49.6% of children undergoing KPE achieved a normal bilirubin post-op within 3 months of surgery, and almost 50% of all children had been transplanted or died by two years after the Kasai. Even the successful clearance of jaundice does not ensure avoidance of early liver transplant [3]. Despite this, the standard of care remains to perform a KPE in all patients with followed by a liver transplantation when it fails [4,5]. In the United States, only patients with advanced liver disease at diagnosis are candidates for a primary liver transplantation (pLT) [6]. pLT is rarely performed but has been associated with excellent survival [7,8].

pLT is not recommended for all patients with BA since a third to a half of the patients may avoid a liver transplant in childhood after a successful KPE [9]. However, it is currently difficult to predict which patients will develop early failure after KPE (<1–2 years postoperatively) and who could, therefore, benefit from pLT. For patients who develop early failure, a pLT may lead to superior outcomes by decreasing the waitlist morbidity and possibly mortality and reducing post-transplant complications [10–12].

Here, we present our institutional experience with pLT for patients with BA and compared them to patients who received a liver transplant early (<2 years) after a failed KPE. We hypothesized that pLT leads to superior post-transplant outcomes to transplant after KPE and is associated with a lower waitlist morbidity and mortality.

2. Material and Methods
2.1. Patient Selection, Definitions and Data Collection

Data were collected retrospectively from our BA and liver transplant databases. Only patients who suffered from early failure after KPE or who received a pLT at our institution between August 1997 and June 2020 were included for this comparative study. Early failure was defined as BA patients who received a liver transplant less than 2 years after KPE. Patient selection is illustrated in Figure 1.

This retrospective study comparing patients with BA who were transplanted either after KPE or with a pLT was approved by our Institutional Review Board (IRB 2013-15357 and 2007-12989). Ultimately, a total of 99 patients were included in the KPE group and 14 patients received a pLT.

Primary liver transplant was done in patients who were diagnosed with BA by biopsy and operative cholangiogram who had signs of advanced liver disease at presentation: portal hypertension defined by the presence of hypersplenism (thrombocytopenia, splenomegaly) or history of variceal bleed, ascites, growth failure or synthetic liver dysfunction (INR ≥ 1.7, Albumin ≤ 3.2 g/dL).

Data collected included: patient's characteristics (sex, prematurity); age and weight at BA diagnosis (for KPE group: age at KPE; for pLT group: age at liver biopsy showing features of BA); transplant waitlist-related data (age at listing, waitlist duration, hospital admissions while listed, number of days admitted, indication for hospital admission, cost of admissions—see below); transplant-related data (age and weight at transplant, natural Pediatric End-stage Liver Disease (PELD) score a transplant for patients listed for transplant after 2002, length of transplant surgery, intraoperative packed red blood cell transfusion requirements, surgical complications, length of post-operative mechanical ventilation, length of intensive care and hospital stay). Patient and graft status at last follow-up as well as retransplantation were also collected.

For the purposes of evaluating the impact of practice changes over time on outcomes, we divided the experience into an early (August 1997–December 2008) and modern (January 2009—June 2020) era. Both the KPE and transplants were done primarily by a single surgeon (RS) in both eras.

Post-operative management did not change substantially from one era to the other for the post-operative KPE care. Intravenous ampicillin and gentamicin were used in all KPE patients post-operatively for 5 days followed by trimethoprim/sulfamethoxazole oral prophylaxis for 6 months. Post-operative steroids were not used routinely in either of the two eras. All KPE were done open and not laparoscopically.

Listing criteria for transplantation in the KPE group included failure to thrive despite optimal nutritional management, recurrent spontaneous bacterial peritonitis despite optimal management of ascites and hepatic synthetic failure as exemplified by vitamin K resistant INR of greater than 1.7 and albumin less the 3.0 g/100 mL.

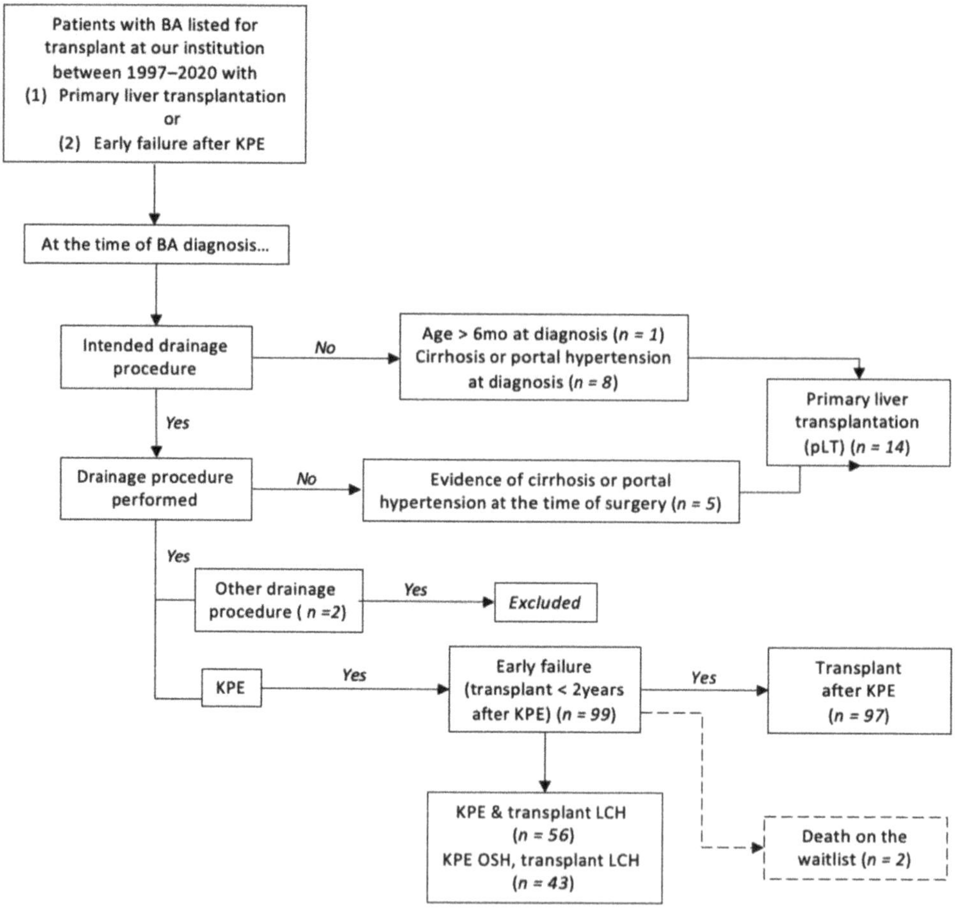

Figure 1. Flowchart describing patient selection (legend: BA: biliary atresia; KPE: Kasai portoenterostomy; LCH: Lurie Children's Hospital; OSH: Outside hospital; pLT: Primary liver transplantation).

Children who achieved at least a 2-year transplant-free survival or who achieved a serum direct bilirubin of <0.2 mg/dL after KPE were not included in the study, since these children met criteria for a successful KPE and were older and bigger than the control group.

No child survived more than two years after a failed KPE without a transplant.

Cost data were obtained through our institution's billing department for patients transplanted at our institution after 2009. In order to ensure the data would be comparable, all cost data were converted into an inflation-adjusted measure for a chosen baseline time period (chosen as the Consumer Price Index (CPI) for 2020). The CPI medical services index (a measure of change over time in the prices of medical services) was utilized to perform this conversion (https://fred.stlouisfed.org/series/CPIMEDSL (accessed on 26 June 2021)). Instead of performing a calculation on a monthly basis, an average of the CPI values for all months in a given year was obtained and then used for calculation using the following formula: Equivalent cost in baseline period = (Cost amount) × ((CPI for baseline time period)/(CPI for time period of the charge)). The adjusted cost of hospital admissions while on the transplant waitlist included the cost of the KPE admission for patients in the KPE group. The cost data are presented in United States dollars (USD).

2.2. Outcomes

Primary outcomes included 1-year and 3-year post-transplant patient and graft survival. Secondary outcomes focused on waitlist morbidity (number of hospital admissions, days admitted while on the wait list, indication for hospital admission and waitlist duration). Additionally, the morbidity at the time of transplant was evaluated, focusing on length of surgery, intra-operative transfusion requirements and post-transplant ICU and hospital length of stay.

2.3. Statistical Analysis

Comparisons were made between the KPE and pLT groups using the independent t-test for continuous variables and the Chi-square test for categorical variables. Additionally, comparisons were made based on the era of management to account for changes and improvement in the management of patients with BA. The same statistical analyses were performed.

The Mann–Whitney U test was used to compare billing data given its non-parametric distribution. Kaplan–Meier survival curves were obtained to compare patient and graft survival. Statistics were performed using the IBM SPSS Statistics program (version 24.0.0.0). A $p < 0.05$ was considered statistically significant.

3. Results

3.1. Pre-Transplant Data: Comparison of Patients Transplanted after pLT or KPE

The incidence of pLT was 12.4% (14/113). Patient's characteristics and pre-transplant waitlist data are presented in Table 1. Patients in the pLT group were significantly older at the time of BA diagnosis (KPE 67.1 ± 25.5 vs. pLT 141.5 ± 46.0 days, $p < 0.001$). Although the time between diagnosis and listing for transplant was shorter in the pLT group (KPE 140.8 ± 102.8 vs. pLT 44.5 ± 44.7 days, $p = 0.001$), the time that was spent on the waitlist was not statistically shorter ($p = 0.6$). Neither the number of hospital admissions nor the total number of days admitted while waiting for transplant were different when comparing groups. Although there was a trend in a lower cumulative adjusted cost of hospital admissions for the pLT group, this difference failed to reach statistical significance (KPE $425,090.00 (285,282.83, 566,405.40) vs. pLT $253,004.10 (95,640.49, 431,530.70), $p = 0.07$). The reasons for and number of hospital admissions were similar in both groups, except for cholangitis. Patients from the KPE group were often admitted for cholangitis, a complication that did not occur in any infant from the pLT group (KPE 31/99, 31.3% vs. pLT 0/14, $p = 0.014$). Two deaths on the waitlist occurred in the KPE group. Although there were none in the pLT group, this difference was not significant ($p = 0.59$).

3.2. Transplant and Survival Data: Comparison between pLT and KPE Groups

Patients who received a pLT were nearly 4 weeks younger at the time of transplant (pLT 287.0 ± 82.7 days versus KPE 311.4 ± 144.0, $p = 0.54$) (Table 2). The groups were comparable in terms of severity of disease at transplant (similar growth failure based on weight z-scores and calculated PELD score). From a surgical standpoint, there was no difference in length of surgery or intraoperative packed red blood cell transfusion requirements. The number of combined returns to the operating room for any surgical complication (bleeding, thrombosis, bowel perforation or biliary complications) or procedures performed in interventional radiology were not different between groups. Post-operatively, the groups were also similar in regards to the duration of mechanical ventilation and both intensive care unit and for overall transplant hospitalization length of stay. The retransplantation rate was not significantly different. There was a trend for a more expensive adjusted cost of transplant admission for patients in the pLT group (KPE $588,887.00 (466,829.20, 902,360.70) vs. pLT $932,675.30 (668,937.90, 1,120,433.90), $p = 0.098$.

Table 1. Pre-transplant comparison of patients transplanted after KPE or as pLT: (*) represents a statistically significant result; (‡) the pre-transplant admission cost comparison only included patients managed since 2009 who received their KPE at our institution (n = 31) and patients from the pLT group (n = 10).

Variables	KPE (n = 99)	pLT (n = 14)	p Value
Age at KPE or diagnosis BA (days) (mean ± sd)	67.1 ± 25.5	141.5 ± 46.0	<0.001 *
Time to listing (days) (mean ± sd)	140.8 ± 102.8	44.5 ± 44.7	0.001 *
Waitlist time (days) (mean ± sd)	105.6 ± 102.8	90.8 ± 66.5	0.6
Hospital admissions while on waitlist (n, mean ± sd)	3.2 ± 3.3	2.6 ± 2.4	0.58
Days admitted while on waitlist (mean ± sd)	24.9 ± 31.2	22.4 ± 17.6	0.78
Adjusted cost of hospital admissions on the waitlist ‡ (median (IQR))	425,090.00 (285,282.83, 566,405.40)	253,004.10 (95,640.49, 431,530.70)	0.07
Admission on the waitlist (n, %): Cholangitis	31 (31.3)	0	0.014 *
Admission on the waitlist (n, %): Infections (other than cholangitis)	41 (41.4)	6 (42.9)	0.92
Admission on the waitlist (n, %): Gastrointestinal bleeding	20 (20.2)	2 (14.3)	0.6
Admission on the waitlist (n, %): Ascites or Spontaneous bacterial peritonitis	25 (25.3)	5 (35.7)	0.41
Admission on the waitlist (n, %): Malnutrition	24 (24.2)	4 (28.6)	0.73
Death on the waitlist (yes) (n, %)	2 (2.0)	0	0.59

Table 2. Post-transplant comparison of patients transplanted after KPE or as pLT. Legend: PELD: Pediatric End-stage Liver Disease; LDLT: Living donor liver transplantation; ICU: intensive care unit.

Variables	KPE (n = 97)	pLT (n = 14)	p Value
Age at transplant (days) (mean ± sd)	311.4 ± 144.0	287.0 ± 82.7	0.54
Calculated PELD score at transplant (mean ± sd)	22 ± 11	27 ± 8	0.15
Type of donor (LDLT) (n, %)	39 (40.2)	4 (28.6)	0.4
Transplant surgery duration (minutes) (mean ± sd)	443.9 ± 98.6	423.1 ± 70.0	0.39
Intraoperative pRBC transfusion (cc/kg) (mean ± sd)	143.9 ± 122.3	136.1 ± 137.2	0.83
Duration of mechanical ventilation (days) (mean ± sd)	7.5 ± 6.6	9.8 ± 9.1	0.27
Length of ICU stay (days) (mean ± sd)	14.2 ± 25.6	14.2 ± 10.5	1
Length of hospital stay (days) (mean ± sd)	31.8 ± 36.0	32.8 ± 15.2	0.92
Return to ICU after transplant (n, %)	15 (15.5)	5 (35.7)	0.065
Surgical take back post-transplant (mean ± sd)	0.7 ± 1.1	1.0 ± 1.0	0.31
Adjusted cost of transplant admission (median (IQR))	588,887.00 (466,829.20, 902,360.70)	932,675.30 (668,937.90, 1,120,433.90)	0.098
Retransplant (yes) (n, %)	8 (8.2)	2 (14.3)	0.46
1-year patient survival from list date (n, %)	93 (93.9)	14 (100.0)	0.35
1-year post-transplant patient survival (n, %)	91 (93.8)	14 (100.0)	0.35
3-year post-transplant patient survival (n, %)	88 (90.7)	13 (92.9)	0.8
1-year post-transplant graft survival (n, %)	88 (90.7)	13 (92.9)	0.78
3-year post-transplant graft survival (n, %)	86 (88.7)	12 (85.7)	0.78

The 1-year patient survival from both listing and after transplantation was 100% for patients who received a pLT, but this was not significantly different from patients who were transplanted after KPE, although two patients in the KPE group died while on the waitlist. There was no statistical difference in 1-year and 3-year graft survival.

3.3. Does the Era Make A Difference? Pre-Transplant Comparison of Patients Transplanted after KPE or pLT Based on Early versus Modern Era

In total, 95 of the 97 transplants were done by a single surgeon (R.S.) and a liver transplant operating room team including liver transplant nurses and anesthesiologists. By era, all 51 in the early and 44/46 in the later era were done by the same single surgeon.

When comparing patients who received a pLT to those who were transplanted after KPE, patients from the KPE group remained significantly younger in both eras at the time of BA diagnosis (early era: KPE 67.9 ± 23.3 vs. pLT 139.4 ± 71.7 days, $p < 0.001$; modern era: KPE 66.1 ± 27.9 vs. pLT 127.9 ± 37.2 days, $p < 0.001$) (Table 3). Although the time between diagnosis and listing was shorter in the pLT group in both eras, it was not significantly different in the early era. However, the difference became significant in the modern era, as patients in the KPE group took longer to be listed than patients in the pLT group (KPE 171.5 ± 110.7 vs. pLT 48.6 ± 40.3 days, $p = 0.002$). The waitlist duration shortened in both groups in the modern era. There was no difference in the number of hospital admissions or days admitted while on the waitlist. Only the number of admissions for cholangitis remained significantly higher in the KPE group.

Table 3. Pre-transplant comparison of patients transplanted after KPE or as pLT based on era: demographics, diagnosis of BA and waitlist-related data. Legend: (*) represents a statistically significant result.

Variables	Early Era (1997–2008)			Modern Era (2009–2020)		
	KPE (n = 51)	pLT (n = 5)	p Value	KPE (n = 48)	pLT (n = 9)	p Value
Age at KPE or diagnosis BA (days) (mean ± sd)	67.9 ± 23.3	139.4 ± 71.7	<0.001 *	66.1 ± 27.9	127.9 ± 37.2	<0.001 *
Time to listing (days) (mean ± sd)	112.1 ± 95.6	63.8 ± 69.3	0.28	171.5 ± 110.7	48.6 ± 40.3	0.002 *
Waitlist time (days) (mean ± sd)	117.8 ± 121.9	130.0 ± 83.1	0.83	92.6 ± 76.7	69.0 ± 47.4	0.38
Number of hospital admissions while on waitlist (n, mean ± sd)	2.8 ± 3.3	2.0 ± 2.0	0.61	3.6 ± 3.4	3 ± 2.4	0.62
Number of days admitted while on waitlist (mean ± sd)	23.1 ± 34.0	22.8 ± 23.9	0.99	26.1 ± 28.3	19.7 ± 16.0	0.53
Admission on the waitlist (n, %): Cholangitis	15 (29.4)	0	0.16	16 (33.3)	0	0.041 *
Admission on the waitlist (n, %): Infections (other than cholangitis)	20 (39.2)	3 (60.0)	0.37	21 (43.8)	3 (33.3)	0.56
Admission on the waitlist (n, %): Gastrointestinal bleeding	11 (21.6)	0 (0)	0.25	9 (18.8)	3 (33.3)	0.81
Admission on the waitlist (n, %): Ascites or Spontaneous bacterial peritonitis	10 (19.6)	1 (20.0)	0.98	14 (29.2)	4 (44.4)	0.37
Admission on the waitlist (n, %): Malnutrition	5 (9.8)	0 (0)	0.46	19 (39.6)	4 (44.4)	0.79
Death on the waitlist (n, %)	0 (0)	0	—	2 (4.2)	0	0.53

3.4. Transplant and Post-Transplant Survival Data: Comparison of Patients Transplanted after KPE or pLT Based on Era

The age at transplant improved in the pLT group in the modern era compared to the KPE group, but the difference remained not significant (KPE 326.4 ± 144.2 vs. pLT 261.3 ± 64.6 days, $p = 0.19$) (Table 4). Patients in the pLT group were significantly sicker at the time of transplant as shown by a higher natural PELD score (KPE 16 ± 8 vs. pLT 23 ± 8, $p = 0.022$). The length of the transplant operation shortened in both groups in the modern era, but the operative times, blood loss, ICU and hospital length of stay were quite similar between the two groups. Post-operatively, in the modern era, there was a trend to longer duration of mechanical ventilation for patients in the pLT group (KPE 7.7 ± 6.8 vs. pLT 12.3 ± 9.2 days, $p = 0.085$). The number of readmissions to the intensive care unit were significantly more frequent in the early era in the pLT group (KPE 8/51, 15.7% vs. pLT 3/5, 60%, $p = 0.017$). While the proportion of ICU readmissions remained higher in the pLT in the modern era, this was no longer significant (KPE 7/46, 15.2 vs. pLT 3/9, 33.3%, $p = 0.2$). Overall, there was no difference in 1-year or 3-year patient and graft survival between groups.

Table 4. Post-transplant comparison of patients transplanted after KPE or as pLT based on era: transplant-related data and post-transplant outcomes. Legend: (*) represents a statistically significant result.

Variables	Early Era (1997–2008)			Modern Era (2009–2020)		
	KPE (n = 51)	pLT (n = 5)	p Value	KPE (n = 46)	pLT (n = 9)	p Value
Age at transplant (days) (mean ± sd)	297.9 ± 144.0	333.2 ± 98.6	0.6	326.4 ± 144.2	261.3 ± 64.6	0.19
Calculated PELD score at transplant (mean ± sd)	17 ± 9	18 ± 0	0.78	16 ± 8	23 ± 8	0.022 *
Type of donor (LDLT) (n, %)	25 (49.0)	1 (20.0)	0.21	14 (30.4)	3 (33.3)	0.86
OR duration (minutes) (mean ± sd)	467.8 ± 89.3	451.2 ± 76.9	0.69	417.4 ± 74.7	407.4 ± 64.3	0.71
Intraoperative pRBC transfusion (cc/kg) (mean ± sd)	162.7 ± 142.1	156.7 ± 176.4	0.93	123.1 ± 92.9	124.7 ± 120.9	0.96
Days on the ventilator (days) (mean ± sd)	7.3 ± 6.4	2.0 ± 2.0	0.64	7.7 ± 6.8	12.3 ± 9.2	0.085
Length of ICU stay (days) (mean ± sd)	15.0 ± 34.1	7.0 ± 2.3	0.67	13.3 ± 10.2	17.6 ± 11.1	0.27
Length of hospital stay (days) (mean ± sd)	32.9 ± 40.1	24.3 ± 18.1	0.1	30.7 ± 31.5	34.7 ± 13.9	0.32
Return to ICU after transplant (n, %)	8 (15.7)	3 (60.0)	0.017 *	7 (15.2)	3 (33.3)	0.2
Retransplant (n, %)	8 (15.7)	2 (40.0)	0.18	1 (2.2)	0 (0)	0.66
1-year patient survival from list date (n, %)	48 (94.1)	5 (100.0)	0.58	45 (93.8)	9 (100.0)	0.45
1-year post-transplant patient survival (n, %)	46 (90.2)	5 (100.0)	0.48	45 (97.8)	9 (100.0)	0.66
3-year post-transplant patient survival (n, %)	44 (86.3)	5 (100.0)	0.39	44 (95.7)	8 (88.9)	0.4
1-year post-transplant graft survival (n, %)	43 (84.3)	4 (80.0)	0.86	45 (97.8)	9 (100.0)	0.66
3-year post-transplant graft survival (n, %)	42 (82.4)	4 (80.0)	0.94	44 (95.7)	8 (88.9)	0.4

3.5. Comparison of Patients Transplanted after KPE Based on Era

There was no difference in age at KPE (early 67.9 ± 23.3 vs. modern 66.1 ± 27.9 days, $p = 0.73$) (Table 5). However, the time to listing became significantly longer in the modern era (early 112.1 ± 95.6 vs. modern 171.5 ± 110.7 days, $p = 0.005$). The number of hospital admissions were similar in the two eras as were reasons for admission except for a higher incidence of hospital admissions for malnutrition (including initiation of tube feeds or parental nutrition) in the modern early (early 5/51, 9.8% vs. modern 19/48, 39.6%, $p = 0.001$). Two deaths occurred on the waitlist in the modern era ($p = 0.14$).

KPE patients were older at transplant in the modern era, although not significantly so (early 297.9 ± 144.0 vs. modern 326.4 ± 144.2 days, $p = 0.21$) (Table 6). The length of transplant surgery shortened by almost an hour in the modern era (early 467.8 ± 89.3 vs. modern 417.4 ± 74.7 min, $p = 0.005$) and blood transfusion requirements diminished, although not significantly (early 162.7 ± 142.1 vs. modern 123.1 ± 92.9 cc/kg, $p = 0.11$). The rate of retransplantation improved significantly (early 8/51, 15.7% vs. modern 1/46, 2.2%, $p = 0.022$), and therefore, the 1-year and 3-year graft survival improved significantly in the modern era.

Table 5. Pre-transplant comparison of patients transplanted after KPE based on era: demographics, diagnosis of BA and waitlist-related data. Legend: (*) represents a statistically significant result.

Variables	KPE		p Value
	Early Era (1997–2008) (n = 51)	Modern Era (2009–2020) (n = 48)	
Age at KPE (days) (mean ± sd)	67.9 ± 23.3	66.1 ± 27.9	0.73
Time to listing (days) (mean ± sd)	112.1 ± 95.6	171.5 ± 110.7	0.005 *
Waitlist time (days) (mean ± sd)	117.8 ± 121.9	92.6 ± 76.7	0.22
Number of hospital admissions while on waitlist (mean ± sd)	2.7 ± 3.3	2.0 ± 2.0	0.17
Number of days admitted while on waitlist (mean ± sd)	23.1 ± 34.0	26.1 ± 28.3	0.64
Admission on the waitlist (n, %): Cholangitis	15 (29.4)	16 (33.3)	0.67
Admission on the waitlist (n, %): Infections (other than cholangitis)	20 (39.2)	21 (43.8)	0.65
Admission on the waitlist (n, %): Gastrointestinal bleeding	11 (21.6)	9 (18.8)	0.73
Admission on the waitlist (n, %): Ascites or Spontaneous bacterial peritonitis	10 (19.6)	14 (29.2)	0.27
Admission on the waitlist (n, %): Malnutrition	5 (9.8)	19 (39.6)	0.001 *
Death on the waitlist (n, %)	0 (0)	2 (4.2)	0.14

Table 6. Post-transplant comparison of patients transplanted after KPE based on era: transplant-related data and post-transplant outcomes. Legend: * represents a statistically significant result.

Variables	KPE		p Value
	Early Era (1997–2008) (n = 51)	Modern Era (2009–2020) (n = 46)	
Age at transplant (days) (mean ± sd)	297.9 ± 144.0	326.4 ± 144.2	0.21
Calculated PELD score at transplant (mean ± sd)	17 ± 9	16 ± 8	0.46
Type of donor (LDLT) (n, %)	25 (49.0)	14 (30.4)	0.06
OR duration (minutes) (mean ± sd)	467.8 ± 89.3	417.4 ± 74.7	0.005 *
Intraoperative pRBC transfusion (cc/kg) (mean ± sd)	162.7 ± 142.1	123.1 ± 92.9	0.11
Days on the ventilator (days) (mean ± sd)	7.3 ± 6.4	7.7 ± 6.8	0.84
Length of ICU stay (days) (mean ± sd)	15.0 ± 34.1	13.3 ± 10.2	0.73
Length of hospital stay (days) (mean ± sd)	32.9 ± 40.1	30.7 ± 31.5	0.73
Return to ICU after transplant (n, %)	8 (15.7)	7 (15.2)	0.95
Retransplant (n, %)	8 (15.7)	1 (2.2)	0.022 *
1-year patient survival from list date (n, %)	48 (94.1)	45 (93.8)	0.94
1-year post-transplant patient survival (n, %)	46 (90.2)	45 (97.8)	0.13
3-year post-transplant patient survival (n, %)	44 (86.3)	44 (95.7)	0.13
1-year graft survival (n, %)	43 (84.3)	45 (97.8)	0.025 *
3-year graft survival (n, %)	42 (82.4)	44 (95.7)	0.044 *

3.6. Results of pLT: Comparison of Patients Who Received a pLT Based on Era

There were no significant differences in demographic variables when comparing patients of the pLT based on era (Table 7). Although both the time to listing (early 63.8 ± 69.3 vs. modern 48.6 ± 40.3 days, $p = 0.61$) and the waitlist duration (early 130.0 ± 83.1 vs. pLT 69.0 ± 47.4 days, $p = 0.1$) were shorter, the number of patients was small and did not reach statistical significance. There was a trend in more admissions for malnutrition in the modern era (early 0/5, 0% vs. modern 4/9, 44.4%, $p = 0.078$).

Table 7. Pre-transplant comparison of patients transplanted after pLT based on era: demographics, diagnosis of BA and waitlist-related data.

Variables	pLT		p Value
	Early Era (1997–2008) (n = 5)	Modern Era (2009–2020) (n = 9)	
Age at diagnosis BA (days) (mean ± sd)	139.4 ± 71.7	127.9 ± 37.2	0.70
Time to listing (days) (mean ± sd)	63.8 ± 69.3	48.6 ± 40.3	0.61
Waitlist time (days) (mean ± sd)	130.0 ± 83.1	69.0 ± 47.4	0.10
Number of hospital admissions while on waitlist (mean ± sd)	3.6 ± 3.4	3 ± 2.4	0.45
Number of days admitted while on waitlist (mean ± sd)	22.8 ± 23.9	19.8 ± 16.0	0.79
Admission on the waitlist (n, %): Cholangitis	0	0	—
Admission on the waitlist (n, %): Infections (other than cholangitis)	3 (60.0)	3 (33.3)	0.33
Admission on the waitlist (n, %): Gastrointestinal bleeding	0 (0)	3 (33.3)	0.15
Admission on the waitlist (n, %): Ascites or Spontaneous bacterial peritonitis	1 (20.0)	4 (44.4)	0.36
Admission on the waitlist (n, %): Malnutrition	0 (0)	4 (44.4)	0.078
Death on the waitlist (n, %)	0	0	—

Although patients in the modern era were transplanted faster, the difference was not significant (age at transplant early 333.2 ± 98.6 vs. modern 261.3 ± 64.6 days, $p = 0.12$) (Table 8). Length of surgery and transfusion requirements improved with time, but also not significantly. Ventilation days, ICU stay and hospital stay were shorter in the early era, but this is due to one early patient being excluded from those analyses, as he was chronically ventilated through a tracheostomy and remained in the ICU until his discharge from the hospital. The rate of retransplantation improved significantly in the modern era (early 2/5, 40.0% vs. 0/9, 0%, $p = 0.04$). The patient and graft survival were similar between eras.

Table 8. Post-transplant comparison of patients transplanted after pLT based on era: transplant-related data and post-transplant outcomes (waitlist). Legend: (*) represents a statistically significant result.

Variables	pLT		p Value
	Early Era (1997–2008) (n = 5)	Modern Era (2009–2020) (n = 9)	
Age at transplant (days) (mean ± sd)	333.2 ± 98.6	261.3 ± 64.6	0.12
Calculated PELD score at transplant (mean ± sd)	18 ± 0	23 ± 8	0.18
Type of donor (LDLT) (n, %)	1 (20.0)	3 (33.3)	0.60
OR duration (minutes) (mean ± sd)	451.2 ± 76.9	407.4 ± 64.3	0.28
Intraoperative pRBC transfusion (cc/kg) (mean ± sd)	156.7 ± 176.4	124.7 ± 120.8	0.69
Days on the ventilator (days) (mean ± sd)	2.0 ± 2.0	12.3 ± 9.2	0.099
Length of ICU stay (days) (mean ± sd)	7.0 ± 2.3	17.6 ± 11.1	0.12
Length of hospital stay (days) (mean ± sd)	24.3 ± 18.1	34.7 ± 13.9	0.28
Return to ICU after transplant (n, %)	3 (60.0)	3 (33.3)	0.33
Retransplant (n, %)	2 (40.0)	0 (0)	0.04 *
1-year patient survival from list date (n, %)	5 (100.0)	9 (100.0)	–
1-year post-transplant patient survival (n, %)	5 (100.0)	9 (100.0)	–
3-year post-transplant patient survival (n, %)	5 (100.0)	8 (88.9)	0.40
1-year post-transplant graft survival (n, %)	4 (80.0)	9 (100.0)	0.18
3-year post-transplant graft survival (n, %)	4 (80.0)	8 (88.9)	0.68

4. Discussion

Primary liver transplant for children with biliary atresia is usually reserved for those children who present with advanced liver disease at the time of diagnosis. Reported incidences of pLT vary between 3–16% [9,13–18], but have been as low as less than 1% in Japan [19,20] and as high as 40% in Brazil [11]. Comparing these incidences is challenging given the different rates of organ donation and organ availability in different cultures and countries. Additionally, some studies compare pLT to all patients transplanted after KPE regardless of the timing of when a patient is ultimately listed for a transplant. Additionally, the denominator for these studies varies: some use the total number of patients with BA managed at their institution (regardless of their management), while others only include patients with BA who were ultimately transplanted. In our institutional experience spanning over 23 years, the overall rate of pLT was 10.7%, comparable to previously published data.

Our study is purposefully limited to the comparison of outcomes in children after pLT to those children who have had unsuccessful KPE and have had to undergo liver transplant within two years of a failed KPE. It does not include comparisons to older children who have had a successful KPE, since we wanted to focus on a population of children who have derived no ostensible benefit from the KPE, and who, with the appropriate, albeit yet unknown selection criteria, might have been spared an unnecessary surgery.

While some studies have reported that transplants after KPE are more complex (higher blood transfusion volumes, longer operative time and increased rate of bowel perforations due to the post-operative adhesions), the differences were actually not statistically significant [12,18,21,22]. Our study showed comparable results between transplant after KPE or pLT. This was felt to be related to the increased surgical experience in transplanting patients after KPE and not to any significant paradigm shifts in the post-operative management either after the KPE or the transplant. The surgical team remained constant over the time span of both eras examined.

Another factor testifying to the increased surgical experience in transplanting complex patients is the statistically lower rate of retransplantation in the modern era in both the KPE and pLT groups.

Patients in the pLT group had a higher PELD score in the modern era and presented at a later age in both eras. Despite these disadvantages, results in the pLT group were comparable to the KPE group. This may explain the trend in a higher transplant admission cost for the pLT group. The authors recognize that the PELD score is an imperfect metric to reflect the severity of disease in children that underestimates pediatric waitlist mortality [23] and that modifications to the scoring are needed to better attest of the status of patients, and potentially decrease the request of exception points. However, one might speculate that if pLT were done in more patients who presented earlier and would normally be considered for a KPE, the overall morbidity would be reduced below what was observed in both groups in the present study. The key is how to select those 30–50% of patients who fail the KPE within two years so they could be spared surgery with no apparent benefit.

A higher PELD score in patients who received a pLT in the modern era did not translate into a higher number of admissions while on the liver transplant waitlist. Conversely, having undergone a previous KPE did not affect the rate of hospital admissions for complications of ESLD except for admissions for cholangitis. However, while all patients in the pLT group were diagnosed and managed at our institution until transplant, 45% of patients in the KPE group had their KPE done at an outside institution. Therefore, hospital admissions that occurred at outside institutions while being active on the transplant waitlist were not captured in our analysis and could explain why the difference in cost of admissions was not significantly lower for the pLT group.

Improvements in both post-transplant medical as well as surgical care has led to excellent survival after liver transplant for pediatric patients with BA [24]. Our experience with pLT showed an excellent 100% patient survival at 1 year from listing and 1 year after transplant, and comparable 3-year patient and graft survival to patients transplanted after

KPE. This was similar to the findings from other published studies [9,25,26]. However, a recent study reported superior long-term survival outcomes for pLT [10]. This study was done by using a large database and based its patient selection on billing codes for diagnosis and surgical procedures. Surprisingly, their rate of pLT was 50% which is much higher than any previously reported rates and calls into question the accuracy of the methods. Additionally, it does not take into account patients who underwent their KPE in another state [27]. While single-center retrospective studies lack the power to show significant association, large database studies lack granularity, accuracy and stringent data verification processes, and their results should, therefore, be interpreted with caution.

It is currently difficult, if not impossible, to predict which patient with BA will experience early failure after KPE. The development of a predictive score based on pre-KPE factors would help identify patients without ESLD at high risk for early failure in whom a pLT could be recommended. Pre-KPE histological criteria have been proposed as a means to predict successful bile drainage after a KPE [28], but it has been difficult to reproduce those results. A Taiwanese study suggested a pLT be discussed with parents of children with BA unless they have no living donor available [26]. Suggesting a higher number of patients may undergo a pLT would raise the question of organ shortage and worsening waitlist mortality. Additionally, the waitlist mortality is already the highest in patients less than 1 year of age [29]. In our study, the only waitlist mortalities occurred in children listed after KPE. The authors believe that if policies were established to ensure the splitting of all liver suitable for split liver transplant (intent-to-split policy), the waitlist mortality could be significantly reduced, as has been shown in other countries [30], despite potentially increasing the number of pLT. Segmental grafts have been shown to have beneficial post-transplant outcomes, including reduced incidence of hepatic artery thrombosis due to the large size of donor vessels [31]. ABO incompatible liver transplantation can also be used safely in infants less than 12 months given the immaturity of their immune system [32]. Lastly, promoting living donation in centers able to perform technical variant graft transplants would help reduce the waitlist mortality.

The Kasai operation remains the treatment of choice at the moment for all babies diagnosed with biliary atresia unless the child demonstrates clear signs of deteriorating liver function. However, in studies from many centers, it has been demonstrated that there is a high failure rate of the KPE even in children with early diagnosis and before the onset of liver failure [7]. Even though our results show no obvious disadvantage in doing the actual transplant operation after a failed KPE, those children will have been subjected to a prior operation that yielded no benefit, with considerable expenditures and with the obvious consequences of suffering through a major operation. The key to adopting a more selective use of the KPE in the treatment of children with BA is to develop accurate and reliable predictors of failure in the approximately 30% of children who need a transplant within 2 years of the KPE. Until the success of the KPE in delaying the need for a transplant approaches 100% success either by immunological or anti-proliferative adjuncts to surgery, a primary liver transplant with a success rate that approaches 100% should be considered in any child who would be predicted to have an unfavorable result after a KPE.

The authors recognize limitations to their study. It is a small retrospective single center study. However, as mentioned earlier, while it lacks the power of a large population sample, it allows for thorough data verification and accuracy when compared to large databases results. The study period extended over 23 years and the management of patients with BA has evolved over time. However, it was not as different as the modern management as other studies who reported and compared the use of other biliary drainage procedure than KPE.

In conclusion, primary liver transplantation leads to similar outcomes when compared to transplant after early failure of a Kasai portoenterostomy with less mortality on the waitlist. It is possible that a larger multicenter retrospective review followed by a prospective study may show the benefits of performing a primary liver transplant in selected children who are predicted to have a poor outcome after a Kasai procedure.

Author Contributions: Conceptualization, R.S.; Methodology, C.P.L., J.P.L., K.A.B. and R.S.; Software, C.P.L. and K.A.B.; Validation, C.P.L., K.A.B. and R.S.; Formal Analysis, C.P.L. and K.A.B.; Investigation, J.P.L., C.P.L. and K.A.B.; Resources, K.A.B. and C.P.L.; Data Curation, J.P.L., C.P.L. and K.A.B.; Writing—Original Draft Preparation, C.P.L.; Writing—Review and Editing, C.P.L., J.P.L., K.A.B. and R.S.; Visualization, R.S.; Supervision, R.S.; Project Administration, R.S. and K.A.B.; Funding Acquisition, R.S. All authors have read and agreed to the published version of the manuscript.

Funding: We acknowledge support from the Robert E. Schneider Foundation in conducting the research for this work.

Institutional Review Board Statement: The study was conducted in accordance with the Declaration of Helsinki and approved by the Institutional Review Board (IRB 2013-15357 and 2007-12989).

Informed Consent Statement: Patient consent was waived because the research study and disclosed patient health information involved no more than a minimal risk to the subjects.

Data Availability Statement: The data that support the findings of this study are available from the corresponding author upon reasonable request.

Acknowledgments: All members who participated in the study were included in the authors.

Conflicts of Interest: The authors have no conflict of interest to declare. The authors have no commercial interest in any product mentioned or concept discussed in this article.

Abbreviations

BA	Biliary atresia
CPI	Consumer price index
ESLD	End-stage liver disease
ICU	Intensive care unit
INR	International normalized ratio
IR	Interventional radiology
KPE	Kasai portoenterostomy
LDLT	Living donor liver transplantation
OSH	Outside hospital
PELD	Pediatric end-stage liver disease
PHIS	Pediatric Health Information System
pLT	Primary liver transplantation
pRBC	Packed red blood cells
USD	United States dollars

References

1. Nizery, L.; Chardot, C.; Sissaoui, S.; Capito, C.; Henrion-Caude, A.; Debray, D.; Girard, M. Biliary atresia: Clinical advances and perspectives. *Clin. Res. Hepatol. Gastroenterol.* **2016**, *40*, 281–287. [CrossRef] [PubMed]
2. Kasai, M.; Suzuki, S. A new operation for "non-correctable" biliary atresia-portoenterostomy. *Shijitsu* **1959**, *13*, 733–739.
3. Shneider, B.L.; Magee, J.C.; Karpen, S.J.; Rand, E.B.; Narkewicz, M.R.; Bass, L.M.; Schwarz, K.; Whitington, P.F.; Bezerra, J.A.; Kerkar, N.; et al. Total Serum Bilirubin within 3 Months of Hepatoportoenterostomy Predicts Short-Term Outcomes in Biliary Atresia. *J. Pediatr.* **2016**, *170*, 211–217. [CrossRef] [PubMed]
4. Otte, J.B.; de Ville de Goyet, J.; Reding, R.; Hausleithner, V.; Sokal, E.; Chardot, C.; Debande, B. Sequential treatment of biliary atresia with Kasai portoenterostomy and liver transplantation: A review. *Hepatology* **1994**, *20*, 41S–48S. [PubMed]
5. Davenport, M.; De Ville de Goyet, J.; Stringer, M.D.; Mieli-Vergani, G.; Kelly, D.A.; McClean, P.; Spitz, L. Seamless management of biliary atresia in England and Wales (1999–2002). *Lancet* **2004**, *363*, 1354–1357. [CrossRef]
6. Superina, R.; Magee, J.C.; Brandt, M.L.; Healey, P.J.; Tiao, G.; Ryckman, F.; Karrer, F.M.; Iyer, K.; Fecteau, A.; West, K.; et al. The anatomic pattern of biliary atresia identified at time of Kasai hepatoportoenterostomy and early postoperative clearance of jaundice are significant predictors of transplant-free survival. *Ann. Surg.* **2011**, *254*, 577–585. [CrossRef]
7. Superina, R. Biliary atresia and liver transplantation: Results and thoughts for primary liver transplantation in select patients. *Pediatr. Surg. Int.* **2017**, *33*, 1297–1304. [CrossRef]
8. Wang, P.; Xun, P.; He, K.; Cai, W. Comparison of liver transplantation outcomes in biliary atresia patients with and without prior portoenterostomy: A meta-analysis. *Dig. Liver Dis.* **2016**, *48*, 347–352. [CrossRef]
9. Chardot, C.; Buet, C.; Serinet, M.O.; Golmard, J.L.; Lachaux, A.; Roquelaure, B.; Gottrand, F.; Broue, P.; Dabadie, A.; Gauthier, F.; et al. Improving outcomes of biliary atresia: French national series 1986–2009. *J. Hepatol.* **2013**, *58*, 1209–1217. [CrossRef]

10. LeeVan, E.; Matsuoka, L.; Cao, S.; Groshen, S.; Alexopoulos, S. Biliary-Enteric Drainage vs Primary Liver Transplant as Initial Treatment for Children with Biliary Atresia. *JAMA Surg.* **2019**, *154*, 26–32. [CrossRef]
11. Neto, J.S.; Feier, F.H.; Bierrenbach, A.L.; Toscano, C.M.; Fonseca, E.A.; Pugliese, R.; Candido, H.L.; Benavides, M.R.; Porta, G.; Chapchap, P. Impact of Kasai portoenterostomy on liver transplantation outcomes: A retrospective cohort study of 347 children with biliary atresia. *Liver Transplant.* **2015**, *21*, 922–927. [CrossRef] [PubMed]
12. Sandler, A.D.; Azarow, K.S.; Superina, R.A. The impact of a previous Kasai procedure on liver transplantation for biliary atresia. *J. Pediatr. Surg.* **1997**, *32*, 416–419. [CrossRef]
13. Davenport, M.; Ong, E.; Sharif, K.; Alizai, N.; McClean, P.; Hadzic, N.; Kelly, D.A. Biliary atresia in England and Wales: Results of centralization and new benchmark. *J. Pediatr. Surg.* **2011**, *46*, 1689–1694. [CrossRef] [PubMed]
14. de Vries, W.; de Langen, Z.J.; Groen, H.; Scheenstra, R.; Peeters, P.M.; Hulscher, J.B.; Verkade, H.J.; Netherlands Study Group of Biliary Atresia and Registry. Biliary atresia in the Netherlands: Outcome of patients diagnosed between 1987 and 2008. *J. Pediatr.* **2012**, *160*, 638–644.e632. [CrossRef] [PubMed]
15. Schreiber, R.A.; Barker, C.C.; Roberts, E.A.; Martin, S.R.; Canadian Pediatric Hepatology Research Group. Biliary atresia in Canada: The effect of centre caseload experience on outcome. *J. Pediatr. Gastroenterol. Nutr.* **2010**, *51*, 61–65. [CrossRef] [PubMed]
16. Wildhaber, B.E.; Majno, P.; Mayr, J.; Zachariou, Z.; Hohlfeld, J.; Schwoebel, M.; Kistler, W.; Meuli, M.; Le Coultre, C.; Mentha, G.; et al. Biliary atresia: Swiss national study, 1994–2004. *J. Pediatr. Gastroenterol. Nutr.* **2008**, *46*, 299–307. [CrossRef]
17. Leonhardt, J.; Kuebler, J.F.; Leute, P.J.; Turowski, C.; Becker, T.; Pfister, E.D.; Ure, B.; Petersen, C. Biliary atresia: Lessons learned from the voluntary German registry. *Eur. J. Pediatr. Surg.* **2011**, *21*, 82–87. [CrossRef]
18. Alexopoulos, S.P.; Merrill, M.; Kin, C.; Matsuoka, L.; Dorey, F.; Concepcion, W.; Esquivel, C.; Bonham, A. The impact of hepatic portoenterostomy on liver transplantation for the treatment of biliary atresia: Early failure adversely affects outcome. *Pediatr. Transplant.* **2012**, *16*, 373–378. [CrossRef]
19. Nio, M.; Ohi, R.; Miyano, T.; Saeki, M.; Shiraki, K.; Tanaka, K.; Japanese Biliary Atresia Registry. Five- and 10-year survival rates after surgery for biliary atresia: A report from the Japanese Biliary Atresia Registry. *J. Pediatr. Surg.* **2003**, *38*, 997–1000. [CrossRef]
20. Uto, K.; Inomata, Y.; Sakamoto, S.; Hibi, T.; Sasaki, H.; Nio, M. A multicenter study of primary liver transplantation for biliary atresia in Japan. *Pediatr. Surg. Int.* **2019**, *35*, 1223–1229. [CrossRef]
21. Millis, J.M.; Brems, J.J.; Hiatt, J.R.; Klein, A.S.; Ashizawa, T.; Ramming, K.P.; Quinones-Baldrich, W.J.; Busuttil, R.W. Orthotopic liver transplantation for biliary atresia. Evolution of management. *Arch. Surg.* **1988**, *123*, 1237–1239. [CrossRef] [PubMed]
22. Wood, R.P.; Langnas, A.N.; Stratta, R.J.; Pillen, T.J.; Williams, L.; Lindsay, S.; Meiergerd, D.; Shaw, B.W., Jr. Optimal therapy for patients with biliary atresia: Portoenterostomy ("Kasai" procedures) versus primary transplantation. *J. Pediatr. Surg.* **1990**, *25*, 153–160. [CrossRef]
23. Chang, C.H.; Bryce, C.L.; Shneider, B.L.; Yabes, J.G.; Ren, Y.; Zenarosa, G.L.; Tomko, H.; Donnell, D.M.; Squires, R.H.; Roberts, M.S. Accuracy of the Pediatric End-stage Liver Disease Score in Estimating Pretransplant Mortality among Pediatric Liver Transplant Candidates. *JAMA Pediatr.* **2018**, *172*, 1070–1077. [CrossRef] [PubMed]
24. Taylor, S.A.; Venkat, V.; Arnon, R.; Gopalareddy, V.V.; Rosenthal, P.; Erinjeri, J.; Anand, R.; Daniel, J.F.; Society of Pediatric Liver Transplantation. Improved Outcomes for Liver Transplantation in Patients with Biliary Atresia Since Pediatric End-Stage Liver Disease Implementation: Analysis of the Society of Pediatric Liver Transplantation Registry. *J. Pediatr.* **2020**, *219*, 89–97. [CrossRef]
25. Cowles, R.A.; Lobritto, S.J.; Ventura, K.A.; Harren, P.A.; Gelbard, R.; Emond, J.C.; Altman, R.P.; Jan, D.M. Timing of liver transplantation in biliary atresia-results in 71 children managed by a multidisciplinary team. *J. Pediatr. Surg.* **2008**, *43*, 1605–1609. [CrossRef]
26. Tiao, M.M.; Yang, C.Y.; Tsai, S.S.; Chen, C.L.; Kuo, H.W. Liver transplantation for biliary atresia in Taiwan: A national study. *Transplant. Proc.* **2008**, *40*, 3569–3570. [CrossRef]
27. Kim, H.B.; Elisofon, S.A. Biliary Atresia: Biliary-Enteric Drainage or Primary Liver Transplant? *Hepatology* **2020**, *71*, 751–752. [CrossRef]
28. Azarow, K.S.; Phillips, M.J.; Sandler, A.D.; Hagerstrand, I.; Superina, R.A. Biliary atresia: Should all patients undergo a portoenterostomy? *J. Pediatr. Surg.* **1997**, *32*, 168–172, discussion 172–164. [CrossRef]
29. Kwong, A.J.; Kim, W.R.; Lake, J.R.; Smith, J.M.; Schladt, D.P.; Skeans, M.A.; Noreen, S.M.; Foutz, J.; Booker, S.E.; Cafarella, M.; et al. OPTN/SRTR 2019 Annual Data Report: Liver. *Am. J. Transplant.* **2021**, *21* (Suppl. 2), 208–315. [CrossRef]
30. Battula, N.R.; Platto, M.; Anbarasan, R.; Perera, M.T.; Ong, E.; Roll, G.R.; Ferraz Neto, B.H.; Mergental, H.; Isaac, J.; Muiesan, P.; et al. Intention to Split Policy: A Successful Strategy in a Combined Pediatric and Adult Liver Transplant Center. *Ann. Surg.* **2017**, *265*, 1009–1015. [CrossRef]
31. Ebel, N.H.; Hsu, E.K.; Dick, A.A.S.; Shaffer, M.L.; Carlin, K.; Horslen, S.P. Decreased Incidence of Hepatic Artery Thrombosis in Pediatric Liver Transplantation Using Technical Variant Grafts: Report of the Society of Pediatric Liver Transplantation Experience. *J. Pediatr.* **2020**, *226*, 195–201. [CrossRef] [PubMed]
32. Egawa, H.; Oike, F.; Buhler, L.; Shapiro, A.M.; Minamiguchi, S.; Haga, H.; Uryuhara, K.; Kiuchi, T.; Kaihara, S.; Tanaka, K. Impact of recipient age on outcome of ABO-incompatible living-donor liver transplantation. *Transplantation* **2004**, *77*, 403–411. [CrossRef] [PubMed]

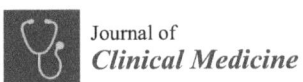
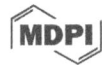

Article

Hepatic Ly6C^{Lo} Non-Classical Monocytes Have Increased Nr4a1 (Nur77) in Murine Biliary Atresia

Sarah Mohamedaly [1,2], Claire S. Levy [1,2], Cathrine Korsholm [3], Anas Alkhani [1,2], Katherine Rosenberg [1,2], Judith F. Ashouri [4] and Amar Nijagal [1,2,5,6,*]

[1] Department of Surgery, University of California, San Francisco, CA 94143, USA
[2] Liver Center, University of California, San Francisco, CA 94143, USA
[3] Department of Comparative Pediatrics and Nutrition, University of Copenhagen, 1870 Frederiksberg, Denmark
[4] Rosalind Russell and Ephraim P. Engleman Rheumatology Research Center, Department of Medicine, University of California, San Francisco, CA 94143, USA
[5] The Pediatric Liver Center, UCSF Benioff Children's Hospital, San Francisco, CA 94143, USA
[6] Eli and Edythe Broad Center of Regeneration Medicine, University of California, San Francisco, CA 94143, USA
* Correspondence: amar.nijagal@ucsf.edu

Abstract: Biliary atresia (BA) is a rapidly progressive perinatal inflammatory disease, resulting in liver failure. Hepatic Ly6C^{Lo} non-classical monocytes promote the resolution of perinatal liver inflammation during rhesus rotavirus-mediated (RRV) BA in mice. In this study, we aim to investigate the effects of inflammation on the transcription factor Nr4a1, a known regulator of non-classical monocytes. Nr4a1-GFP reporter mice were injected with PBS for control or RRV within 24 h of delivery to induce perinatal liver inflammation. GFP expression on myeloid immune populations in the liver and bone marrow (BM) was quantified 3 and 14 days after injection using flow cytometry. Statistical significance was determined using a student's t-test and ANOVA, with a p-value < 0.05 for significance. Our results demonstrate that non-classical monocytes in the neonatal liver exhibit the highest mean fluorescence intensity (MFI) of Nr4a1 (Ly6C^{Lo} MFI 6344 vs. neutrophils 3611 p < 0.001; macrophages 2782; p < 0.001; and Ly6C^{Hi} classical monocytes 4485; p < 0.0002). During inflammation, hepatic Ly6C^{Lo} non-classical monocytes showed a significant increase in Nr4a1 expression intensity from 6344 to 7600 (p = 0.012), while Nr4a1 expression remained unchanged on the other myeloid populations. These findings highlight the potential of using Nr4a1 as a regulator of neonatal hepatic Ly6C^{Lo} non-classical monocytes to mitigate perinatal liver inflammation.

Keywords: perinatal liver inflammation; innate immune system; monocytes; biliary atresia; cholangiopathy

Citation: Mohamedaly, S.; Levy, C.S.; Korsholm, C.; Alkhani, A.; Rosenberg, K.; Ashouri, J.F.; Nijagal, A. Hepatic Ly6C^{Lo} Non-Classical Monocytes Have Increased Nr4a1 (Nur77) in Murine Biliary Atresia. J. Clin. Med. 2022, 11, 5290. https://doi.org/10.3390/jcm11185290

Academic Editor: Claus Petersen

Received: 28 July 2022
Accepted: 3 September 2022
Published: 8 September 2022

Publisher's Note: MDPI stays neutral with regard to jurisdictional claims in published maps and institutional affiliations.

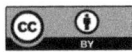

Copyright: © 2022 by the authors. Licensee MDPI, Basel, Switzerland. This article is an open access article distributed under the terms and conditions of the Creative Commons Attribution (CC BY) license (https://creativecommons.org/licenses/by/4.0/).

1. Introduction

Biliary atresia (BA) is a perinatal hepatic inflammatory disease that results in rapid obliteration of the biliary tree, leading to cirrhosis and requiring liver transplantation. The etiology of BA is not fully understood, but multiple factors including genetic predisposition, immune dysregulation, toxins, and infections are thought to ultimately result in an inflammatory cascade within the liver [1]. Although a well-controlled acute inflammatory response is essential for the resolution of tissue injury, a dysregulated inflammatory response can lead to the development of pathological inflammation and devastating long-term consequences [2]. Thus, understanding how perinatal hepatic inflammation is propagated is an essential prerequisite for developing therapeutic targets that can interrupt this inflammatory cascade and alleviate the need for liver transplantation in patients with BA.

The innate immune system, particularly through the actions of monocytes, plays a crucial role in the initiation and resolution of inflammation [3–6]. There are two main subtypes of monocytes: Ly6C^{Hi} classical monocytes are pro-inflammatory [3,7,8], and

Ly6C^{Lo} non-classical monocytes are pro-reparative [9–12]. In a murine model of BA, we have demonstrated that the relative abundance of Ly6C^{Lo} non-classical monocytes promotes the resolution of periportal liver inflammation and confers protection to liver disease in neonates [12]. However, the development and differentiation of Ly6C^{Lo} non-classical monocytes in neonatal mice are not well understood. In adult murine bone marrow, the transcription factor Nr4a1 has been shown to play a critical role in mediating the differentiation and survival of Ly6C^{Lo} non-classical monocytes [13]. Nr4a1 is an orphan nuclear receptor and a member of the Nr4a family of intracellular transcription factors [14,15]. The Nr4a1 family is widely expressed across various tissues, and its diverse scope of actions includes DNA repair, cell proliferation, differentiation, apoptosis, migration, metabolism, and inflammation [14,16]. Such diverse roles stem from the fact that Nr4a1 activity is tissue- and environment-specific [17–19].

Given the importance of Ly6C^{Lo} non-classical monocytes in promoting the resolution of perinatal liver inflammation, and our current understanding of Nr4a1 as a monocyte regulator in the adult murine bone marrow, we sought to investigate the effects of inflammation on Nr4a1 expression in a murine model of BA. Understanding the factors that regulate non-classical monocytes during perinatal inflammation is particularly important, because the early dysregulation of monocyte development can contribute to detrimental sequelae of BA.

2. Materials and Methods

Mice. BALB/c wildtype mice were obtained from the National Cancer Institute (Wilmington, MA) and Jackson labs (Bar Harbor, ME). Nr4a1-GFP reporter mice were originally described by Zikherman et al. [20] and were backcrossed onto the BALB/c background for >12 generations. All mouse experiments were approved by the UCSF Institutional Animal Care and Use Committee, and animals received humane care in accordance with the criteria outlined in the Guide for the Care and Use of Laboratory Animals. Mice were euthanized by decapitation (pups < 7 days old) or carbon dioxide inhalation (pups $\geq$ 7 days of age).

Creation of single-cell suspensions from fetal and neonatal livers. The liver and bone marrow were isolated from euthanized mice. To create single-cell suspensions, livers were weighed upon extraction and washed in cold PBS over ice for 5 min. Using sterile fine surgical scissors, livers were cut into small pieces to facilitate mechanical dissociation in cold PBS (for pups at 3 days of life) and in 2.5 mg/mL Liberase (Roche, Indianapolis, IN, USA, 05401119001) homogenization buffer (for pups at 14 days of life). Once the liver was completely homogenized, the cell suspension was passed through a 100 µm cell strainer to remove any undigested tissue or debris and to create SCS. Neonatal bone marrow was extracted by harvesting the sacral spine, pelvic bone, both femurs and tibias from each pup and washing them in cold PBS over ice for 5 min followed by crushing the bones using a pestle and mortar and washing the cells using cold PBS once the bones were completely crushed. Washed cells were then passed through a 100 µm cell strainer to remove any undigested bone or debris and to create an SCS. Both the liver and BM SCS were then incubated in 1 mL of ACK Lysis buffer (Gibco, Waltham, MA, USA, A10492-01) over ice to remove red blood cells, followed by manual cell counting to determine cell count and viability. Cells were also stained using Ghost Live/Dead stain (Tonbo, San Diego, CA, USA, 13-0870-T100) to determine cell viability in analysis.

Flow cytometry. Liver and bone marrow single-cell suspensions were stained using the following antibodies: Cd11c, clone N418 (Biolegend, San Diego, CA, USA, 117339); Ly6C, clone HK1.4 (Biolegend, 128035); MHCII, clone M5/114.15.2 (eBioscience, Waltham, MA, USA, 48-5321-82); Cd45, clone 30-F11 (eBioscience, 56-0451-82); Cd11b, clone M1/70 (eBioscience, 47-0112-82); Cd64, clone X54-5/7.1 (BD Biosciences, Franklin Lakes, NJ, USA, 741024); Ly6g, clone 1A8 (BD Biosciences, 560601); Fc block Cd16/Cd32, clone 2.4G2 (BD Biosciences, 553142); Ly6g, RB6-8c5 (Tonbo, San Diego, CA, USA, 60-5931); Ghost

(Tonbo, 13-0870-T100). Flow cytometric data were acquired on a BD LSRII Fortessa X20 and analyzed using FlowJo (v10.8.1 Franklin Lakes, NJ, USA).

Postnatal model of perinatal inflammation. Rhesus rotavirus (RRV) and Cercopithecus aethiops kidney epithelial (MA104) cells were obtained from Dr. Henry Greenberg (Stanford University, Palo Alto, CA, USA). The virus was grown and titered in MA104 cells. To induce postnatal hepatic inflammation, P0 pups were injected intraperitoneally with 1.5×10^6 focus-forming units (ffu) 24 h after delivery. Controls were injected with PBS using the same technique.

Data analysis. To compare the two groups, the unpaired t-test with Welch's correction, the non-parametric Mann–Whitney test, and the Chi-square test were used, respectively, for normally distributed variables, non-normally distributed variables, and proportions. A one-way ANOVA with Tukey's multiple comparisons test was used to compare multiple groups. Myeloid populations after Ab-mediated depletion were quantified by dividing the number of live cells of interest by organ weight. Graphpad Prism 9.0 (San Diego, CA, USA) was used to generate graphs and perform statistical analysis.

3. Results

$Ly6C^{Lo}$ non-classical monocytes reside in the neonatal liver. We quantified the proportion of mature myeloid populations in the neonatal liver and bone marrow under homeostatic conditions. Using flow cytometry, we identified neutrophils (Ly6G+, MHCII−), macrophages (CD64+, CD11b+/−), and monocytes (CD64− CD11b+). We further separated monocytes into $Ly6C^{Hi}$ classical and $Ly6C^{Lo}$ non-classical monocytes (Figure 1a). Monocytes, particularly $Ly6C^{Lo}$ non-classical monocytes, were abundant in the liver but not in the bone marrow (Figure 1b). This finding was similar to that derived in our previous work, demonstrating the relative abundance of $Ly6C^{Lo}$ non-classical monocytes in the late-gestation fetus [12].

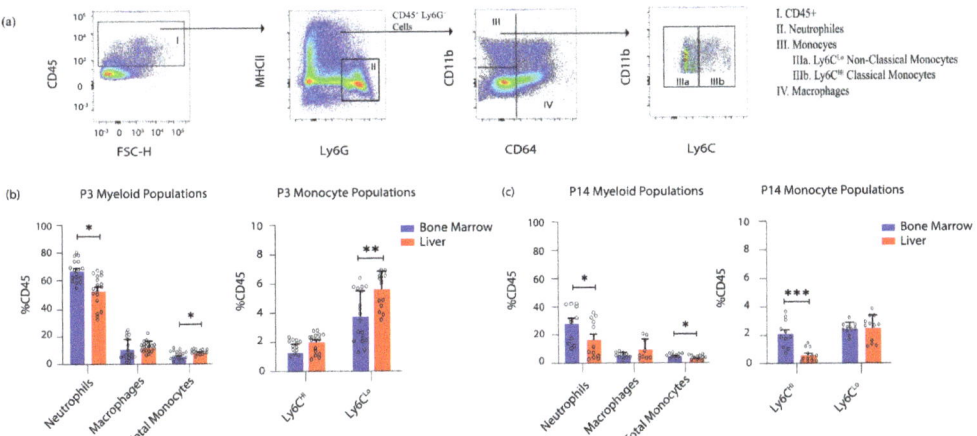

Figure 1. Pro-reparative $Ly6C^{Lo}$ non-classical monocytes reside in the liver at the early neonatal timepoint. (**a**) Myeloid populations including neutrophils, macrophages, $Ly6C^{Hi}$ classical monocytes and $Ly6C^{Lo}$ non-classical monocytes identified by flow cytometry. (**b**) Myeloid populations at an early neonatal timepoint (P3) as a proportion of all CD45% leukocytes. The neonatal liver ($n = 19$) harvests significantly more monocytes, particularly $Ly6C^{Lo}$ non-classical monocytes, compared to the BM ($n = 18$) (BM 3.76% vs liver 5.62%; $p = 0.0015$). (**c**) At the juvenile timepoint (P14) the liver ($n = 12$) no longer harvests monocytic populations. $Ly6C^{Hi}$ classical monocytes predominately reside in the BM ($n = 11$) at this point (BM 2.11% vs liver 0.58%, $p < 0.0001$). * $p \leq 0.05$; ** $p \leq 0.01$; *** $p \leq 0.001$.

In P3 pups, monocytes comprised ~8% of all CD45+ leukocytes in the liver, compared to ~6% in the bone marrow ($p = 0.018$). $Ly6C^{Lo}$ non-classical monocytes were the predominant monocyte subset in the liver (5.62% vs. 3.76% for bone marrow, $p = 0.001$) (Figure 1b). Higher proportions of neutrophils were seen in the bone marrow than in the liver (69.78% vs. 53.43%, $p = 0.002$), whereas macrophages comprised ~12% in both organs. In juvenile mice, monocytes no longer predominated in the liver at P14; instead, these were seen in higher proportions in the bone marrow (4.59% vs. liver 3.1%, $p = 0.01$) (Figure 1c). Ly6C^{Hi} classical monocytes were seen in higher proportions in the bone marrow (2.11% vs. liver 0.58%, $p < 0.0001$), whereas Ly6C^{Lo} non-classical monocytes comprised ~2.5% of all leukocytes in both organs at this timepoint (Figure 1c). Monocytes overall, and specifically Ly6C^{Lo} non-classical monocytes, were present in higher proportions in the P3 liver than in the bone marrow, and made up a smaller proportion of total leukocytes in P14 mice than in neonates (Figure 1c).

Nr4a1 expression is highest in Ly6C^{Lo} non-classical monocytes compared to other myeloid populations in the neonatal liver. We characterized Nr4a1 expression in mature myeloid populations under homeostatic conditions in the neonatal liver and bone marrow. To quantify the expression of Nr4a1, we used a reporter mouse in which the expression of enhanced green fluorescent protein (GFP) is under the control of the Nr4a1 regulatory region [20]. We observed that high proportions of all myeloid populations expressed Nr4a1 (%GFP-positive cells) in both the neonatal liver and the bone marrow (Figure 2a–d). In particular, significantly higher proportions of neutrophils, macrophages, and Ly6C^{Hi} classical monocytes in the neonatal bone marrow expressed Nr4a1 compared to the neonatal liver (Neutrophils: 80.03% vs. 66.52%; $p = 0.02$. Macrophages: 53.46% vs. 33.83%; $p < 0.001$. Ly6C^{Hi} classical monocytes: 66.13% vs. 56.51%; $p = 0.03$) (Figure 2a–c). In contrast, relatively equal proportions of Ly6C^{Lo} non-classical monocytes expressed Nr4a1 in both the neonatal bone marrow and liver (66.60% vs. 68.42%; $p = 0.67$) (Figure 2d).

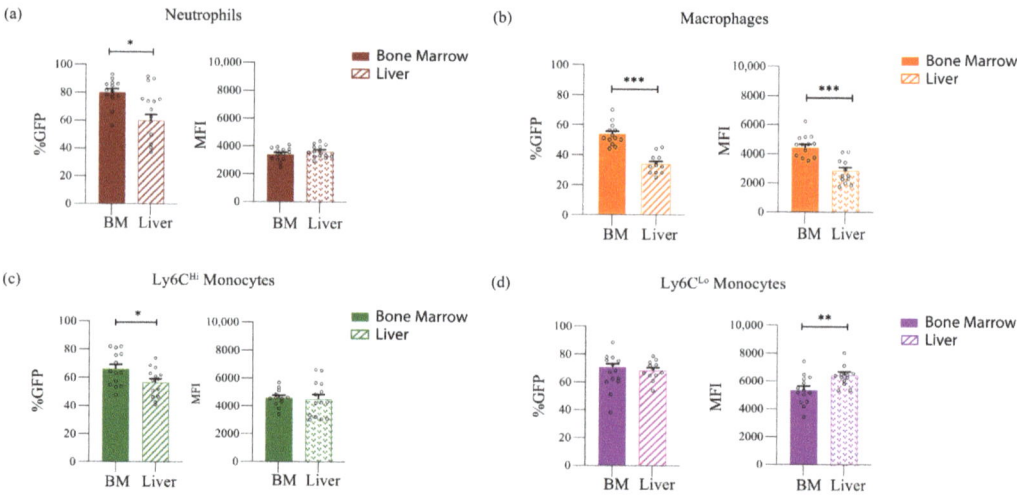

Figure 2. Cont.

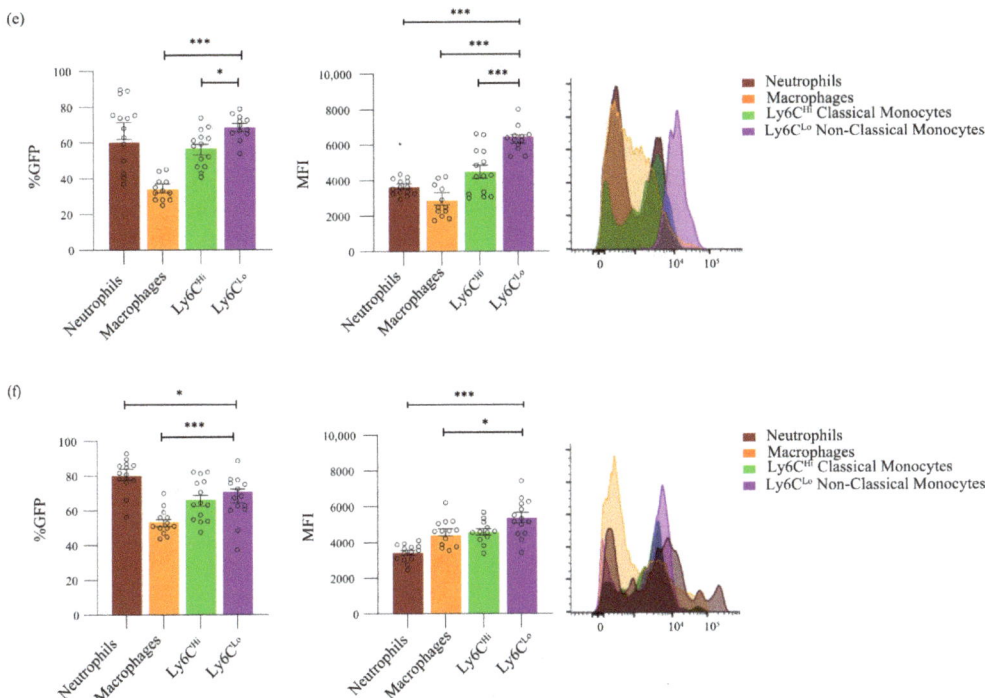

Figure 2. Ly6C^{Lo} **non-classical monocytes exhibit the highest expression of Nr4a1.** (**a**) Nr4a1 expression on neutrophils as %GFP positive ($n = 14$; BM 80.03% vs liver 66.52%; $p = 0.02$). Both organs exhibit similar intensity of expression, represented as Mean Fluorescence Intensity (MFI) (BM 3408 vs liver 3611; $p = 0.25$). (**b**) Neonatal BM macrophages show higher expression of Nr4a1 compared to the liver ($n = 14$; BM %GFP 53.46% vs liver 33.83; $p < 0.001$) (BM MFI 4554 vs liver 2782; $p < 0.0001$). (**c**) Higher proportion of Ly6CHi classical monocytes exhibit Nr4a1 expression in the neonatal BM ($n = 14$; BM 66.13% vs Liver 56.51; $p = 0.03$); however, MFI is similar between both organs (BM 4575 vs liver 4485; $p = 0.82$). (**d**) High proportions of Ly6C^{Lo} non-classical monocytes exhibit Nr4a1 expression in both organs ($n = 14$; BM 66.60 vs liver 68.42%; $p = 0.67$); however, Ly6C^{Lo} non-classical monocytes in the neonatal liver show a higher intensity of expression (BM MFI 5338 vs liver 6344; $p = 0.009$). (**e**) Among the myeloid populations in the neonatal liver, Ly6C^{Lo} non-classical monocytes exhibit the highest expression of Nr4a1 compared to neutrophils (MFI 6344 vs 3611, respectively; $p < 0.0001$), macrophages (MFI 6344 vs 2782, respectively; $p < 0.001$), and Ly6C^{Hi} classical monocytes (MFI 6344 vs 4485, respectively; $p < 0.0002$). (**f**) Ly6C^{Lo} non-classical monocytes also exhibit the highest expression of Nr4a1 in the neonatal BM; however, the degree of intensity is significantly lower than in the liver. * $p \leq 0.05$; ** $p \leq 0.01$; *** $p \leq 0.001$.

Although Nr4a1 was expressed in moderately high proportions by neutrophils (Figure 2a), macrophages (Figure 2b) and monocyte subsets (Figure 2c,d), we evaluated the mean fluorescent intensity of Nr4a1 to quantify the level of Nr4a1 expression. Ly6C^{Lo} non-classical monocytes had significantly higher expression of Nr4a1 compared to populations in both the liver and the bone marrow (Figure 2e,f). Among the myeloid populations in the neonatal liver, Ly6C^{Lo} non-classical monocytes showed the highest intensity of Nr4a1 expression compared to neutrophils (MFI 6344 vs. 3611; $p < 0.001$), macrophages (MFI 6344 vs. 2782; $p < 0.001$), and Ly6C^{Hi} classical monocytes (MFI 6344 vs. 4485; $p < 0.0002$) (Figure 2e). Ly6C^{Lo} non-classical monocytes also exhibited the highest intensity of Nr4a1 expression in the neonatal bone marrow compared to other myeloid populations (Figure 2f); however, the Nr4a1 expression was significantly higher in liver Ly6C^{Lo} non-classical monocytes than in bone marrow Ly6C^{Lo} non-classical monocytes (MFI 6344 vs. 5338; $p = 0.009$) (Figure 2d). These results demonstrate that although Nr4a1 was present in high proportions in most myeloid populations, the expression was highest in Ly6C^{Lo} non-classical monocytes in the neonatal liver.

Perinatal liver inflammation leads to increased expression of Nr4a1 in hepatic Ly6C^{Lo} non-classical monocytes. Having shown that Nr4a1 expression is environment-specific, we next quantified the proportion of mature myeloid populations, and characterized their Nr4a1 expression in the setting of inflammation in the neonatal bone marrow (Figure 3) and liver (Figure 4). We used the well-established murine model of BA, which involves the infection of neonatal pups with Rhesus rotavirus. The injection of RRV during the first 24 h of life results in weight loss, jaundice, and death in the majority of neonatal pups by 21 days [12,21–24]. The characteristic histologic findings after RRV infection include periportal inflammation, which is apparent within 3 days. Our thorough analysis of the immune cells involved in the pathogenesis of RRV-mediated inflammation has demonstrated a limited role for the adaptive immune system and type 2 immunity in the pathogenesis of RRV, and has implicated Ly6C^{Lo} non-classical monocytes in the resolution of murine BA [12].

In the neonatal bone marrow, the neutrophil population decreased during inflammation (WT 67.44% vs. RRV 46.49%; $p = 0.004$), whereas other myeloid populations remained unchanged (Figure 3a,b). Nr4a1 expression remained stable in neutrophils (Figure 3c), decreased in macrophages (WT 4416 vs. RRV 3739; $p = 0.04$) (Figure 3d) and Ly6C^{Lo} non-classical monocytes (WT 5338 vs. RRV 4089; $p = 0.003$) (Figure 3f), and increased in Ly6C^{Hi} classical monocytes (MFI WT 4575 vs. RRV 6259; $p = 0.0002$) (Figure 3e).

In the neonatal liver, the levels of hepatic macrophages decreased during inflammation (WT 11.76% vs. RRV 6.53%; $p < 0.0001$), as did Ly6C^{Lo} non-classical monocytes (WT 4.96% vs. RRV 3.12%; $p = 0.037$) (Figure 4a–c), but the proportions of hepatic neutrophils and Ly6C^{Hi} classical monocytes were unchanged (Figure 4a). Despite these decreases in hepatic macrophages and Ly6C^{Lo} non-classical monocytes, inflammatory conditions resulted in an increase in Nr4a1 expression in those myeloid populations. The proportion of macrophages expressing Nr4a1 increased to 45.73% (WT 33.38%, $p = 0.0078$), and the intensity of Nr4a1 expression also increased from 2848 to 3752 ($p = 0.013$) (Figure 4e). Approximately 70% of all hepatic Ly6C^{Lo} non-classical monocytes expressed Nr4a1 under homeostatic and inflammatory conditions, but the intensity of Nr4a1 expression increased significantly from 6344 to 7600 during inflammation ($p = 0.012$) (Figure 4g). Nr4a1 expression remained unchanged in hepatic neutrophils and Ly6C^{Hi} classical monocytes Figure 4d,f.

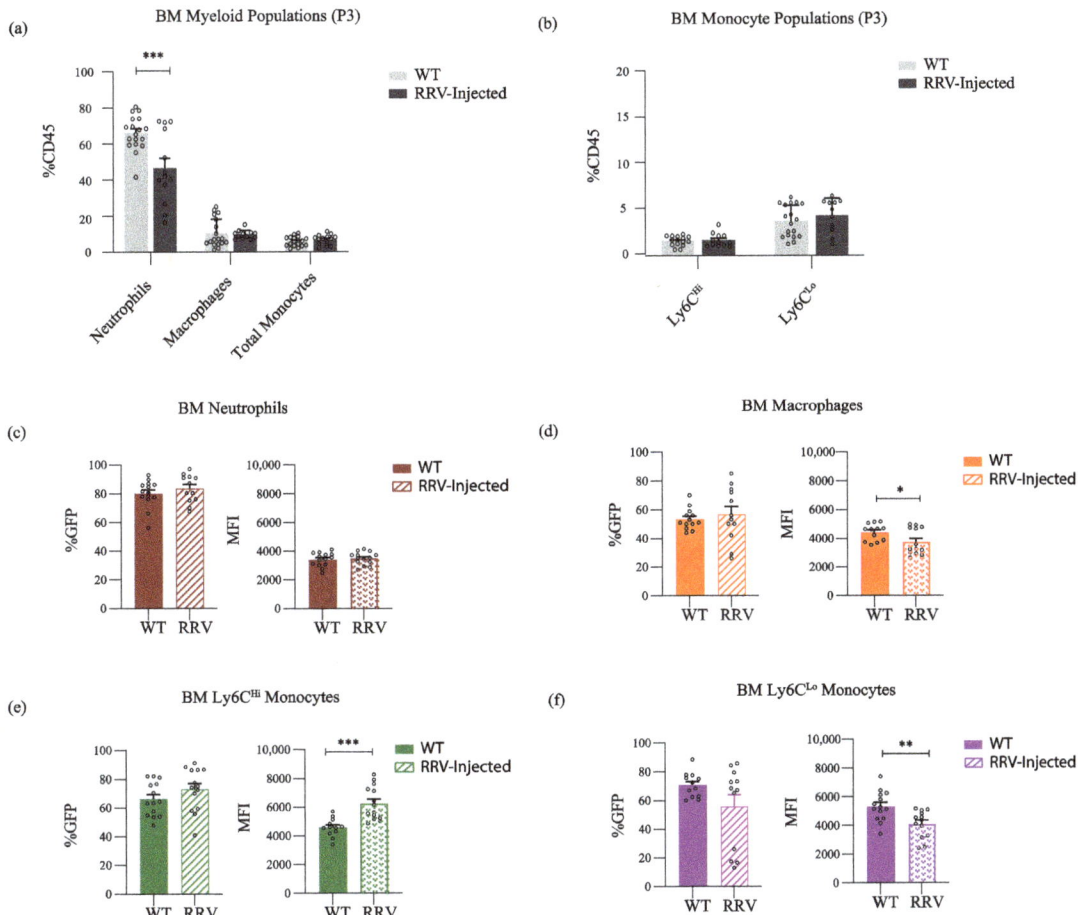

Figure 3. BM Ly6C^{Lo} non-classical monocytes decrease their Nr4a1 expression in the setting of inflammation. (**a**,**b**) Myeloid populations and monocyte subsets at (P3) as a proportion of all CD45% leukocytes under homeostatic (n = 18) and inflammatory (n = 14) conditions in the neonatal BM. (**c**–**f**) %GFP and intensity of Nr4a1 expression (MFI) on myeloid populations in the BM under homeostatic conditions (n = 14) and in the setting of inflammation (n = 14). * $p \leq 0.05$; ** $p \leq 0.01$; *** $p \leq 0.001$.

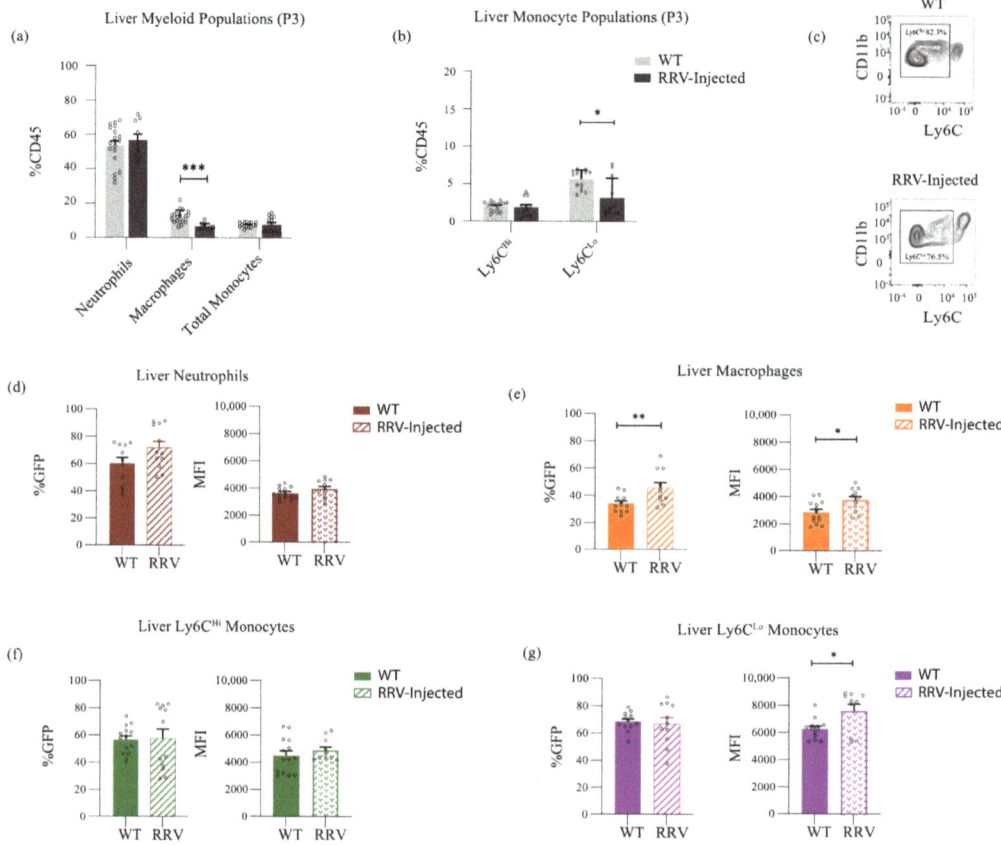

Figure 4. Ly6C^{Lo} non-classical monocytes increase Nr4a1 expression in the setting of inflammation. (**a,b**) Myeloid populations and monocyte subsets at (P3) as a proportion of all CD45% leukocytes under homeostatic ($n = 19$) and inflammatory ($n = 13$) conditions in the neonatal liver. (**c**) Reduction of Ly6C^{Lo} non-classical monocyte population in the liver by flow cytometry. (**d–g**) Intensity of Nr4a1 expression (MFI) is increased on macrophages and Ly6C^{Lo} non-classical monocytes in the setting of inflammation (WT $n = 14$, RRV $n = 12$). * $p \leq 0.05$; ** $p \leq 0.01$; *** $p \leq 0.001$.

4. Discussion

In this study, we hypothesized that Nr4a1 is important for Ly6C^{Lo} non-classical monocyte differentiation, and is therefore a key regulator of perinatal liver inflammation. Our results demonstrate that in the liver and bone marrow, Nr4a1 expression was highest among hepatic neonatal Ly6C^{Lo} non-classical monocytes compared to neutrophils, macrophages, and Ly6C^{Hi} classical monocytes. In a murine model of BA, although the levels of hepatic Ly6C^{Lo} non-classical monocytes decreased, their expression of Nr4a1 increased significantly. However, in the bone marrow, Nr4a1 expression decreased significantly during inflammation, but increased in Ly6C^{Hi} classical monocytes. Collectively, these results support the idea that Nr4a1 is an important transcription factor for the pro-reparative response mediated by hepatic Ly6C^{Lo} non-classical monocytes during inflammation in murine BA.

Ly6C^{Lo} non-classical monocytes have been shown to promote a pro-reparative response in the setting of inflammation, and specifically promote the resolution of periportal liver inflammation to confer protection to liver disease in murine neonates [9–12]. In our study, we demonstrate that the liver acts as a reservoir for Ly6C^{Lo} non-classical monocytes in neonatal mice before the physiologic homing process of hematopoietic cells to the bone marrow. While the homing process is a well-described phenomenon, the normal physiology and development of the murine hematopoietic system shortly before and after birth are not yet fully elucidated [25–27]. Hematopoietic cells have been examined extensively in the murine fetus [28–30]; however, mature cells at later stages of development, particularly in perinatal pups, have not been examined as thoroughly [31,32]. Hematopoietic cells are believed to migrate to the fetal liver at approximately day 10 post-coitus, and at or near birth, cells then migrate from the liver to the bone marrow, where they remain throughout the animal's adult life [25–27]. Our results demonstrate that by postnatal day 14, the myeloid populations predominately reside in the bone marrow, and the liver no longer maintains a significant proportion of monocytes. Not only does this finding clarify the timing of the homing process from the liver to the bone marrow, but it also highlights that the neonatal liver initially maintains a high proportion of the pro-reparative Ly6C^{Lo} non-classical monocytes, raising the possibility that these cells may confer resistance to perinatal injury.

Previous studies have demonstrated the importance of Nr4a1 in the differentiation and survival of the pro-reparative Ly6C^{Lo} non-classical monocytes [13,33]. Monocyte subsets arise from a common monocyte progenitor (cMoP) in the adult murine bone marrow, but the intricacies of this development remain poorly understood due to the challenges of lineage tracing [33]. The most accepted hypothesis currently supports the idea that cMoPs give rise to Ly6C^{Hi} classical monocytes, which can then differentiate into Ly6C^{Lo} non-classical monocytes [33–38]. Multiple transcription factors such as PU.1, C/EBP-β and IRF8 have been implicated at various stages of monocyte development [39]; however, Nr4a1 has been most notably shown to regulate the differentiation of Ly6C^{Lo} non-classical monocytes in the adult murine bone marrow [13]. The relationship between Nr4a1 and Ly6C^{Lo} non-classical monocytes in the perinatal period is largely unknown. Our results demonstrate that Nr4a1 expression is highest among Ly6C^{Lo} non-classical monocytes in the neonatal liver under homeostatic and inflammatory conditions. Despite the decrease in the proportion of Ly6C^{Lo} non-classical monocytes in the liver during inflammation, the intensity of Nr4a1 expression in this pro-reparative subset significantly increased in response to inflammation. These data suggest that a small population of Nr4a1^{Hi}Ly6C^{Lo} monocytes may play a functional role during murine BA. Moreover, our data suggest that Nr4a1 may play a role in the regulation of both Ly6C^{Lo} monocytes and macrophages during inflammation. Though further work will be needed to specifically define the separate roles of Ly6C^{Lo} monocytes and macrophages, our data highlight the potential implications of using Nr4a1 as a regulator of neonatal hepatic Ly6C^{Lo} non-classical monocytes to mitigate inflammatory injuries.

Further investigation is needed to determine the functional significance of Nr4a1 in myeloid immune responses during perinatal liver inflammation. Previous studies have shown that Nr4a1-deficient mice have significantly fewer Ly6C^{Lo} non-classical monocytes circulating in their blood or spleen, or patrolling the endothelium [13]. Moreover, the few Ly6C^{Lo} non-classical monocytes present in the bone marrow of Nr4a1-deficient mice were found to be arrested in the S phase of the cell cycle, and rapidly underwent apoptosis [13]. Given that the patterns of Nr4a1 expression in neonatal pups in our study are similar to those in studies of adult bone marrow [13], we anticipate that neonatal mice deficient in Nr4a1 will also have significantly fewer Ly6C^{Lo} non-classical monocytes, and will therefore not be able to mitigate perinatal liver inflammation effectively. Further studies of the relationship between Nr4a1 and pro-reparative Ly6C^{Lo} non-classical monocytes are needed before potential therapeutic targets can be developed to halt BA and other inflammatory diseases.

5. Conclusions

In conclusion, our results demonstrate that the transcription factor Nr4a1 is expressed at its highest level in Ly6C^{Lo} non-classical monocytes in the neonatal mouse liver. Furthermore, in response to inflammation, these levels decreased in Ly6C^{Lo} non-classical monocytes in the bone marrow, but increased in Ly6C^{Lo} non-classical monocytes in the liver. These findings highlight the potential implications of using Nr4a1 as a regulator of neonatal hepatic Ly6C^{Lo} non-classical monocytes to mitigate perinatal liver inflammation.

Author Contributions: Conceptualization, A.N. and S.M.; methodology, S.M., C.S.L., A.A. and K.R.; formal analysis, S.M.; validation, S.M; investigation, S.M.; resources, S.M., C.S.L., C.K., A.A., K.R. J.F.A. and A.N.; data curation, S.M., C.S.L., C.K., A.N. and K.R.; writing—original draft preparation, A.N. and S.M.; writing—review and editing, A.N. and S.M.; visualization, A.N. and S.M.; supervision, A.N.; project administration, A.N. and S.M.; funding acquisition, A.N. and S.M. All authors have read and agreed to the published version of the manuscript.

Funding: C.K. was supported by a fellowship from the Lundbeck Foundation's Danish-American Research Exchange Program, administered by Innovation Center Denmark, Silicon Valley. Additional funding was provided by the NIH FAVOR T32 training grant (5T32AI125222-05, S.M.), National Institute of Health grant K08AR072144 (J.F.A.), Nora Eccles Treadwell Foundation (J.F.A.), UCSF Center for the Rheumatic Diseases (J.F.A.), American Pediatric Surgical Association Foundation Jay Grosfeld, MD Scholar Award (A.N.), an American College of Surgeons Faculty Research Fellowship (A.N.), a UCSF Liver Center Pilot Award (NIH P30 DK026743, A.N.), the UCSF Parnassus Flow Cytometry Core (DRC Center Grant NIH P30 DK063720), and core resources of the UCSF Liver Center (P30 DK026743).

Institutional Review Board Statement: The animal study protocol was approved by the Institutional Review Board of University of California, San Francisco (protocol code AN183751-02E, 17 March 2022).

Informed Consent Statement: Not applicable.

Data Availability Statement: The data presented in this study are available on request from the corresponding author.

Acknowledgments: The authors would like to thank Henry Greenberg (Stanford University, CA) for providing MA104 cells and Rhesus rotavirus. The authors would also like to thank Pamela Derish for her critical review of the manuscript.

Conflicts of Interest: The authors declare no conflict of interest. The funders had no role in the design of the study; in the collection, analyses, or interpretation of data; in the writing of the manuscript; or in the decision to publish the results.

References

1. Hartley, J.L.; Davenport, M.; Kelly, D.A. Biliary atresia. *Lancet* **2009**, *374*, 1704–1713. [CrossRef]
2. Czaja, A.J. Hepatic inflammation and progressive liver fibrosis in chronic liver disease. *World J. Gastroenterol.* **2014**, *20*, 2515–2532. [CrossRef] [PubMed]
3. Brempelis, K.J.; Crispe, I.N. Infiltrating monocytes in liver injury and repair. *Clin. Transl. Immunol.* **2016**, *5*, e113. [CrossRef] [PubMed]
4. Liaskou, E.; Wilson, D.V.; Oo, Y.H. Innate immune cells in liver inflammation. *Mediat. Inflamm.* **2012**, *2012*, 949157. [CrossRef]
5. Robinson, M.W.; Harmon, C.; O'Farrelly, C. Liver immunology and its role in inflammation and homeostasis. *Cell Mol. Immunol.* **2016**, *13*, 267–276. [CrossRef]
6. Sander, L.E.; Sackett, S.D.; Dierssen, U.; Beraza, N.; Linke, R.P.; Muller, M.; Blander, J.M.; Tacke, F.; Trautwein, C. Hepatic acute-phase proteins control innate immune responses during infection by promoting myeloid-derived suppressor cell function. *J. Exp. Med.* **2010**, *207*, 1453–1464. [CrossRef]
7. Lee, P.Y.; Nelson-Maney, N.; Huang, Y.; Levescot, A.; Wang, Q.; Wei, K.; Cunin, P.; Li, Y.; Lederer, J.A.; Zhuang, H.; et al. High-dimensional analysis reveals a pathogenic role of inflammatory monocytes in experimental diffuse alveolar hemorrhage. *JCI Insight* **2019**, *4*, e129703. [CrossRef]
8. Olingy, C.E.; San Emeterio, C.L.; Ogle, M.E.; Krieger, J.R.; Bruce, A.C.; Pfau, D.D.; Jordan, B.T.; Peirce, S.M.; Botchwey, E.A. Non-classical monocytes are biased progenitors of wound healing macrophages during soft tissue injury. *Sci. Rep.* **2017**, *7*, 447. [CrossRef]

9. Gao, Y.; Zhou, J.; Qi, H.; Wei, J.; Yang, Y.; Yue, J.; Liu, X.; Zhang, Y.; Yang, R. LncRNA lncLy6C induced by microbiota metabolite butyrate promotes differentiation of Ly6C(high) to Ly6C(int/neg) macrophages through lncLy6C/C/EBPbeta/Nr4A1 axis. *Cell Discov.* **2020**, *6*, 87. [CrossRef]
10. Guilliams, M.; Mildner, A.; Yona, S. Developmental and Functional Heterogeneity of Monocytes. *Immunity* **2018**, *49*, 595–613. [CrossRef]
11. Morias, Y.; Abels, C.; Laoui, D.; Van Overmeire, E.; Guilliams, M.; Schouppe, E.; Tacke, F.; deVries, C.J.; De Baetselier, P.; Beschin, A. Ly6C- Monocytes Regulate Parasite-Induced Liver Inflammation by Inducing the Differentiation of Pathogenic Ly6C+ Monocytes into Macrophages. *PLoS Pathog.* **2015**, *11*, e1004873. [CrossRef] [PubMed]
12. Alkhani, A.; Levy, C.S.; Tsui, M.; Rosenberg, K.A.; Polovina, K.; Mattis, A.N.; Mack, M.; Van Dyken, S.; Wang, B.M.; Maher, J.J.; et al. Ly6c(Lo) non-classical monocytes promote resolution of rhesus rotavirus-mediated perinatal hepatic inflammation. *Sci. Rep.* **2020**, *10*, 7165. [CrossRef] [PubMed]
13. Hanna, R.N.; Carlin, L.M.; Hubbeling, H.G.; Nackiewicz, D.; Green, A.M.; Punt, J.A.; Geissmann, F.; Hedrick, C.C. The transcription factor NR4A1 (Nur77) controls bone marrow differentiation and the survival of Ly6C- monocytes. *Nat. Immunol.* **2011**, *12*, 778–785. [CrossRef] [PubMed]
14. Herring, J.A.; Elison, W.S.; Tessem, J.S. Function of Nr4a Orphan Nuclear Receptors in Proliferation, Apoptosis and Fuel Utilization Across Tissues. *Cells* **2019**, *8*, 1373. [CrossRef]
15. Martinez-Gonzalez, J.; Badimon, L. The NR4A subfamily of nuclear receptors: New early genes regulated by growth factors in vascular cells. *Cardiovasc. Res.* **2005**, *65*, 609–618. [CrossRef]
16. Pawlak, A.; Strzadala, L.; Kalas, W. Non-genomic effects of the NR4A1/Nur77/TR3/NGFIB orphan nuclear receptor. *Steroids* **2015**, *95*, 1–6. [CrossRef] [PubMed]
17. Maxwell, M.A.; Muscat, G.E. The NR4A subgroup: Immediate early response genes with pleiotropic physiological roles. *Nucl. Recept. Signal.* **2006**, *4*, e002. [CrossRef]
18. Mohan, H.M.; Aherne, C.M.; Rogers, A.C.; Baird, A.W.; Winter, D.C.; Murphy, E.P. Molecular pathways: The role of NR4A orphan nuclear receptors in cancer. *Clin. Cancer Res.* **2012**, *18*, 3223–3228. [CrossRef]
19. Pearen, M.A.; Muscat, G.E. Minireview: Nuclear hormone receptor 4A signaling: Implications for metabolic disease. *Mol. Endocrinol.* **2010**, *24*, 1891–1903. [CrossRef]
20. Zikherman, J.; Parameswaran, R.; Weiss, A. Endogenous antigen tunes the responsiveness of naive B cells but not T cells. *Nature* **2012**, *489*, 160–164. [CrossRef]
21. Liu, Y.J.; Li, K.; Yang, L.; Tang, S.T.; Wang, X.X.; Cao, G.Q.; Li, S.; Lei, H.Y.; Zhang, X. Dendritic Cells Regulate Treg-Th17 Axis in Obstructive Phase of Bile Duct Injury in Murine Biliary Atresia. *PLoS ONE* **2015**, *10*, e0136214. [CrossRef]
22. Riepenhoff-Talty, M.; Schaekel, K.; Clark, H.F.; Mueller, W.; Uhnoo, I.; Rossi, T.; Fisher, J.; Ogra, P.L. Group A rotaviruses produce extrahepatic biliary obstruction in orally inoculated newborn mice. *Pediatr. Res.* **1993**, *33*, 394–399. [CrossRef]
23. Shivakumar, P.; Campbell, K.M.; Sabla, G.E.; Miethke, A.; Tiao, G.; McNeal, M.M.; Ward, R.L.; Bezerra, J.A. Obstruction of extrahepatic bile ducts by lymphocytes is regulated by IFN-gamma in experimental biliary atresia. *J. Clin. Investig.* **2004**, *114*, 322–329. [CrossRef] [PubMed]
24. Shivakumar, P.; Sabla, G.E.; Whitington, P.; Chougnet, C.A.; Bezerra, J.A. Neonatal NK cells target the mouse duct epithelium via Nkg2d and drive tissue-specific injury in experimental biliary atresia. *J. Clin. Investig.* **2009**, *119*, 2281–2290. [CrossRef] [PubMed]
25. Clapp, D.W.; Dumenco, L.L.; Hatzoglou, M.; Gerson, S.L. Fetal liver hematopoietic stem cells as a target for in utero retroviral gene transfer. *Blood* **1991**, *78*, 1132–1139. [CrossRef] [PubMed]
26. Keller, G.; Lacaud, G.; Robertson, S. Development of the hematopoietic system in the mouse. *Exp. Hematol.* **1999**, *27*, 777–787. [CrossRef]
27. Wolber, F.M.; Leonard, E.; Michael, S.; Orschell-Traycoff, C.M.; Yoder, M.C.; Srour, E.F. Roles of spleen and liver in development of the murine hematopoietic system. *Exp. Hematol.* **2002**, *30*, 1010–1019. [CrossRef]
28. Cumano, A.; Ferraz, J.C.; Klaine, M.; Di Santo, J.P.; Godin, I. Intraembryonic, but not yolk sac hematopoietic precursors, isolated before circulation, provide long-term multilineage reconstitution. *Immunity* **2001**, *15*, 477–485. [CrossRef]
29. Golub, R.; Cumano, A. Embryonic hematopoiesis. *Blood Cells Mol. Dis.* **2013**, *51*, 226–231. [CrossRef]
30. McGrath, K.E.; Frame, J.M.; Palis, J. Early hematopoiesis and macrophage development. *Semin. Immunol.* **2015**, *27*, 379–387. [CrossRef]
31. Ema, H.; Nakauchi, H. Expansion of hematopoietic stem cells in the developing liver of a mouse embryo. *Blood* **2000**, *95*, 2284–2288. [CrossRef] [PubMed]
32. Ito, T.; Tajima, F.; Ogawa, M. Developmental changes of CD34 expression by murine hematopoietic stem cells. *Exp. Hematol.* **2000**, *28*, 1269–1273. [CrossRef]
33. Hettinger, J.; Richards, D.M.; Hansson, J.; Barra, M.M.; Joschko, A.C.; Krijgsveld, J.; Feuerer, M. Origin of monocytes and macrophages in a committed progenitor. *Nat. Immunol.* **2013**, *14*, 821–830. [CrossRef] [PubMed]
34. Dal-Secco, D.; Wang, J.; Zeng, Z.; Kolaczkowska, E.; Wong, C.H.; Petri, B.; Ransohoff, R.M.; Charo, I.F.; Jenne, C.N.; Kubes, P. A dynamic spectrum of monocytes arising from the in situ reprogramming of CCR2+ monocytes at a site of sterile injury. *J. Exp. Med.* **2015**, *212*, 447–456. [CrossRef] [PubMed]
35. Geissmann, F.; Jung, S.; Littman, D.R. Blood monocytes consist of two principal subsets with distinct migratory properties. *Immunity* **2003**, *19*, 71–82. [CrossRef]

36. Ginhoux, F.; Jung, S. Monocytes and macrophages: Developmental pathways and tissue homeostasis. *Nat. Rev. Immunol.* **2014**, *14*, 392–404. [CrossRef]
37. Sunderkotter, C.; Nikolic, T.; Dillon, M.J.; Van Rooijen, N.; Stehling, M.; Drevets, D.A.; Leenen, P.J. Subpopulations of mouse blood monocytes differ in maturation stage and inflammatory response. *J. Immunol.* **2004**, *172*, 4410–4417. [CrossRef]
38. Yona, S.; Kim, K.W.; Wolf, Y.; Mildner, A.; Varol, D.; Breker, M.; Strauss-Ayali, D.; Viukov, S.; Guilliams, M.; Misharin, A.; et al. Fate mapping reveals origins and dynamics of monocytes and tissue macrophages under homeostasis. *Immunity* **2013**, *38*, 79–91. [CrossRef]
39. Auffray, C.; Sieweke, M.H.; Geissmann, F. Blood monocytes: Development, heterogeneity, and relationship with dendritic cells. *Annu. Rev. Immunol.* **2009**, *27*, 669–692. [CrossRef]

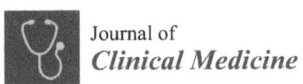

Article

Identification of Early Clinical and Histological Factors Predictive of Kasai Portoenterostomy Failure

Caroline P. Lemoine [1], Hector Melin-Aldana [2], Katherine A. Brandt [1] and Riccardo Superina [1,*]

[1] Division of Transplant and Advanced Hepatobiliary Surgery, Ann & Robert H. Lurie Children's Hospital of Chicago, Northwestern University Feinberg School of Medicine, Chicago, IL 60611, USA
[2] Department of Pathology, Ann & Robert H. Lurie Children's Hospital of Chicago, Northwestern University Feinberg School of Medicine, Chicago, IL 60611, USA
* Correspondence: rsuperina@luriechildrens.org; Tel.: +312-227-4040; Fax: +312-227-9387

Abstract: Background: It is impossible to predict which patients with biliary atresia (BA) will fail after Kasai portoenterostomy (KPE). We evaluated the predictive nature of pre-KPE clinical and histological factors on transplant-free survival (TFS) and jaundice clearance. Methods: A retrospective review of patients who received a KPE at our institution (1997–2018) was performed. Primary outcomes were two-year TFS, five-year TFS, and jaundice clearance 3 months after KPE. $p < 0.05$ was considered significant. Results: Fifty-four patients were included in this study. The two-year TFS was 35.1%, five-year TFS was 24.5%, and 37% patients reached a direct bilirubin (DB) $\leq$ 2.0 mg/dL 3 months post KPE. The median age at biopsy was younger in the five-year TFS (39.0 (24.5–55.5) vs. 56.0 days (51.0–67.0), $p = 0.011$). Patients with DB $\leq$ 1.0 mg/dL 3 months after KPE were statistically younger at biopsy (DB $\leq$ 1.0 44.0 (26.0–56.0) vs. DB > 1.0 56.0 days (51.0–69.0), $p = 0.016$). Ductal plate malformation was less frequent in the five-year TFS (16/17, 94.1%, vs. 1/17, 5.9%, $p = 0.037$). Portal fibrosis (19/23, 82.6%, vs. 4/23, 17.4%, $p = 0.028$) and acute cholangitis (6/7, 85.7%, vs. 1/7, 14.3%, $p = 0.047$) occurred less frequently in two-year TFS. Conclusion: Older age at biopsy, acute cholangitis, portal fibrosis, and ductal plate malformation were associated with lower native liver survival. Evaluation in a larger study population is needed to validate these results.

Keywords: biliary atresia; Kasai portoenterostomy; liver histology; transplant-free survival

1. Introduction

Biliary atresia (BA) is characterized by progressive fibrosing and scarring of the bile ducts preventing bile excretion by the liver. If untreated, it leads to the development of biliary cirrhosis and death in infancy [1,2]. The Kasai portoenterostomy (KPE) is the gold standard for the treatment of BA. The success of this procedure is determined by its ability to clear jaundice. The reported jaundice clearance rate is 55–60% [3]. Even with successful bile drainage, half of children with BA will need a liver transplant (LT) by age 2. Infants whose total bilirubin level remains above 2.0 mg/dL 3 months after KPE have been shown to be at risk for early disease progression [4].

The standard of care remains to perform a KPE first and a secondary liver transplant (LT) if it fails [5,6]. In the USA, only patients with advanced liver disease at diagnosis are considered for primary LT. Although rarely performed (0.1–11%), it is associated with good survival and outcomes [2,7,8]. Despite this, surgeons are reluctant to perform a primary LT, since it is estimated that approximately one third of all patients with BA may not require a LT. It is currently very difficult to predict which patients will survive long term with their native liver ("success") from those who will need a LT within the first two years of life ("failure"). Identification of "early failure" patients could lead to avoiding an unnecessary KPE, with earlier listing and LT, decreasing the wait list morbidity and mortality.

Many groups have tried to identify clinical and histological predictive factors of post-KPE failure [9–12], but few groups have tried identifying pre-KPE factors that could

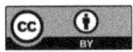

predict native liver survival after KPE [13]. We aim to confirm the predictive value of those previously reported histology findings and to identify additional predictive histological and clinical factors.

2. Methods

2.1. Patient Selection and Data Collection

Institutional Review Board approval was obtained (IRB 2007-12989, study approved 31 August 2018). Since the surgical technique and number of KPEs per year per surgeon have been shown to influence outcomes after KPE, only patients whose KPE was performed by our institution's pediatric hepatobiliary surgeon (RS) were included (August 1997–December 2018). Fifty patients were excluded because of the following reasons: pre-KPE biopsy slides were not available for review, they underwent a primary LT, they did not have a liver biopsy before the KPE, or they had <2 years followup. Fifty-four patients were ultimately included in this study.

2.2. Outcomes and Clinical Factors

Primary outcomes were defined as two-year and five-year transplant free survival (TFS) and clearance of jaundice at 3 months after KPE (direct bilirubin (DB) ≤ 2.0 or ≤ 1.0 mg/dL). Clinical factors that were available pre-KPE were evaluated: age at diagnosis of jaundice, age at liver biopsy, and DB at the time of liver biopsy.

2.3. Histological Factors

Azarow et al. evaluated the predictive nature of pre-KPE liver biopsy histologic findings on post KPE outcomes [13]. These factors were evaluated, as well as those from the "Histological assessment for cholestasis in infancy" developed by the Biliary Atresia Research Consortium (BARC) [14]. The list of the histologic features that were reviewed is presented in Table 1.

Table 1. List of histologic factors reviewed on liver biopsies as potential predictive factors of outcomes (Legend: BARC: Biliary Atresia Research Consortium).

	Histologic Findings	**Source**
Portal tracts	Portal fibrosis	BARC
	Portal inflammation	BARC
	Portal edema	BARC
Bile ducts	Bile in zone 1	Azarow et al. [13]
	Bile duct proliferation	BARC
	Bile duct damage	BARC
	Acute cholangitis	BARC/Azarow et al. [13]
	Portal ductular reaction	BARC
	Ductal plate malformation	BARC
	Focal necrosis	Azarow et al. [13]
	Bridging necrosis	BARC/Azarow et al. [13]
Hepatocytes	Hepatocellular cholestasis	BARC
	Lobular inflammation	BARC/Azarow et al. [13]
	Multinucleated giant hepatocytes	BARC
	Syncytial giant cells	Azarow et al. [13]
	Individually necrotic hepatocytes	BARC
	Hepatocellular rosettes	BARC

All 54 pre KPE liver biopsies were reviewed blindly by our institutional pediatric liver pathologist (HMA) and two pediatric hepatobiliary surgeons (CL, RS). Participants were unaware of the patient's identity and KPE outcome. To reduce interobserver variation, all features were evaluated with a tertiary (0 = absent/mild, 1 = moderate, 2 = severe, or 0 = absent/minimally present, 1 = present, 2 = prominent) and a binary system (0 = absent/mild, 1 = moderate/severe, or 0 = absent/minimally present, 1 = present/prominent), except for the ductal plate malformation (DPM) and bile in zone 1 (binary scoring system only).

2.4. Statistical Analysis

The Chi-square test and Fisher's exact test were used for univariate analyses of categorical variables, while linear logistic regression was used for continuous variables. Statistics were performed using the IBM SPSS Statistics program (version 24.0.0.0). A $p < 0.05$ was considered statistically significant. A $p < 0.1$ was used to account for the limitations from the small sample size in observing statistical trends.

3. Results

3.1. Descriptive Statistics and Outcomes

The patients' characteristics are presented in Table 2. Fifty-four patients met the inclusion criteria and were included in this study (fifty patients were excluded). The median gestational age was 39 weeks (range 28–42); seven patients were born prematurely. Most patients were diagnosed with jaundice on the first day of life (range 0–78). In 26 patients, an alternative explanation for jaundice was mentioned. Only one patient had a biliary atresia splenic malformation. The predictive value of this factor was therefore not evaluated. The median age at the time of initial hepatology evaluation was 51 days (range 3–81), while the median age at liver biopsy was 55.5 days (range 19–152). The median DB level was 5.3 mg/dL (2.5–14.7). All patients underwent a KPE (median age 59 days (range 22–153)).

Table 2. Descriptive statistics of the study population (Legend: KPE: Kasai portoenterostomy; (‡) One patient was both breastfed and thought to have a perinatal infection; (§) Non-corrected age for prematurely born patients).

Variable	Results ($n = 54$)
Sex (n, male, %)	26 (48.1)
Gestational age (weeks, median, range)	39 (28–42)
Prematurity (n, yes, %)	7 (13.0)
Age at onset of jaundice (days, median, range)	1 (0–78)
Potential explanation for jaundice (n, yes, %)	26 (48.1) ‡
• Breastfeeding	20 (37)
• Perinatal infection	5 (9.3)
• Galactosemia	1 (1.9)
• Total parenteral nutrition	1 (1.9)
• ABO incompatibility	0 (0)
Biliary atresia splenic malformation (n, yes, %)	1 (1.9)
Age at biopsy (days, median, range) §	55.5 (19.0–152.0)
Aspartate aminotransferase at biopsy (IU/L, median, range)	168.5 (48–451)
Alanine aminotransferase at biopsy (IU/L, median, range)	110 (20–375)
Direct bilirubin at biopsy (mg/dL, median, range)	5.3 (2.5–14.7)
Age at KPE (days, median, range) §	59.0 (22.0–153.0)

The median DB level 3 months after KPE was 4.1 mg/dL (0.1–13.9). Nineteen patients (37.3%) reached a DB ≤ 2.0 3 months after KPE, while 14 (27.5%) achieved a DB ≤ 1.0. The two-year TFS was 35.2% (19/54). The five-year TFS was 24.5% (12/49). Of note, the 19 patients who reached a DB ≤ 1.0 were not the same as those who had a two-year TFS.

3.2. Univariate Analysis of Clinical and Histological Factors Based on Individual Outcome

Clinical and histological factors that either reached statistical significance or displayed a trend in predicting any outcome are presented in Table 3 (binary scoring system) and Table 4 (tertiary scoring system). Representative histology slides of these features are shown in Figure 1. Other histology findings that were evaluated in the statistical model are presented in the Supplemental Tables S1 and S2 (Table S1 shows the univariate analysis using the binary scoring system, Table S2 shows the results of the univariate analysis using the tertiary scoring system).

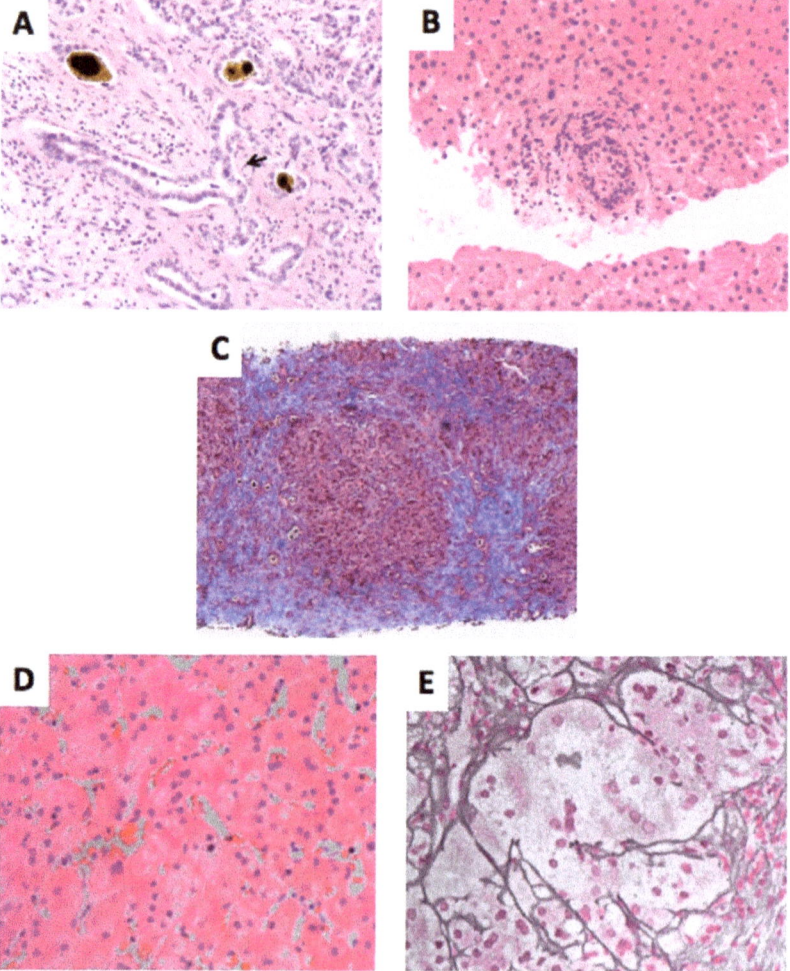

Figure 1. Histology findings found to be statistically significant ($p < 0.05$: (**A–C**)) or a statistical trend ($p < 0.1$: (**D,E**)) with either TFS or DB level at 3 months after KPE using univariate analysis. (Legend: (**A**): DPM; (**B**): acute cholangitis; (**C**): portal fibrosis; (**D**): multinucleated giant cells; (**E**): syncytial giant cells) ((**A**): Cytokeratin-19 stain; (**B,D**): hematoxylin and eosin stain; (**C**): Trichrome Masson stain; (**E**): reticulin stain).

Table 3. Univariate analysis of clinical and histologic factors, binary scoring system. (Legend: DB: Direct bilirubin; KPE: Kasai portoenterostomy; (*): p value < 0.05 statistically significant; (†): p value < 0.1, statistical trend).

Variables		2-Year Transplant-Free Survival			5-Year Transplant-Free Survival			DB ≤ 2 at 3 Months after KPE			DB ≤ 1 at 3 Months after KPE		
		No (n = 35)	Yes (n = 19)	p-Value	No (n = 37)	Yes (n = 12)	p-Value	No (n = 32)	Yes (n = 19)	p-Value	No (n = 37)	Yes (n = 14)	p-Value
Age at biopsy (days, median, IQR)		55.0 (51.0, 67.0)	48.0 (26.0, 64.0)	0.14	56.0 (51.0, 67.0)	39.0 (24.0, 55.5)	0.011 *	55.0 (45.5, 68.0)	55.0 (29.0, 63.0)	0.19	56.0 (51.0, 69.0)	44.0 (26.0, 56.0)	0.016 *
Ductal plate malformation (n, %)	0	20 (57.1)	15 (42.9)	0.11	21 (65.6)	11 (34.4)	0.037 *	20 (58.8)	14 (41.2)	0.41	23 (67.6)	11 (32.4)	0.33
	1	15 (78.9)	4 (21.1)		16 (94.1)	1 (5.9)		12 (70.6)	5 (29.4)		14 (82.4)	3 (17.6)	
Acute cholangitis (n, %)	0	14 (53.8)	12 (46.2)	0.10	14 (63.6)	8 (36.4)	0.081 †	12 (50.0)	12 (50.0)	0.076 †	15 (62.5)	9 (37.5)	0.13
	1	21 (75.0)	7 (25.0)		23 (85.2)	4 (14.8)		20 (74.1)	7 (25.9)		22 (81.5)	5 (18.5)	
Multinucleated giant cells (n, %)	0	15 (53.6)	13 (46.4)	0.073 †	16 (66.7)	8 (33.3)	0.16	16 (61.5)	10 (38.5)	0.86	17 (65.4)	9 (34.6)	0.24
	1	20 (76.9)	6 (23.1)		21 (84.0)	4 (16.0)		16 (64.0)	9 (36.0)		20 (80.0)	5 (20.0)	

Table 4. Univariate analysis of clinical and histologic factors, tertiary scoring system. (Legend: DB: Direct bilirubin; KPE: Kasai portoenterostomy; (*): p value < 0.05 statistically significant; (†): p value < 0.1, statistical trend).

Variables		2-Year Transplant-Free Survival			5-Year Transplant-Free Survival			DB ≤ 2 at 3 Months after KPE			DB ≤ 1 at 3 Months after KPE		
		No (n = 35)	Yes (n = 19)	p-Value	No (n = 37)	Yes (n = 12)	p-Value	No (n = 32)	Yes (n = 19)	p-Value	No (n = 37)	Yes (n = 14)	p-Value
Age at biopsy (days, median, IQR)		55.0 (51.0, 67.0)	48.0 (26.0, 64.0)	0.14	56.0 (51.0, 67.0)	39.0 (24.0, 55.5)	0.011 *	55.0 (45.5, 68.0)	55.0 (29.0, 63.0)	0.19	56.0 (51.0, 69.0)	44.0 (26.0, 56.0)	0.016 *
Portal fibrosis (n, %)	0	1 (25.0)	3 (75.0)	0.028 *	1 (33.3)	2 (66.7)	0.072 †	2 (40.0)	3 (60.0)	0.40	2 (40.0)	3 (60.0)	0.066 †
	1	15 (55.6)	12 (44.4)		16 (69.6)	7 (30.4)		15 (60.0)	10 (40.0)		17 (68.0)	8 (32.0)	
	2	19 (82.6)	4 (17.4)		20 (87.0)	3 (13.0)		15 (71.4)	6 (28.6)		18 (85.7)	3 (14.3)	
Acute cholangitis (n, %)	0	10 (45.5)	12 (54.5)	0.047 *	10 (55.6)	8 (44.4)	0.038 *	11 (52.4)	10 (47.6)	0.30	12 (57.1)	9 (42.9)	0.063 †
	1	19 (76.0)	6 (24.0)		20 (83.3)	4 (16.7)		15 (65.2)	8 (34.8)		18 (78.3)	5 (21.7)	
	2	6 (85.7)	1 (14.3)		7 (100)	0 (0.0)		6 (85.7)	1 (14.3)		7 (100)	0 (0.0)	
Syncytial giant cells (n, %)	0	16 (55.2)	13 (44.8)	0.28	17 (68.0)	8 (32.0)	0.21	15 (57.7)	11 (42.3)	0.29	16 (61.5)	10 (38.5)	0.085 †
	1	12 (75.0)	4 (25.0)		12 (75.0)	4 (25.0)		10 (58.8)	7 (41.2)		13 (76.5)	4 (23.5)	
	2	7 (77.8)	2 (22.2)		8 (100)	0 (0.0)		7 (87.5)	1 (12.5)		8 (100)	0 (0.0)	

3.2.1. Two-Year Transplant-Free Survival

Fifty-four patients were included in the two-year TFS analysis. There were no clinical factors that could predict the two-year TFS. The median age at the onset of jaundice was similar. The median age at biopsy and median DB at biopsy were higher in the LT group but did not reach statistical significance (55 days (IQR 51.0, 67.0) vs. 48 days (IQR 26.0, 64.0), $p = 0.14$). Using the binary scoring system of the histologic features, none reached statistical significance. The multinucleated giant cells on liver biopsy showed a trend in failure after KPE (76.9% vs. 23.1%, $p = 0.073$). When using the tertiary scoring system, portal fibrosis (82.6% vs. 17.4%, $p = 0.028$) and acute cholangitis (85.7% vs. 14.3%, $p = 0.047$) were found to be statistically significant. Severe portal fibrosis, severe acute cholangitis, and moderate acute cholangitis were more prevalent in the two-year LT group.

3.2.2. Five-Year Transplant Free Survival

Forty-nine patients were included in the five-year TFS analysis. The median age at biopsy was significantly lower in the five-year TFS group (56 days (IQR 51.0, 67.0) vs. 39 (IQR 24.0, 55.5), $p = 0.011$). DB at the time of liver biopsy was lower in the five-year TFS group, but not significant (0 days (IQR 0.0, 7.0) vs. 10 days (IQR 0.0, 14.5), $p = 0.63$). When evaluating liver biopsies with the binary scoring system, the presence of DPM was associated with failure (94.1% vs. 5.9%, $p = 0.037$). Acute cholangitis showed a trend towards KPE failure (85.2% vs. 14.8%, $p = 0.081$). Using the tertiary scoring system, severe acute cholangitis reached statistical significance for failure (100.0% vs. 0.0%, $p = 0.038$). Severe portal fibrosis was associated with a trend in KPE failure (87.0% vs. 13.0%, $p = 0.072$).

3.2.3. Clearance of Jaundice Three Months after KPE

When evaluating patients who reached a DB ≤ 2.0 ($n = 19$), only the presence of acute cholangitis on the binary scoring system showed a trend towards failure (74.1% vs. 25.9%, $p = 0.076$). Fourteen patients successfully reached a DB ≤ 1.0 3 months after KPE. They were statistically younger at liver biopsy (44 days (IQR 26.0, 56.0) vs. 56 days (IQR 51.0, 69.0), $p = 0.016$). None of the histologic factors reached statistical significance with the binary scoring system. With the tertiary scoring system, three histologic features showed a trend towards failure: severe portal fibrosis (85.7% vs. 14.3%, $p = 0.066$), severe acute cholangitis (100.0% vs. 0.0%, $p = 0.063$), and numerous syncytial giant cells (100.0% vs. 0.0%, $p = 0.085$).

4. Discussion

While the KPE was a groundbreaking development in the management of infants with BA, for most patients it remains a palliative procedure serving as a bridge to LT [15]. Reported native liver survival in Western countries varies between 20% and 56%, although the length of followup varies greatly, making comparisons difficult. [7] Most of the research aimed at identifying the predictive factors of BA outcomes focused on intra- or postoperative factors. We sought to identify predictive factors of "early failure post-KPE" relying on preoperative clinical and histological factors. Our results suggest that older age at biopsy, DPM, moderate to severe portal fibrosis, and acute cholangitis are predictive factors of failure. Additionally, multinucleated giant cells and syncytial giant cells could be associated with a lower native liver survival.

Younger age at KPE is frequently cited as a favorable factor to achieve TFS and resolution of jaundice [16–19]. Patients who receive a KPE at a younger age undergo a diagnostic liver biopsy at a younger age, explaining how the younger age at biopsy was associated with five-year TFS and achieving a DB ≤ 1.0 3 months after KPE in our study. The ability to diagnose BA on early liver biopsy has been questioned, as "typical BA findings" may not be present early or in premature infants [20,21]. However, a recent meta-analysis showed there was no difference in the accuracy of liver biopsy in patients younger or older than 60 days [22]. In our study, nearly half of the patients had an "alternative explanation" for their jaundice. Pediatric gastroenterologists recommend investigating jaundice if it persists 3 weeks after birth [23]. Earlier identification of direct hyperbilirubinemia could lead to earlier liver biopsy and improved post KPE outcomes. Therefore, when a liver biopsy shows features suggestive of BA, an operative cholangiogram should be performed promptly to allow patients to undergo a KPE at the youngest possible age, possibly allowing jaundice clearance and survival with their native liver.

The presence of moderate or severe acute cholangitis on liver biopsy was the only histologic feature found to be associated with all three outcomes investigated in this study. This is the first report of the predictive nature of acute cholangitis on pre-KPE liver biopsy. Infection and inflammation in already abnormal bile ducts may lead to unrecoverable intrinsic injury despite KPE. In the BARC assessment, interobserver agreement was the poorest in the histologic features of inflammation such as cholangitis [14]. The BARC scoring system uses a 4-tier score. Reducing it to a binary or tertiary scoring system, as we suggest, may improve pathologists' agreement.

The presence of fibrosis on liver biopsy is a controversial predictor of post-KPE outcome [24,25]. Studies have reported fibrosis as a predictor of poor outcomes as it could compromise bile outflow [26–30]. Webb et al. reported that the absence of bridging fibrosis on liver biopsy was the only factor significantly associated with improved five-year TFS [31]. Another group showed that high-grade fibrosis was an indicator of poor postoperative prognosis even when KPE was performed in young patients [27]. Our experience is concordant with these groups.

DPM has been thought to represent an interruption of the normal remodeling process of the biliary tract during fetal life [32]. Its incidence in patients with BA has been reported between 20 and 50% [33]. DPM is considered a marker of antenatal onset of disease leading to a longer duration of liver injury and has been associated with a lower jaundice clearance rate 3 months after KPE and a shorter interval to LT [27,30,33–36]. Low et al. reported that all their BA patients with DPM on biopsy had a poor outcome [33]. Safwan et al. reported that 69% of patients in their study who underwent a primary LT had evidence of DPM on biopsy, and DPM was associated with a shorter native-liver survival after KPE [35]. In our cohort, thirty-five percent of patients had DPM identified on their pre KPE liver biopsy, and the presence of DPM was associated with a lower five-year TFS.

Multinucleated hepatocytes are individual hepatocytes containing three or more nuclei [14]. Syncytial giant cells were originally described as large conglomerate of hepatocytes containing up to 30 nuclei [37]. Azarow et al. reported that both were associated with poor KPE outcomes [13]. Vazquez et al. reported the same association but on KPE surgical specimens [38]. A recent study concluded that the presence of hepatitis-like features was an indicator of poor short-term jaundice clearance [39]. These findings correlate with ours, where multinucleated giant cells were associated with a lower two-year TFS, and syncytial giant cells were associated with a lower jaundice clearance post-KPE.

The authors recognize the limitations of this study. First, it is a retrospective single institution study with a small sample size. This is explained by the exclusion of 50 additional patients due to liver biopsy performed at other institutions being unavailable for review; the absence of a preoperative biopsy; primary LT; and other types of biliary drainage procedure. Second, the liver biopsies were reviewed by a single pathologist. Since this pathologist reviews all liver biopsies performed at our institution, it did not appear helpful to have other pathologists participate in the review, especially since interobserver agreement between expert pediatric liver pathologists can be challenging [14].

5. Conclusions

In conclusion, a combination of clinical factors (younger age at biopsy) and the presence of histologic factors on the diagnostic liver biopsy (presence of severe acute cholangitis, portal fibrosis, and ductal plate malformation) of infants with BA can likely predict early failure after KPE and would identify patients who could benefit from a primary LT. A positive predictive score with a high degree of sensitivity and specificity that combines elements of both clinical and histological parameters could be used to stream patients at high risk for early failure into a primary transplant arm rather than having them undergo an operation that could be futile and that would complicate any probably future liver transplant. A larger multicenter study will be needed to externally validate the findings of this study. It will also allow the evaluation of other pertinent clinical and histologic factors, as a larger study population may generate stronger results to be incorporated in a predictive score of BA outcomes.

Supplementary Materials: The following supporting information can be downloaded at: https://www.mdpi.com/article/10.3390/jcm11216523/s1, Table S1: Additional data to Table 3: Univariate analysis of clinical and histologic factors using the binary scoring system; Table S2: Additional data to Table 4: Univariate analysis of clinical and histologic factors using the tertiary scoring system.

Author Contributions: Conceptualization, R.S.; Methodology, C.P.L., H.M.-A., K.A.B. and R.S.; Software, C.P.L. and K.A.B.; Validation, C.P.L., K.A.B. and R.S.; Formal Analysis, C.P.L. and K.A.B.; Investigation, C.P.L., H.M.-A., K.A.B. and R.S.; Resources, K.A.B. and C.P.L.; Data Curation, C.P.L., H.M.-A. and K.A.B.; Writing—Original Draft Preparation, C.P.L.; Writing—Review and Editing, C.P.L., H.M.-A., K.A.B. and R.S.; Visualization, R.S.; Supervision, R.S.; Project Administration, R.S.; K.A.B.; Funding Acquisition, R.S. All authors have read and agreed to the published version of the manuscript.

Funding: We acknowledge support from the Robert E. Schneider Foundation in conducting the research for this work.

Institutional Review Board Statement: The study was conducted in accordance with the Declaration of Helsinki, and approved by the Institutional Review Board (or Ethics Committee) of the Ann & Robert H Lurie Children's Hospital of Chicago (IRB 2007-12989, study approved 31 August 2018).

Informed Consent Statement: Patient consent was waived because the research study and disclosed patient health information involved no more than a minimal risk to the subjects.

Data Availability Statement: The data that support the findings of this study are available from the corresponding author upon reasonable request.

Conflicts of Interest: The authors declare no conflict of interest.

Abbreviations

BA	Biliary atresia
BARC	Biliary atresia research consortium
DB	Direct bilirubin
KPE	Kasai portoenterostomy
LT	Liver transplantation
TB	Total bilirubin
TFS	Transplant-free survival

References

1. Karrer, F.M.; Price, M.R.; Bensard, D.D.; Sokol, R.J.; Narkewicz, M.R.; Smith, D.J.; Lilly, J.R. Long-term results with the Kasai operation for biliary atresia. *Arch. Surg.* **1996**, *131*, 493–496. [CrossRef]
2. Superina, R. Liver transplantation for biliary atresia: Does the insurance type really make a difference? *Liver Transplant.* **2013**, *19*, 470–471. [CrossRef]
3. Lakshminarayanan, B.; Davenport, M. Biliary atresia: A comprehensive review. *J. Autoimmun.* **2016**, *73*, 1–9. [CrossRef]
4. Shneider, B.L.; Magee, J.C.; Karpen, S.J.; Rand, E.B.; Narkewicz, M.R.; Bass, L.M.; Schwarz, K.; Whitington, P.F.; Bezerra, J.A.; Kerkar, N.; et al. Total Serum Bilirubin within 3 Months of Hepatoportoenterostomy Predicts Short-Term Outcomes in Biliary Atresia. *J. Pediatr.* **2016**, *170*, 211–217.e2. [CrossRef]
5. Davenport, M.; Goyet, J.D.V.D.; Stringer, M.; Mieli-Vergani, G.; Kelly, D.; McClean, P.; Spitz, L. Seamless management of biliary atresia in England and Wales (1999–2002). *Lancet* **2004**, *363*, 1354–1357. [CrossRef]
6. Otte, J.-B.; Goyet, J.D.V.D.; Reding, R.; Hausleithner, V.; Sokal, E.; Chardot, C.; Debande, B. Sequential treatment of biliary atresia with kasai portoenterostomy and liver transplantation: A review. *Hepatology* **1994**, *20*, S41–S48. [CrossRef]
7. Superina, R. Biliary atresia and liver transplantation: Results and thoughts for primary liver transplantation in select patients. *Pediatr. Surg. Int.* **2017**, *33*, 1297–1304. [CrossRef]

8. Wang, P.; Xun, P.; He, K.; Cai, W. Comparison of liver transplantation outcomes in biliary atresia patients with and without prior portoenterostomy: A meta-analysis. *Dig. Liver Dis.* **2016**, *48*, 347–352. [CrossRef]
9. Chen, G.; Zheng, S.; Sun, S.; Xiao, X.; Ma, Y.; Shen, W.; Chen, L.; Song, Z. Early surgical outcomes and pathological scoring values of older infants (≥90 d old) with biliary atresia. *J. Pediatr. Surg.* **2012**, *47*, 2184–2188. [CrossRef]
10. Sun, S.; Zheng, S.; Lu, X.; Chen, G.; Ma, Y.; Chen, L.; Dong, K. Clinical and pathological features of patients with biliary atresia who survived for more than 5 years with native liver. *Pediatr. Surg. Int.* **2018**, *34*, 381–386. [CrossRef]
11. Goda, T.; Kawahara, H.; Kubota, A.; Hirano, K.; Umeda, S.; Tani, G.; Ishii, T.; Tazuke, Y.; Yoneda, A.; Etani, Y.; et al. The most reliable early predictors of outcome in patients with biliary atresia after Kasai's operation. *J. Pediatr. Surg.* **2013**, *48*, 2373–2377. [CrossRef] [PubMed]
12. Ihn, K.; Ho, I.G.; Chang, E.Y.; Han, S.J. Correlation between gamma-glutamyl transpeptidase activity and outcomes after Kasai portoenterostomy for biliary atresia. *J. Pediatr. Surg.* **2018**, *53*, 461–467. [CrossRef]
13. Azarow, K.S.; Phillips, M.J.; Sandler, A.D.; Hagerstrand, I.; Superina, R.A. Biliary atresia: Should all patients undergo a portoenterostomy? *J. Pediatr. Surg.* **1997**, *32*, 168–172; discussion 164–172. [CrossRef]
14. Russo, P.; Magee, J.C.; Boitnott, J.; Bove, K.E.; Raghunathan, T.; Finegold, M.; Haas, J.; Jaffe, R.; Kim, G.E.; Magid, M.; et al. Design and Validation of the Biliary Atresia Research Consortium Histologic Assessment System for Cholestasis in Infancy. *Clin. Gastroenterol. Hepatol.* **2011**, *9*, 357–362.e2. [CrossRef] [PubMed]
15. Hartley, J.L.; Davenport, M.; Kelly, D.A. Biliary atresia. *Lancet* **2009**, *374*, 1704–1713. [CrossRef]
16. Superina, R.; Magee, J.C.; Brandt, M.L.; Healey, P.J.; Tiao, G.; Ryckman, F.; Karrer, F.M.; Iyer, K.; Fecteau, A.; West, K.; et al. The Anatomic Pattern of Biliary Atresia Identified at Time of Kasai Hepatoportoenterostomy and Early Postoperative Clearance of Jaundice Are Significant Predictors of Transplant-Free Survival. *Ann. Surg.* **2011**, *254*, 577–585. [CrossRef]
17. Lien, T.-H.; Chang, M.-H.; Wu, J.-F.; Chen, H.-L.; Lee, H.-C.; Chen, A.-C.; Tiao, M.-M.; Wu, T.-C.; Yang, Y.-J.; Lin, C.-C.; et al. Effects of the infant stool color card screening program on 5-year outcome of biliary atresia in taiwan. *Hepatology* **2011**, *53*, 202–208. [CrossRef]
18. Schreiber, R.A.; Barker, C.C.; Roberts, E.A.; Martin, S.R.; Alvarez, F.; Smith, L.; Butzner, J.D.; Wrobel, I.; Mack, D.; Moroz, S.; et al. Biliary Atresia: The Canadian Experience. *J. Pediatr.* **2007**, *151*, 659–665.e1. [CrossRef]
19. Serinet, M.-O.; Wildhaber, B.E.; Broué, P.; Lachaux, A.; Sarles, J.; Jacquemin, E.; Gauthier, F.; Chardot, C. Impact of Age at Kasai Operation on Its Results in Late Childhood and Adolescence: A Rational Basis for Biliary Atresia Screening. *Pediatrics* **2009**, *123*, 1280–1286. [CrossRef]
20. Ferry, G.D.; Selby, M.L.; Udall, J.; Finegold, M.; Nichols, B. Guide to Early Diagnosis of Biliary Obstruction in Infancy. *Clin. Pediatr.* **1985**, *24*, 305–311. [CrossRef]
21. Mowat, A.P.; Psacharopoulos, H.T.; Williams, R. Extrahepatic biliary atresia versus neonatal hepatitis. Review of 137 prospectively investigated infants. *Arch. Dis. Child.* **1976**, *51*, 763–770. [CrossRef]
22. Lee, J.Y.; Sullivan, K.; El Demellawy, D.; Nasr, A. The value of preoperative liver biopsy in the diagnosis of extrahepatic biliary atresia: A systematic review and meta-analysis. *J. Pediatr. Surg.* **2016**, *51*, 753–761. [CrossRef]
23. Fawaz, R.; Baumann, U.; Ekong, U.; Fischler, B.; Hadzic, N.; Mack, C.L.; McLin, V.A.; Molleston, J.P.; Neimark, E.; Ng, V.L.; et al. Guideline for the Evaluation of Cholestatic Jaundice in Infants: Joint Recommendations of the North American Society for Pediatric Gastroenterology, Hepatology, and Nutrition and the European Society for Pediatric Gastroenterology, Hepatology, and Nutrition. *J. Pediatr. Gastroenterol. Nutr.* **2017**, *64*, 154–168. [CrossRef]
24. Bhatnagar, V.; Agarwala, S.; Gupta, S.D.; Baruah, R.R. Correlation of pre- and post-operative liver function, duct diameter at porta hepatis, and portal fibrosis with surgical outcomes in biliary atresia. *J. Indian Assoc. Pediatr. Surg.* **2015**, *20*, 184–188. [CrossRef]
25. Czubkowski, P.; Cielecka-Kuszyk, J.; Rurarz, M.; Kaminska, D.; Markiewicz-Kijewska, M.; Pawlowska, J. The limited prognostic value of liver histology in children with biliary atresia. *Ann. Hepatol.* **2015**, *14*, 902–909. [CrossRef]
26. Weerasooriya, V.S.; White, F.V.; Shepherd, R. Hepatic fibrosis and survival in biliary atresia. *J. Pediatr.* **2004**, *144*, 123–125. [CrossRef]
27. Muthukanagarajan, S.J. Diagnostic and Prognostic Significance of Various Histopathological Features in Extrahepatic Biliary Atresia. *J. Clin. Diagn. Res.* **2016**, *10*, EC23–EC27. [CrossRef]
28. Arii, R.; Koga, H.; Arakawa, A.; Miyahara, K.; Lane, G.J.; Okazaki, T.; Urao, M.; Yamataka, A. How valuable is ductal plate malformation as a predictor of clinical course in postoperative biliary atresia patients? *Pediatr. Surg. Int.* **2010**, *27*, 275–277. [CrossRef]
29. Salzedas-Netto, A.; Chinen, E.; de Oliveira, D.; Pasquetti, A.; Azevedo, R.; Patricio, F.D.S.; Cury, E.; Gonzalez, A.; Vicentine, F.; Martins, J. Grade IV Fibrosis Interferes in Biliary Drainage After Kasai Procedure. *Transplant. Proc.* **2014**, *46*, 1781–1783. [CrossRef]
30. Russo, P.; Magee, J.C.; Anders, R.A.; Bove, K.E.; Chung, C.; Cummings, O.W.; Finegold, M.J.; Finn, L.S.; Kim, G.E.; Lovell, M.A.; et al. Key Histopathologic Features of Liver Biopsies That Distinguish Biliary Atresia From Other Causes of Infantile Cholestasis and Their Correlation With Outcome. *Am. J. Surg. Pathol.* **2016**, *40*, 1601–1615. [CrossRef]
31. Webb, N.L.; Jiwane, A.; Ooi, C.; Nightinghale, S.; Adams, S.E.; Krishnan, U. Clinical significance of liver histology on outcomes in biliary atresia. *J. Paediatr. Child Health* **2017**, *53*, 252–256. [CrossRef] [PubMed]
32. Raynaud, P.; Tate, J.; Callens, C.; Cordi, S.; Vandersmissen, P.; Carpentier, R.; Sempoux, C.; Devuyst, O.; Pierreux, C.E.; Courtoy, P.; et al. A classification of ductal plate malformations based on distinct pathogenic mechanisms of biliary dysmorphogenesis. *Hepatology* **2011**, *53*, 1959–1966. [CrossRef] [PubMed]

33. Low, Y.; Vijayan, V.; Tan, C.E. The prognostic value of ductal plate malformation and other histologic parameters in biliary atresia: An immunohistochemical study. *J. Pediatr.* **2001**, *139*, 320–322. [CrossRef] [PubMed]
34. Shimadera, S.; Iwai, N.; Deguchi, E.; Kimura, O.; Ono, S.; Fumino, S.; Higuchi, K. Significance of ductal plate malformation in the postoperative clinical course of biliary atresia. *J. Pediatr. Surg.* **2008**, *43*, 304–307. [CrossRef] [PubMed]
35. Safwan, M.; Ramachandran, P.; Vij, M.; Shanmugam, N.; Rela, M. Impact of ductal plate malformation on survival with native liver in children with biliary atresia. *Pediatr. Surg. Int.* **2015**, *31*, 837–843. [CrossRef] [PubMed]
36. Roy, P.; Chatterjee, U.; Ganguli, M.; Banerjee, S.; Chatterjee, S.; Basu, A. A histopathological study of liver and biliary remnants with clinical outcome in cases of extrahepatic biliary atresia. *Indian J. Pathol. Microbiol.* **2010**, *53*, 101–105. [CrossRef]
37. Phillips, M.J.; Blendis, L.M.; Poucell, S.; Patterson, J.; Petric, M.; Roberts, E.; Levy, G.A.; Superina, R.A.; Greig, P.D.; Cameron, R.; et al. Syncytial Giant-Cell Hepatitis. *N. Engl. J. Med.* **1991**, *324*, 455–460. [CrossRef]
38. Vazquez-Estevez, J.; Stewart, B.; Shikes, R.H.; Hall, R.J.; Lilly, J.R. Biliary atresia: Early determination of prognosis. *J. Pediatr. Surg.* **1989**, *24*, 48–51. [CrossRef]
39. Suda, K.; Muraji, T.; Ohtani, H.; Aiyoshi, T.; Sasaki, T.; Toma, M.; Yanai, T. Histological significance of hepatitis-like findings in biliary atresia: An analysis of 34 Japanese cases. *Pediatr. Int.* **2019**, *61*, 364–368. [CrossRef]

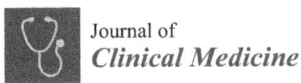

Article

Surgical and Medical Aspects of the Initial Treatment of Biliary Atresia: Position Paper

Mark Davenport [1,*], Omid Madadi-Sanjani [2], Christophe Chardot [3], Henkjan J. Verkade [4], Saul J. Karpen [5] and Claus Petersen [2]

1. Department of Paediatric Surgery, Kings College Hospital, London SE5 9RS, UK
2. Klinik für Kinderchirurgie, Medizinische Hochschule Hannover, Carl-Neuberg-Str. 1, 30625 Hannover, Germany
3. Chirurgie Pédiatrique—Transplantation, Hôpital Necker—Enfants Maladies, Université Paris Descartes, 149 Rue de Sèvres, 75015 Paris, France
4. Center for Liver, Digestive and Metabolic Diseases, Universitair Medisch Centrum, 9713 AV Groningen, The Netherlands
5. Center for Advanced Pediatrics, 1400 Tullie Circle SE 2nd Floor, Atlanta, GA 30329, USA
* Correspondence: markdav2@ntlworld.com

Abstract: Biliary atresia, a fibro-obliterative disease of the newborn, is usually initially treated by Kasai portoenterostomy, although there are many variations in technique and different options for post-operative adjuvant medical therapy. A questionnaire on such topics (e.g., open vs. laparoscopic; the need for liver mobilisation; use of post-operative steroids; use of post-operative anti-viral therapy, etc.) was circulated to delegates ($n = 43$) of an international webinar (Biliary Atresia and Related Diseases—BARD) held in June 2021. Respondents were mostly European, but included some from North America, and represented 18 different countries overall. The results of this survey are presented here, together with a commentary and review from an expert panel convened for the meeting on current trends in practice.

Keywords: biliary atresia; Kasai operation; adjuvant therapy; corticosteroids; cytomegalovirus; ursodeoxycholic acid

1. Introduction

Biliary atresia (BA) is an obliterative condition of the biliary tract that typically presents with jaundice and pale stools during neonatal life [1,2]. All affected infants have conjugated hyperbilirubinemia, often evident in the first days of life [3], along with elevated liver enzymes, but may present little in the way of conclusive diagnostic signs, at least in the first few weeks of life. Although diagnosis can be strongly suggested by a range of secondary investigations including abdominal ultrasound, radionuclide imaging, and liver biopsy, it is usually confirmed only at surgical exploration and intraoperative cholangiography.

This investigative strategy has changed little over the past few years, although there is emerging interest in newer and potentially more specific biochemical markers such as MMP-7 [4]. To date, the early studies have been Asian in origin and retrospective [5], with conflicting cut-off values. Other possible diagnostic methods, again still very much in the investigative phase, include the use of AI algorithms in the interpretation of ultrasound data [6].

It is possible to screen for cases of BA, and this has been national strategy in Taiwan and Japan, based on relatively low-tech stool-colour cards. More recently, particularly in Texas, whole blood sampling with measurement of conjugated bilirubin has been trialled [7].

The definitive management of this condition is entirely surgical, usually with an initial attempt at restoration of bile flow and preservation of the native liver (Kasai portoenterostomy—KPE) in the first few months of life. If this fails or is felt to be futile, liver transplant may be carried out. In 1959, Morio Kasai, a Japanese surgeon working in Sendai, described his original experience with what has become known as KPE [8]. Over the subsequent two decades, this operation and its principle—radical excision of the extrahepatic ducts with a biliary reconstruction in the porta hepatis—gradually became accepted for infants with BA, although many modifications (e.g., Roux loop stomas and intussusception valves) were attempted along the way [9,10]. It is also possible to perform a KPE laparoscopically, although this is controversial and has not been widely adopted outside certain high-volume Asian centres [11,12].

The first ever liver transplant in a child born with BA was reported in 1963 by Thomas Starzl and a team from Denver, CO, USA [13]. Although actually unsuccessful, it prompted the first wave of liver transplant centres to be set up during the 1960s, which demonstrated the validity of the surgical technique. Nonetheless, the lack of effective immunosuppression precluded longer-term success and a moratorium was declared. Liver transplantation was re-invigorated in the 1980s with the discoveries of cyclosporin and subsequently tacrolimus, leading to its widespread adoption throughout the world.

The aim of this paper is to review the current diagnostic strategies of BA, and to provide a review of current operative techniques and the role of post-operative adjuvant therapy for KPE, aligned to a survey of current practice. The future direction of clinical research was also explored.

2. Methods

An online survey was conducted among members of the European reference network RARE-LIVER, and members of the faculty of the Biliary Atresia and Related Diseases (BARD) network (Supplementary File S1). Questions were drafted in multiple choice format by members of the working group, all of whom were experienced paediatric hepatologists and hepatobiliary surgeons. The survey was performed via an online tool (SurveyMonkey, Survey Monkey Inc., now Momentive Inc.) and was completed anonymously. Respondents could not be traced back to any participating centre. The results of the questionnaire were subsequently discussed by an online panel during the 2021 online Biliary Atresia and Related Diseases (BARD) conference.

3. Results

Completed forms were analysed from 43 respondents (with 22 self-declared as surgeons) from centres distributed across 18 countries.

3.1. Diagnostic Strategy

In patients with BA, the age at which KPE is performed is negatively related to the success rate of the surgery, in terms both of clearance of jaundice and survival with native liver [14,15]. However, neonatal cholestasis can be caused by a multitude of other conditions and diseases other than BA, for which surgery is not indicated. It has been estimated that BA accounts for 25–40% of neonatal cholestasis [16]. Accordingly, the initial diagnostic strategy in infants with neonatal cholestasis aims to rapidly identify whether a condition other than biliary atresia is the cause of the cholestasis. The workup of neonatal cholestasis has been summarised in the joint guidelines of the North American Society for Pediatric Gastroenterology, Hepatology, and Nutrition (NASPGHAN) and the European Society for Paediatric Gastroenterology, Hepatology, and Nutrition (ESPGHAN); the reader is directed there for details [16]. The causes of neonatal cholestasis can be categorized in anatomical extrahepatic obstructions of bile flow (such as choledochal malformations, cholelithiasis), genetic diseases, either multisystemic (Alagille syndrome, cystic fibrosis, galactosemia, mitochondrial diseases, and others) or exclusively hepatic (alpha-1-antitrypsin deficiency, bile acid synthesis defects, canalicular membrane transport protein defects, and others), endocrinologic disorders (hypocortisolism, hypothyroidism), or as secondary to other diseases (e.g., sepsis, congenital viral infection). Over recent years, the possibilities for genetic analyses have increased [17,18]. The time needed for genetic analysis has so far precluded it from being a prerequisite before intraoperative cholangiography and, in case of BA, KPE surgery. Since the turn-around time for genetic analyses has decreased over the past decade, this may change in future. Early candidates would then be expected to be infants referred in the very first weeks of life, who may not yet have acholic stools.

Generally, the diagnostic strategy for neonatal cholestasis aims at demonstrating or excluding the most frequent non-BA causes. The workup as indicated in the guidelines includes (re)checking of newborn blood-screening results (galactosemia, hypothyroidism, cystic fibrosis), and blood analyses including measurement of white blood counts, differential alpha-1-antitrypsin level and phenotype, thyroid hormone and TSH, bile acid concentration, cortisol, glucose, lactate, and metabolic parameters. Urine analysis is aimed at reducing substances (galactitol), and bacterial or viral infections (including CMV PCR). Imaging of the liver is performed by ultrasound for anatomical abnormalities (choledochal malformations, cholelithiasis) and by X-ray for evidence of multisystem disease (such as in Alagille syndrome, or butterfly vertebrae). On indication such as a cardiac murmur, a cardiac ultrasound doppler is performed for detection of congenital malformations, such as pulmonary artery stenosis in Alagille syndrome. Most (but not all) centres perform a percutaneous liver biopsy as a final step in the diagnostic analysis. In case of sufficient histological indications compatible with biliary obstruction, particularly if combined with ductular reaction and fibrosis, the decision is frequently made to perform intraoperative cholangiography, followed by KPE, based on positive cholangiography or macroscopic absence of extrahepatic bile ducts. The diagnostic use of hepatobiliary scintigraphy for the discrimination of biliary atresia is no longer advocated, partly because of relatively low specificity [19] which fails to abolish the need for liver biopsy and, if suspicious, an intraoperative cholangiogram.

3.2. Surgical Strategy (Based on 42 Completed Questionnaires)

Confirmation of the actual diagnosis is the first step in the operation, and 80% of respondents indicated that they would do this using a small right upper quadrant incision centred over the anticipated position of the gallbladder; 20% would utilize less invasive techniques for this step. Cholangiography was regarded as "obligatory" at this stage by 60% of practitioners surveyed, by 33% only when inspection of the hepatoduodenal ligament was inconclusive, and by 7% when an ERCP was not available or was inconclusive. The use of indocyanine green is becoming more prevalent in adult biliary surgery, and one respondent stated that they would use this diagnostically during KPE. Following confirmation of the diagnosis, 95% would then look for other features of syndromic BA (e.g., polysplenia).

There was only a single respondent who would perform the KPE laparoscopically, all others opting for a conventional open technique. With this in mind, the degree of liver mobilisation prior to porta hepatis was then investigated. Total mobilisation (i.e., division of suspensory ligaments on both right and left) would be performed by 33%, partial mobilisation (i.e., division of only falciform and left triangular ligaments) by 43%, and no additional mobilisation by 24%.

Surgical loupe magnification was used by 90% of respondents during dissection of the porta hepatis, with most carrying out sharp dissection using a knife (78%) and avoiding bipolar diathermy (52%).

Deliberate exposure of the Rex recessus was sought by 52%, and was regarded as optional by 14%. Most surgeons (67%) aimed for an extended dissection of the porta hepatis (beyond the division of the portal vein), with the remainder actively avoiding this.

The preferred length of the retrocolic Roux loop was 25–50 cm for 90% of respondents, but 5% aimed for less than this while 5% aimed for more. A single respondent stated that they would create an intussusception valve within the loop. Most surgeons would use a hand-sewn (86%), end-to-side technique (67%) for the jejunojejunostomy.

All surgeons performed an end-to-side portoenterostomy using either an interrupted (48%) or running stitch (43%) or both (9%), and usually using 6/0 sutures (57%). The total time for the KPE was assessed at 120–240 min (76%) and for those performing it laparoscopically >240 min (71%).

Post-operatively, most respondents felt that prophylactic antibiotics should be prescribed for >1 week (82%) and the regimen should include ursodeoxycholic acid (94%). Respondents were split between use of steroids (50%) and no one used immunoglobulins, farnesoid X receptor agonists, or ileal bile acid transporter (IBAT) inhibitors.

4. Discussion

The main aim of this paper is to present the breadth of current surgical techniques and practice for biliary atresia as performed in a predominantly European and North American setting. We did not seek to debate actual indications or limitations such as the late-presenting infant or the possible role of liver transplantation as a primary procedure.

4.1. Surgical Strategy

Our survey confirms an important observation which bears repeating, that the Kasai portoenterostomy is not a single, uniform operation performed every time by each surgeon in the same way. Rather, it is simply a principle of extrahepatic dissection and excision with (nowadays) a Roux loop reconstruction and anastomosis high in the porta hepatis. It might be questioned whether the details matter, and in some respects they probably do not. Visualisation of the biliary tree is an axiom of diagnosis, but can be achieved as easily by laparoscopy as by an exploratory right upper quadrant incision. Similarly, despite textbook adherence to the concept of cholangiography, in most cases the gallbladder is so atrophic as to be without a lumen and hence the siting of a catheter is not possible. Alternatively, about 20% of cases have a gallbladder that is structurally normal (evident on ultrasound) but is filled with clear mucus. Cholangiography is essentially redundant here, in that it will inevitably show a patent common bile duct into the duodenum but no sign of a more proximal biliary tree. Some centres, particularly in France, would consider a portocholecystostomy (i.e., the gallbladder opened and anastomosed to the transected portal plate) for BA to make use of this feature [20]. This option effectively abolishes the risk of post-operative cholangitis, although has a higher revision rate for leaks and obstruction.

In those centres with a less stringent, less discriminatory pre-surgical workup, the proportion of non-BA cases coming to surgical exploration is likely to be higher and cholangiography to exclude BA will performed more frequently. Cholangiography is also important in cases of cystic BA, where it may or may not show connections to the residual intrahepatic ducts and is able to distinguish cystic BA from cystic choledochal malformation—a much more benign condition.

4.1.1. Role of Laparoscopy

Laparoscopic KPE remains unpopular in Europe and North America, although some of the early reports arose from European centres [21–23]. More recently, more reports and interest have arisen in the larger Asian centres, including in China [11,24]. However, no report has shown or even implied its superiority to the more conventional open approach, and indeed it is difficult to see a real rationale for this technique beyond the cosmetic. Certainly, in terms of the primary objective—clearance of jaundice and preservation of the native liver—it clearly has no advantage.

4.1.2. Degree of Liver Mobilisation

The need for liver mobilisation in the open technique continues to be contentious, but exteriorization was favoured by 75% of respondents, although it is clear that this can be achieved by less than complete mobilisation, dividing only the falciform ± left triangular ligaments—the most popular technique. The degree of dissection in the porta hepatis has changed over the years. It is clear from Kasai's original descriptions that he was relatively conservative in leaving residual biliary tissue in the porta and performing the Roux loop anastomosis to form an ovoid section. His successor in Sendai, Ryoji Ohi, and other Japanese surgeons [25] adopted more radical dissection to widen the resultant portoenterostomy and incorporate the interstices behind the bifurcation of the portal vein on the left into the Rex recessus (facilitated by dividing the bridge between the third and fourth segments), and on the right up to and sometimes into Rouviere's fosse (containing the posterior branches of the right hepatic artery and right portal vein). The majority (67%) of our surgical group seem to favour this latter approach. Interestingly, Ohi's successor in Sendai, Masaki Nio, reverted somewhat to a less extensive dissection more in keeping with the original [26]. Nowadays the only group of surgeons who have reverted to Kasai's original approach have been those who do this operation entirely laparoscopically, as it is evident that radical dissection is only effectively possible as an open technique [27].

4.1.3. Roux Loop

Use of a retrocolic Roux loop was standard for all respondents, with the only debate being about how long it should be. The clear majority aim for 40 cm with only one respondent aiming for a short (<25 cm) loop and one deliberately measuring it as >50 cm. There is little firm evidence on this matter presented in the literature. Most recently, a Chinese centre prospectively randomized 166 infants, comparing standard length with a short length (13–20 cm) [28]; there was no difference in incidence of cholangitis (43% vs. 47%) or clearance of jaundice (45% vs. 50%).

A single surgeon favoured modification of the Roux limb by creation of an "intussusception valve". These were briefly in vogue during the 1990s [9] as they were thought to prevent reflux and hence reduce cholangitis. A small-scale prospective trial from Tokyo involving 20 infants showed no difference in outcome [29] and interest seemed to wane. However, more recently this technique has become popular, at least in China where a recent questionnaire-based survey showed it was being used in half of their centres [30]. It is unclear whether this is in any way evidence-based.

A range of different techniques were reported for the jejunojejunostomy, including end-to-side, end-to-end, hand-sewn, and stapled. By contrast, the actual portoenterostomy anastomosis was invariably end-to-side and fashioned by most contributors using a relatively fine (6/0) absorbable suture (PDS).

4.2. Post Operative Adjuvant Therapy

Biliary atresia affects both intra- and extra-hepatic bile ducts, and KPE primarily treats only the extra-hepatic component. Many medications have been advocated to treat the intra-hepatic bile duct damage, though few with any substantial evidence base.

The liver in the BA infant prior to KPE is subject to substantial cholestatic injury with subsequent fibroinflammatory and necrotic pathophysiological adaptations [31]. KPE provides surgical relief of the extrahepatic obstruction, which is key for the BA liver to begin the process attempt to restore normal homeostasis, including reduction of retained bile acids [32], and subsequent activity related to the presence of activated profibrotic and inflammatory mechanisms [33–35]. However, despite KPE, the majority of infants with BA present ongoing cholestasis and progression of liver disease, underlying the expectation of continued inherent developmental cholangiopathy in these patients. In brief, the expected early results of KPE are native liver survival (NLS) at age 2 of ~45–65%, with significant variability between centres and countries e.g., [36–41]. Moreover, progressive liver disease is ongoing in BA during childhood, leading ultimately to NLS rates of ~25% by the beginnings of adulthood [39,41–43]. Thus, with progression of disease and the rapid progression of subsequent liver disease there is a need for medical therapies aimed at improving outcomes after KPE, in order to reduce the risk of death and the need for liver transplant [44]. Among the adjuvant therapies that are generally accepted internationally are antibiotics to address the risk of cholangitis, and ursodeoxycholic acid (UDCA) to act as a potential choleretic and to improve the hydrophilicity of the bile acid pool [44,45]. UDCA and antibiotics both received strong support in our survey (>80% of 33 respondents).

The use of corticosteroids post-KPE is among the more controversial aspects of treatment. Large studies have supported its use [46], including a recent randomised trial from Shanghai [47]. However, there have also been studies indicating no discernible benefit according to the available evidence [48]. Despite this gap in therapeutic support for steroids post-KPE, along with evidence of an increase in side effects and impaired growth among patients receiving steroids [49]; half (17/34) of respondents to the survey reported their use. This is a crucial issue, as use of corticosteroids post-KPE varies widely around the globe—from 0–100%. Clearly, more investigations are needed.

There are currently two ongoing international investigational studies exploring the efficacy of intestinal bile acid transporter (IBAT) inhibitors post-KPE. These studies are focussed on maralixibat (Phase 2, NCT 04524390; EMBARK), assessing a short-term outcome of reduction in total bilirubin at 6 months, and odevixibat (Phase 3 NCT 04336722; BOLD), with a clinical outcome measure of improvement of NLS at 2 years. The rationale for IBAT inhibition seeks to address one of the causes of liver damage in cholestatic diseases such as BA, by reducing the obligate intrahepatic bile acid levels [50]. IBAT inhibitors are approved in many countries for relief of pruritus in children with Alagille syndrome and PFIC [50–52].

Intriguingly, there was support for determining coexistent CMV infection at the time of KPE, which should lead to consideration for antiviral treatment [53], with the potential to improve post-KPE outcomes. Other considerations for improving outcomes that have yet to be studied include varying methods of feeding infants (e.g., breast milk versus formula), the role of parenteral nutrition, and appropriate roles for fat-soluble vitamin monitoring and supplementation.

At least three-quarters of BA patients will need LT in their lifetime [39,54,55]. KPE is essentially palliative in nature and is typically only the first step of treatment. One element that was not addressed in our survey was the prevention of complications evident at the time of transplantation (i.e., reducing post-operative intra-abdominal adhesion). It has been shown [56,57] that duration of total hepatectomy, bleeding, and prognosis of liver transplantation were adversely impacted when KPE was performed in a centre that does not perform liver transplantation. Operative details which may reduce adhesions include avoidance of unnecessary exposure of the intestines outside the abdomen, avoidance of abdominal drains, and possibly the use of anti-adhesion adjuncts such as hyaluronic acid (Seprafilm™, Baxter Inc., Deerfield, IL, USA) and hydrogels (CoSeal™, Baxter Inc., Deerfeield, IL, USA) around the liver. Both are in current use in European centres, though without evidential support.

The obvious limitation of this study is that it is divorced from any report of actual outcomes, and remains opinion-based. Nevertheless, it reflects the views of a large body of surgeons and clinicians involved in the care of these infants.

5. Conclusions and Future Directions

In conclusion, the lack of uniform approach and absence of registries hampers progress in untangling the nuances of the Kasai operation and determining the role of adjuvant therapies for this complex and perplexing disease. It also seems very unlikely that sufficiently powered randomized trials will be available to arrive at a clear answer. Nevertheless, we look forward to a time in the near future when testing of existing and novel therapies will be readily available to help guide clinicians and parents to achieve optimal outcomes. Furthermore, we note the emergence of possible biomarkers which may better refine the diagnostic (e.g., MMP-7) [58] or prognostic processes (e.g., secretin receptor expression) [59].

Supplementary Materials: The following supporting information can be downloaded at: https://www.mdpi.com/article/10.3390/jcm11216601/s1. Supplementary File S1: Questionnaire.

Author Contributions: Conceptualization, M.D. and C.P.; Data curation, M.D., O.M.-S. and C.C.; Formal analysis, M.D. and O.M.-S.; Writing—original draft, M.D.; Writing—review & editing, M.D.,

O.M.-S., C.C., H.J.V., S.J.K. and C.P. All authors have read and agreed to the published version of the manuscript.

Funding: This research received no external funding.

Institutional Review Board Statement: Not applicable.

Informed Consent Statement: Not applicable.

Data Availability Statement: Not applicable.

Acknowledgments: Members of the Biliary Atresia Working Group. Biliary Atresia Working Group: S. Harpavat, Houston, USA; M. Samyn, London, UK; R. Superina, Chicago, USA; M. Pakarinen, Helsinki, Finland; S. Karpen, Atlanta, USA; H. Verkade, Groningen, Netherlands; C. Mack, Denver, USA; K. Wang, Los Angeles, USA; K. Schwarz, San Diego, USA; J. Hulscher, Groningen, Netherlands; C. Chardot, Paris, France; M. Davenport, London, UK; E. Sturm, Tübingen, Germany; R. Schreiber, Vancouver, Canada; S. Scholz, Pittsburgh, USA; J. Bezerra, Cincinnatti, USA.

Conflicts of Interest: The authors declare no conflict of interest.

References

1. Nizery, L.; Chardot, C.; Sissaoui, S.; Capito, C.; Henrion-Caude, A.; Debray, D.; Girard, M. Biliary atresia: Clinical advances and perspectives. *Clin. Res. Hepatol. Gastroenterol.* **2016**, *40*, 281–287. [CrossRef] [PubMed]
2. Scottoni, F.; Davenport, M. Biliary atresia: Potential for a new decade. *Semin. Pediatr. Surg.* **2020**, *29*, 150940. [CrossRef] [PubMed]
3. Harpavat, S.; Finegold, M.J.; Karpen, S.J. Patients with biliary atresia have elevated direct/conjugated bilirubin levels shortly after birth. *Pediatrics* **2011**, *128*, e1428–e1433. [CrossRef] [PubMed]
4. Jiang, J.; Wang, J.; Shen, Z.; Lu, X.; Chen, G.; Huang, Y.; Dong, R.; Zheng, S. Serum MMP-7 in the diagnosis of biliary atresia. *Pediatrics* **2019**, *144*, e20190902. [CrossRef]
5. Wu, J.F.; Jeng, Y.M.; Chen, H.L.; Ni, Y.-H.; Hsu, H.-Y.; Chang, M.-H. Quantification of serum matrix metallopeptide 7 levels may assist in the diagnosis and predict the outcome for patients with biliary atresia. *J. Pediatr.* **2019**, *208*, 30–37.e1. [CrossRef] [PubMed]
6. Hsu, F.R.; Dai, S.T.; Chou, C.M.; Huang, S.Y. The application of artificial intelligence to support biliary atresia screening by ultrasound images: A study based on deep learning models. *PLoS ONE* **2022**, *17*, e0276278. [CrossRef]
7. Harpavat, S.; Garcia-Prats, J.A.; Anaya, C.; Brandt, M.L.; Lupo, P.J.; Finegold, M.J.; Obuobi, A.; Elhennawy, A.A.; Jarriel, W.S.; Shneider, B.L. Diagnostic yield of newborn screening for biliary atresia using direct or conjugated bilirubin measurements. *JAMA* **2020**, *323*, 1141–1150. [CrossRef]
8. Kasai, M.; Suzuki, S. A new operation for "non-correctable" biliary atresia—Portoenterostomy. *Shijitsu* **1959**, *13*, 733–739. (In Japanese)
9. Saeki, M.; Nakano, M.; Hagane, K.; Shimizu, K. Effectiveness of an intussusceptive antireflux valve to prevent ascending cholangitis after hepatic portojejunostomy in biliary atresia. *J. Pediatr. Surg.* **1991**, *26*, 800–803. [CrossRef]
10. Ohya, T.; Miyano, T.; Kimura, K. Indication for portoenterostomy based on 103 patients with Suruga II modification. *J. Pediatr. Surg.* **1990**, *25*, 801–804. [CrossRef]
11. Sun, X.; Diao, M.; Wu, X.; Cheng, W.; Ye, M.; Li, L. A prospective study comparing laparoscopic and conventional Kasai portoenterostomy in children with biliary atresia. *J. Pediatr. Surg.* **2016**, *51*, 374–378. [CrossRef] [PubMed]
12. Li, B.; Chen, B.W.; Xia, L.S. Experience of treating biliary atresia with laparoscopic-modified Kasai and laparoscopic conventional Kasai: A cohort study. *ANZ J. Surg.* **2021**, *91*, 1170–1173. [CrossRef] [PubMed]
13. Starzl, T.E.; Marchioro, T.L.; Vonkailla, K.N.; Hermann, G.; Brittain, R.S.; Waddell, W.R. Homotransplantation of the liver in humans. *Surg. Gynecol. Obste.* **1963**, *117*, 659–676.
14. Chardot, C.; Buet, C.; Serinet, M.O.; Golmard, J.L.; Lachaux, A.; Roquelaure, B.; Gottrand, F.; Broué, P.; Dabadie, A.; Gauthier, F.; et al. Improving outcomes of biliary atresia: French national series 1986–2009. *J. Hepatol.* **2013**, *58*, 1209–1217. [CrossRef]
15. Serinet, M.O.; Wildhaber, B.E.; Broué, P.; Lachaux, A.; Sarles, J.; Jacquemin, E.; Gauthier, F.; Chardot, C. Impact of age at Kasai operation on its results in late childhood and adolescence: A rational basis for biliary atresia screening. *Pediatrics* **2009**, *123*, 1280–1286. [CrossRef] [PubMed]
16. Fawaz, R.; Baumann, U.; Ekong, U.; Fischler, B.; Hadzic, N.; Mack, C.L.; McLin, V.A.; Molleston, J.P.; Neimark, E.; Ng, V.L.; et al. Guideline for the Evaluation of Cholestatic Jaundice in Infants: Joint Recommendations of the North American Society for Pediatric Gastroenterology, Hepatology, and Nutrition and the European Society for Pediatric Gastroenterology, Hepatology, and Nutrition. *J. Pediatr. Gastroenterol. Nutr.* **2017**, *64*, 154–168.
17. Nicastro, E.; Di Giorgio, A.; Marchetti, D.; Barboni, C.; Cereda, A.; Iascone, M.; D'Antiga, L. Diagnostic yield of an algorithm for neonatal and infantile cholestasis integrating Next-Generation Sequencing. *J. Pediatr.* **2019**, *211*, 54–62.e4. [CrossRef]
18. Ibrahim, S.H.; Kamath, B.M.; Loomes, K.M.; Karpen, S.J. Cholestatic liver diseases of genetic etiology: Advances and controversies. *Hepatology* **2022**, *75*, 1627–1646. [CrossRef]

19. Kianifar, H.R.; Tehranian, S.; Shojaei, P.; Adinehpoor, Z.; Sadeghi, R.; Kakhki, V.R.D.; Keshtgar, A.S. Accuracy of hepatobiliary scintigraphy for differentiation of neonatal hepatitis from biliary atresia: Systematic review and meta-analysis of the literature. *Pediatr. Radiol.* **2013**, *43*, 905–919. [CrossRef]
20. Hery, G.; Gonzales, E.; Bernard, O.; Fouquet, V.; Gauthier, F.; Branchereau, S. Hepatic portocholecystostomy: 97 cases From a single institution. *J. Pediatr. Gastroenterol. Nutr.* **2017**, *65*, 375–379. [CrossRef]
21. Ayuso, L.; Vila-Carbó, J.J.; Lluna, J.; Hernández, E.; Marco, A. Intervención de Kasai por vía laparoscópica: Presente y futuro del tratamiento de la atresia de vías biliares. Laparoscopic Kasai portoenterostom: Present and future of biliary atresia treatment. *Cir. Pediatr.* **2008**, *21*, 23–26. (In Spanish) [PubMed]
22. von Sochaczewski, C.O.; Petersen, C.; Ure, B.M.; Osthaus, A.; Schubert, K.-P.; Becker, T.; Lehner, F.; Kuebler, J.F. Laparoscopic versus conventional Kasai portoenterostomy does not facilitate subsequent liver transplantation in infants with biliary atresia. *J. Laparoendosc. Adv. Surg. Tech. A* **2012**, *22*, 408–411. [CrossRef] [PubMed]
23. Ure, B.M.; Kuebler, J.F.; Schukfeh, N.; Engelmann, C.; Dingemann, J.; Petersen, C. Survival with the native liver after laparoscopic versus conventional Kasai portoenterostomy in infants with biliary atresia: A prospective trial. *Ann. Surg.* **2011**, *253*, 826–830. [CrossRef] [PubMed]
24. Ji, Y.; Zhang, X.; Chen, S.; Li, Y.; Yang, K.; Zhou, J.; Xu, Z. Medium-term outcomes after laparoscopic revision of laparoscopic Kasai portoenterostomy in patients with biliary atresia. *Orphanet J. Rare Dis.* **2021**, *16*, 193. [CrossRef]
25. Toyosaka, A.; Okamoto, E.; Okasora, T.; Nose, K.; Tomimoto, Y.; Seki, Y. Extensive dissection at the porta hepatis for biliary atresia. *J. Pediatr. Surg.* **1994**, *29*, 896–899. [CrossRef]
26. Nio, M.; Wada, M.; Sasaki, H.; Kazama, T.; Tanaka, H.; Kudo, H. Technical Standardization of Kasai Portoenterostomy in Biliary Atresia. *J. Pediatr. Surg.* **2016**, *51*, 2105–2108. [CrossRef]
27. Nakamura, H.; Koga, H.; Miyano, G.; Okawada, M.; Doi, T.; Yamataka, A. Does the level of transection of the biliary remnant affect outcome after laparoscopic Kasai portoenterostomy for biliary atresia? *J. Laparoendosc. Adv. Surg. Tech. A* **2017**, *27*, 744–747. [CrossRef]
28. Xiao, H.; Huang, R.; Chen, L.; Diao, M.; Li, L. The application of a shorter loop in Kasai portoenterostomy reconstruction for Ohi Type III Biliary Atresia: A Prospective Randomized Controlled Trial. *J. Surg. Res.* **2018**, *232*, 492–496. [CrossRef]
29. Ogasawara, Y.; Yamataka, A.; Tsukamoto, K.; Okada, Y.; Lane, G.J.; Kobayashi, T.; Miyano, T. The intussusception antireflux valve is ineffective for preventing cholangitis in biliary atresia: A prospective study. *J. Pediatr. Surg.* **2003**, *38*, 1826–1829. [CrossRef]
30. Zheng, Q.; Zhang, S.; Ge, L.; Jia, J.; Gou, Q.; Zhao, J.; Zhan, J. Investigation into multi-centre diagnosis and treatment strategies of biliary atresia in mainland China. *Pediatr. Surg. Int.* **2020**, *36*, 827–833. [CrossRef]
31. Russo, P.; Magee, J.C.; Anders, R.A.; Bove, K.E.; Chung, C.; Cummings, O.W. Childhood Liver Disease Research Network (ChiLDReN). Key histopathologic features of liver biopsies that distinguish biliary atresia from other causes of infantile cholestasis and their correlation with outcome: A multicenter study. *Am. J. Surg. Pathol.* **2016**, *40*, 1601–1615. [CrossRef] [PubMed]
32. Abukawa, D.; Nakagawa, M.; Iinuma, K.; Nio, M.; Ohi, R.; Goto, J. Hepatic and serum bile acid compositions in patients with biliary atresia: A microanalysis using gas chromatography-mass spectrometry with negative ion chemical ionization detection. *Tohoku J. Exp. Med.* **1998**, *185*, 227–237. [CrossRef] [PubMed]
33. Asai, A.; Miethke, A.; Bezerra, J.A. Pathogenesis of biliary atresia: Defining biology to understand clinical phenotypes. *Nat. Rev. Gastroenterol. Hepatol.* **2015**, *12*, 342–352. [CrossRef] [PubMed]
34. Hukkinen, M.; Kerola, A.; Lohi, J.; Jahnukainen, T.; Heikkilä, P.; Pakarinen, M.P. Very low bilirubin after portoenterostomy improves survival of the native liver in patients with biliary atresia by deferring liver fibrogenesis. *Surgery* **2019**, *165*, 843–850. [CrossRef] [PubMed]
35. Moyer, K.; Kaimal, V.; Pacheco, C.; Mourya, R.; Xu, H.; Shivakumar, P.; Chakraborty, R.; Rao, M.; Magee, J.C.; Bove, K.; et al. Staging of biliary atresia at diagnosis by molecular profiling of the liver. *Genome Med.* **2010**, *2*, 33. [CrossRef]
36. Verkade, H.J.; Bezerra, J.A.; Davenport, M.; Schreiber, R.A.; Mieli-Vergani, G.; Hulscher, J.B.; Sokol, R.J.; Kelly, D.A.; Ure, B.; Whitington, P.F.; et al. Biliary atresia and other cholestatic childhood diseases: Advances and future challenges. *J. Hepatol.* **2016**, *65*, 631–642. [CrossRef]
37. Sasaki, H.; Tanaka, H.; Nio, M. Current management of long-term survivors of biliary atresia: Over 40 years of experience in a single center and review of the literature. *Pediatr. Surg. Int.* **2017**, *33*, 1327–1333. [CrossRef]
38. De Vries, W.; de Langen, Z.J.; Groen, H.; Scheenstra, R.; Peeters, P.M.; Hulscher, J.B.; Verkade, H.J. Netherlands Study Group of Biliary Atresia and Registry (NeSBAR). Biliary atresia in the Netherlands: Outcome of patients diagnosed between 1987 and 2008. *J. Pediatr.* **2012**, *160*, 638–644.e2. [CrossRef]
39. Fanna, M.; Masson, G.; Capito, C.; Girard, M.; Guerin, F.; Hermeziu, B.; Lachaux, A.; Roquelaure, B.; Gottrand, F.; Broue, P.; et al. Management of biliary atresia in France 1986 to 2015: Long-term Results. *J. Pediatr. Gastroenterol. Nutr.* **2019**, *69*, 416–424. [CrossRef]
40. Petersen, C.; Madadi-Sanjani, O. Registries for Biliary Atresia and Related Disorders. *Eur. J. Pediatr. Surg.* **2015**, *25*, 469–473.
41. Davenport, M.; Ong, E.; Sharif, K.; Alizai, N.; McClean, P.; Hadzic, N.; Kelly, D.A. Biliary atresia in England and Wales: Results of centralization and new benchmark. *J. Pediatr. Surg.* **2011**, *46*, 1689–1694. [CrossRef] [PubMed]
42. Parolini, F.; Boroni, G.; Milianti, S.; Tonegatti, L.; Armellini, A.; Magne, M.G.; Pedersini, P.; Torri, F.; Orizio, P.; Benvenuti, S.; et al. Biliary atresia: 20–40-year follow-up with native liver in an Italian centre. *J. Pediatr. Surg.* **2019**, *54*, 1440–1444. [CrossRef] [PubMed]

43. Kumagi, T.; Drenth, J.P.; Guttman, O.; Ng, V.; Lilly, L.; Therapondos, G.; Hiasa, Y.; Michitaka, K.; Onji, M.; Watanabe, Y.; et al. Biliary atresia and survival into adulthood without transplantation: A collaborative multicentre clinic review. *Liver Int.* **2012**, *32*, 510–518. [CrossRef] [PubMed]
44. Li, Y.; Bezerra, J.A. Novel approaches to the treatment of biliary atresia. *Clin. Liver Dis.* **2016**, *8*, 145–149. [CrossRef]
45. Qiu, J.L.; Shao, M.Y.; Xie, W.F.; Li, Y.; Yang, H.D.; Niu, M.M.; Xu, H. Effect of combined ursodeoxycholic acid and glucocorticoid on the outcome of Kasai procedure: A systematic review and meta-analysis. *Medicine* **2018**, *97*, e12005. [CrossRef]
46. Davenport, M.; Parsons, C.; Tizzard, S.; Hadzic, N. Steroids in biliary atresia: Single surgeon, single centre, prospective study. *J. Hepatol.* **2013**, *59*, 1054–1058. [CrossRef]
47. Lu, X.; Jiang, J.; Shen, Z.; Chen, G.; Wu, Y.; Xiao, X.; Yan, W.; Zheng, S. Effect of adjuvant steroid therapy in type 3 biliary atresia: A single-center, open-label, randomized controlled trial. *Ann. Surg.* 2022; *ahead of print*. [CrossRef]
48. Bezerra, J.A.; Spino, C.; Magee, J.C.; Shneider, B.L.; Rosenthal, P.; Wang, K.S. Childhood Liver Disease Research and Education Network (ChiLDREN). Use of corticosteroids after hepatoportoenterostomy for bile drainage in infants with biliary atresia: The START randomized clinical trial. *JAMA* **2014**, *311*, 1750–1759. [CrossRef]
49. Alonso, E.M.; Ye, W.; Hawthorne, K.; Venkat, V.; Loomes, K.M.; Mack, C.L.; Hertel, P.M.; Karpen, S.J.; Kerkar, N.; Molleston, J.P.; et al. ChiLDReN Network. Impact of steroid therapy on early growth in infants with biliary atresia: The Multicenter Steroids in Biliary Atresia Randomized Trial. *J. Pediatr.* **2018**, *202*, 179–185.e4. [CrossRef]
50. Karpen, S.J.; Kelly, D.; Mack, C.; Stein, P. Ileal bile acid transporter inhibition as an anticholestatic therapeutic target in biliary atresia and other cholestatic disorders. *Hepatol. Int.* **2020**, *14*, 677–689. [CrossRef]
51. Deeks, E.D. Odevixibat: First Approval. *Drugs* **2021**, *81*, 1781–1786. [CrossRef] [PubMed]
52. Shirley, M. Maralixibat: First Approval. *Drugs* **2022**, *82*, 71–76. [CrossRef] [PubMed]
53. Parolini, F.; Hadzic, N.; Davenport, M. Adjuvant therapy of cytomegalovirus IgM + ve associated biliary atresia: Prima facie evidence of effect. *J. Pediatr. Surg.* **2019**, *54*, 1941–1945. [CrossRef]
54. Jain, V.; Burford, C.; Alexander, E.C.; Sutton, H.; Dhawan, A.; Joshi, D.; Davenport, M.; Heaton, N.; Hadzic, N.; Samyn, M. Prognostic markers at adolescence in patients requiring liver transplantation for biliary atresia in adulthood. *J. Hepatol.* **2019**, *71*, 71–77. [CrossRef] [PubMed]
55. Lykavieris, P.; Chardot, C.; Sokhn, M.; Gauthier, F.; Valayer, J.; Bernard, O. Outcome in adulthood of biliary atresia: A study of 63 patients who survived for over 20 years with their native liver. *Hepatology* **2005**, *41*, 366–371. [CrossRef] [PubMed]
56. Kohaut, J.; Guérin, F.; Fouquet, V.; Gonzales, E.; de Lambert, G.; Martelli, H.; Jacquemin, E.; Branchereau, S. First liver transplantation for biliary atresia in children: The hidden effects of non-centralization. *Pediatr. Transplant.* **2018**, *4*, e13232. [CrossRef]
57. Betalli, P.; Cheli, M.; Colusso, M.M.; Casotti, V.; Alberti, D.; Ferrari, A.; Starita, G.; Lucianetti, A.; Pinelli, D.; Colledan, M.; et al. Association between Kasai portoenterostomy at low caseload centres and transplant complications in children with biliary atresia. *J. Pediatr. Surg.* **2022**, *10*, 223–228. [CrossRef]
58. Yang, L.; Zhou, Y.; Xu, P.P.; Mourya, R.; Lei, H.-Y.; Cao, G.-Q.; Xiong, X.-L.; Xu, H.; Duan, X.-F.; Wang, N.; et al. Diagnostic accuracy of serum matrix metalloproteinase-7 for biliary atresia. *Hepatology* **2018**, *68*, 2069–2077. [CrossRef]
59. Godbole, N.; Nyholm, I.; Hukkinen, M.; Davidson, J.R.; Tyraskis, A.; Lohi, J.; Heikkilä, P.; Eloranta, K.; Pihlajoki, M.; Davenport, M.; et al. Liver secretin receptor predicts portoenterostomy outcomes and liver injury in biliary atresia. *Sci. Rep.* **2022**, *12*, 7233. [CrossRef]

Article

The Impact of a CMV Infection on the Expression of Selected Immunological Parameters in Liver Tissue in Children with Biliary Atresia

Maria Janowska [1,*], Joanna B. Bierła [2], Magdalena Kaleta [2,3], Aldona Wierzbicka-Rucińska [4], Piotr Czubkowski [5], Ewelina Kanarek [6], Bożena Cukrowska [2], Joanna Pawłowska [5] and Joanna Cielecka-Kuszyk [2]

[1] Department of Pediatric Surgery and Organ Transplantation, The Children's Memorial Health Institute, 04-730 Warsaw, Poland
[2] Department of Pathomorphology, The Children's Memorial Health Institute, 04-730 Warsaw, Poland
[3] Teva Pharmaceuticals, 00-113 Warsaw, Poland
[4] Department of Biochemistry, Radioimmunology and Experimental Medicine, The Children's Memorial Health Institute, 04-730 Warsaw, Poland
[5] Department of Gastroenterology, Hepatology, Nutritional Disorders and Pediatrics, The Children's Memorial Health Institute, 04-730 Warsaw, Poland
[6] Histocompatibility Laboratory, The Children's Memorial Health Institute, 04-730 Warsaw, Poland
* Correspondence: m.janowska@ipczd.pl

Abstract: The pathogenesis of biliary atresia (BA) is still not clear. The aim of this study was to evaluate the expression of selected immunological parameters in liver tissue in BA children based on CMV/EBV infection status. Eight of thirty-one children with newly diagnosed BA were included in this prospective study and assigned to two groups (I with active infection, II without active or past infection). All studies were performed on surgical liver biopsies. To visualize CD8+ T cells and CD56 expression, immunohistochemical staining was performed. The viral genetic material in the studied groups was not found, but CMV infection significantly affected the number of CD8+ lymphocytes in both the portal area and the bile ducts. The average number of CD8+ cells per mm^2 of portal area in Groups I and II was 335 and 200 ($p = 0.002$). The average number of these cells that infiltrated the epithelium of the bile duct per mm^2 in Group I and II was 0.73 and 0.37 ($p = 0.0003$), respectively. Expression of CD56 in the bile ducts corresponded to the intensity of the inflammatory infiltrate of CD8+ cells. Our results suggest that active CMV infection induces an increased infiltration of CD8+ lymphocytes, which could play a role in BA immunopathogenesis. Increased CD56 expression can be a sign of a newly formed bile structure often without lumen, suggesting inhibition of the maturation process in BA.

Keywords: biliary atresia; cytomegalovirus; cytotoxic T cells

1. Introduction

Biliary atresia (BA) is a progressive cholangiopathy of unclear etiology affecting extra- and intrahepatic bile ducts. It is the most common cause of neonatal cholestasis and is the main indication for liver transplantation in children. The nature of the disease is the obstruction of the biliary outflow from the liver due to progressive inflammation, fibrosis, and proliferation of the intrahepatic bile ducts [1]. Despite many years of research, the etiopathogenesis of the disease is still not fully understood. It is suggested that BA is not a single disease, but rather a phenotypic expression of various specific entities developing as a result of a combination of external (e.g., viruses, toxins), immunological and genetic factors [2,3].

Reports on the temporal–regional concentration of BA cases may support the theory of damage to the bile ducts due to the action of a viral factor in the prenatal period. Of the large list of viruses studied in the pediatric population with BA, cytomegatovirus

(CMV) seems to be the most likely causative factor [4]. Fisher et al. demonstrated a higher prevalence of anti-CMV antibodies in mothers of children with BA, a higher concentration of CMV-IgM in infants, and the presence of viral DNA in the liver in half of the studied patients with this disease [5]. Xu Y et al. detected CMV DNA in 60% of a large cohort of Chinese patients [6]. In turn, Brindley et al., in 56% of BA patients (out of a group of 16 patients), observed a significant increase in liver T cells producing interferon-gamma in response to CMV, compared to the control groups. This suggests a previous CMV infection [7]. Davenport et al. found a correlation between CMV infection at diagnosis and the presence of higher parameters of cholestasis, hepatitis and fibrosis, and the need for liver transplantation in a group of 210 CMV IgM (+) children with BA [8]. In 2009, the Hannover Group published the results of a biopsy study of 74 BA patients. Research on the amount of RNA/DNA of hepatotropic viruses showed their presence in nearly 50% of patients (reovirus—33%, CMV—11%, adenovirus—1%, enterovirus—1.5%). It has been suggested that viral infection can play a role in the activation of immune deregulation and loss of tolerance to bile epithelial antigens. The question remains whether viruses are an integral part of the destructive inflammatory process of the biliary tract or if they are of minor importance [9]. The aim of the present study was to evaluate the expression of selected immunological parameters in liver tissue in BA children with active CMV/EBV (Epstein–Barr virus) infection and in children without such an infection.

2. Materials and Methods

2.1. Patients

After receiving approval from the local ethics committee, we prospectively recruited children with BA who underwent Kasai portoenterostomy between 2014 and 2019. All the patients had complete obliteration of the bile ducts, and none of them presented biliary atresia splenic malformation (BASM) syndrome. In all cases, the surgical liver biopsies were performed during portoenterostomy to obtain tissue for analysis. Age of HPE was presented in weeks and corrected in premature patients.

Liver biochemistry (total and direct bilirubin, aspartate aminotransferase (AST), alanine aminotransferase (ALT), γ-glutamyltranspeptidase (GGT)) and coagulation features (INR) at the time of diagnosis were available from the prospectively maintained database.

All 31 patients were tested for CMV/EBV infection (serum-specific antibodies of immunoglobulins (Ig) M and IgG, and RT-PCR). None of the patients had active EBV infection. Patients with active CMV infection (4 out of 31 children with positive IgM antibodies or/and positive RT-PCR) were selected for Group I. Patients without an active history of CMV/EBV infection (4 out of 31 children with negative IgM and IgG antibodies and RT-PCR) were selected for Group II. Patients' different virological status (6/31: CMV IgM-IgG+ EBV IgM-IgG-; 9/31: CMV IgM-IgG+ EBV IgM-IgG+; 8/31: CMV IgM-,IgG- EBV IgM-IgG+) did not qualify the subject for any of the above groups.

2.2. Determination of EBV and CMV Infection Status

The virological status of patients was based on serological and molecular tests performed prior to hepatoportoenterostomy. Serum IgM and IgG CMV antibodies were measured by a microparticle chemiluminescent immunoassay at the same time. A result was considered positive when serum antibody titers exceeded the cutoff of 1.0 for IgM and 6.0 for IgG. To confirm CMV infection, molecular examination by RT-PCR (urine or serum) was performed. Serological tests for specific IgM and IgG antibodies against viral capsid antigens (VCA) of the EBV virus and antibodies against Epstein–Barr nuclear antigens (EBNA) in the class IgG were performed using an enzyme-linked immunosorbent assay. Serum EBV VCA IgM positivity was defined as serum levels above the cutoff value of 1.0 index.

2.3. In Situ Hybridization Technique

The 3μm formalin-fixed paraffin-embedded (FFPE) tissue sections after 16 h at 56 °C were dewaxed twice in Xylen, rehydrated through descending ethanol (100%, 90%, 70%) series, and then rinsed in ultrapure water at room temperature. Preparations were digested in a previously prepared 0.3% endogenous peroxidase with proteinase K (QUIAGEN, Germantown, MD, USA) at a concentration level of 0.3 mg/mL. The hybridization was performed with Histosonda EBER (Cenbimo, Lugo, Spain) and Histosonda Cytomegalovirus CMV (Cenbimo, Lugo, Spain) probes for EBV and CMV, respectively. Slides were incubated for 1 h at 62 °C in ThermoBrite (Abott Molecular, Chicago, IL, USA) for both CMV and EBV. After hybridization, the slides were first incubated with monoclonal mouse anti-digoxin antibody (Cenbimo, Lugo, Spain), and then with labeledpolymerhorseradish peroxidase (HRP) anti-mouse immunoglobulins (Dako EnVision+ System–HRP, Santa Clara, CA, USA). As the substrate, HRP3-amino-9-ethylcarbazole containing hydrogen peroxide was used (Dako EnVision+ System–HRP, Santa Clara, CA, USA). The washed slides were stained with Mayer's hematoxylin(O.KINDLERMikroskopischeGläser EUKITT, Freiburg, Germany) and sealed with coverslip and Dako Faramount Aqueous Mounting Medium (Dako, Santa Clara, CA, USA). As positive controls for EBV and CMV, in situ hybridization sections from CMV- or EBV-infected liver tissue were used. The negative controls were performed without the specific hybridization probe.

2.4. Immunohistochemistry

The immunohistochemistry (IHC) staining reaction was performed on FFPE tissue samples. IHC was performed on the Ventana BenchMark ULTRA IHC/ISH autostaining system using primary antibodies anti-CD8 (Ventana anti-CD8, clone SP57, rabbit monoclonal primary antibody) and anti-CD56 (Cell Marque, clone MRQ-42, rabbit monoclonal antibody) after antigen retrieval in Cell Conditioning 1 buffer followed by detection with the Ultra View HRP system (Roche/Ventana).

2.5. Morphometric Analyses

IHC slides were scanned by an Hamamatsu NanoZoomer 2.0 RS scanner (Hamamatsu Photonics, Hamamatsu, Japan) at a magnification of 40× and 20× for morphometric analyses of CD8 and CD56 expression, respectively. Next, morphometric analyses were performed with the use of a Cell^P program (Olympus). To analyze CD8+ cells, the three portal areas were selected for each slide. The surface of the total portal areas and all bile ducts in every portal area were measured. The number of CD8+ cells was counted and calculated per 1 μm^2 of both the portal area and the bile duct area. Results were presented as an arithmetical mean ± standard deviation (SD).

To analyze anti-CD56 immunostaining, five regions within the portal area with positive CD56 expression were selected for each slide. The results were presented as a percentage of the area with CD56 expression in selected regions in relation to the entire area of the scanned image under 20× magnification (this area was 147,978.43 μm^2). The method of analysis is illustrated in Figure 1. The threshold parameters were set using the HSI color space model in the following way: hue (H) 90°, saturation (S) 256°, intensity value (I) 123°.

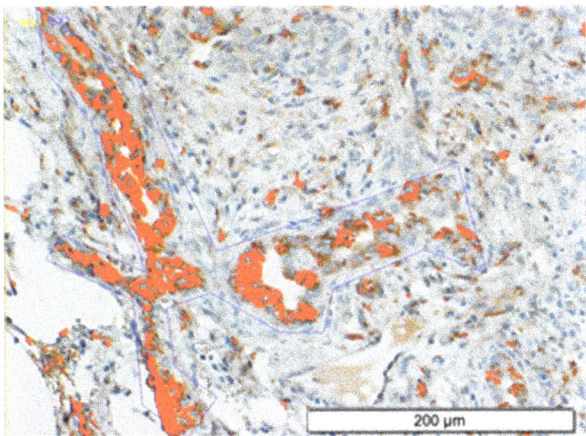

Figure 1. An example of estimation of the expression of CD56 in the portal area of the chosen regions (20× magnification, 147,978.43 μm^2).

2.6. Statistical Analyses

The data were analyzed using the Stata Program version 12.1. The Student's *t* test and the Mann–Whitney U test were performed to compare the two sets of data depending on the group size and the type of distribution. The Shapiro–Wilk test was used to check if the distribution was normal. A *p* value < 0.05 was considered statistically significant.

2.7. Ethics

The approval of the Bioethics Committee at The Children's Memorial Health Institute was obtained (number of ethical approval 17/KBE/2017). Written informed consent was obtained from the parents or the legal guardians.

3. Results

3.1. Patients' Characteristics

Thirty-one Caucasian children (fourteen female, seventeen male) aged 13.1 weeks (range 3,4–31 weeks) with newly diagnosed BA were included in the study. The patients' general biochemical and anthropological characteristics are presented in Table 1.

Table 1. The patients' general biochemical and anthropological characteristics before the HPE.

	Hbd (Weeks)	Age of HPE (Weeks) *	Total Bilirubin (mg/dL)	Direct Bilirubin (mg/dL)	ALT (U/L)	AST (U/L)	GGTP (U/L)	INR
Q1	36	8.1	6.44	5.8	82	134	302	1.03
median	39	11.0	8.74	7.22	128	177	457	1.07
Q3	39.5	13.9	10.39	9.11	175	248.5	784	1.1

ALT—alanine aminotransferase; AST—aspartate aminotransferase; GGTP—γ-glutamyl transpeptidase; INR—International Normalized Ratio; Q—quartile; Hbd—hebdomas—week of pregnancy; HPE—hepatoportoenterostomy. * Age corrected in premature patients.

Of all these patients, eight were selected for further study and divided into two groups: Group I (*n* = 4, 4 male, 0 female; aged 16 weeks [range 10–28 weeks]), with an active CMV infection, and Group II (*n* = 4, 4 female, 0 male; aged 21 weeks [range 12–31 weeks]), without a past and/or active CMV/EBV infection (Table 2).

Table 2. Biochemical, anthropological and clinical characteristics of the patients from Group I and Group II before the HPE.

	Patient	Sex	Hbd (Weeks)	Age of HPE (Weeks) *	Total Bilirubin (mg/dL)	Direct Bilirubin (mg/dL)	ALT (U/L)	AST (U/L)	GGTP (U/L)	INR	Age of LTx (Weeks) *	Time between LTx and HPE (Weeks)
Group I	1	M	40	12	6.31	7.01	88	143	820	1	29	17
	2	M	40	13	8.34	7.47	128	202	1616	1.05		
	3	M	40	10	9.37	7.92	225	358	314	1.08	38	28
	4	M	27	15	11.66	10.24	271	439	450	1.28	28	13
Group II	5	F	38	12	9.46	8.27	176	228	1652	1.08	43	29
	6	F	39	11	5.91	5.24	104	177	358	1.07	41	30
	7	F	26	11	10.5	9.3	544	685	204	1.15	166	155
	8	F	24	15	14.44	12.62	271	326	754	1.07	dq	

ALT—alanine aminotransferase; AST—aspartate aminotransferase; dq—disqualified from LTx; GGTP—γ-glutamyl transpeptidase; Hbd—hebdomas—week of pregnancy; HPE—hepatoportoenterostomy; INR—International Normalized Ratio; LTx liver—transplantation. * Age corrected in premature patients.

Six of eight selected patients underwent LTx (liver transplantation) (three patients in Group I and three patients in Group II). The mean age of LTx patients in Group I was 32 weeks (20 weeks from HPE); in Group II it was 83 weeks (71 weeks from HPE). In Group II, one patient was disqualified from LTx due to neurological complications of prematurity. The patient died in the second year of its life. In Group I, one patient was listed for LTx at the age of 5. Table 2 shows biochemical, anthropological and clinical characteristics of the patients from Group I and Group II.

CMV and EBV infection status was confirmed by the assessment of specific IgM and IgG concentrations and the RT-PCR method in all the children (Table 3). The in situ hybridization technique did not show genetic material of either EBV or CMV in the liver tissues of the study patients. Figure 2 shows a negative in situ hybridization result for the CMV of a patient in Group I.

Table 3. Virological status of CMV infection in the study groups: Group I with active CMV infection and Group II without active CMV infection.

	Patient	CMV		
		IgM (AU/mL)	IgG (AU/mL)	PCR
Group I	1	0.57	59.7	(+)
	2	7.5	41.5	(+)
	3	0.79	715.2	(+)
	4	8.9	1181	(+)
Group II	5	0.23	3.0	(−)
	6	0.13	1.5	(−)
	7	0.15	0.53	(−)
	8	0.25	0.4	(−)

CMV IgM: positive >= 1.0; negative < 1.0. CMV IgG: positive >= 6.0; negative < 6.0.

3.2. Histopathology

Histopathology of the liver showed fibrosis, bile clusters in the bile ducts, ductular proliferation and mild/moderate inflammation in all cases (Figure 3a). The presence of periductal and ductal inflammation was documented by H&E staining within the portal tracts: inflammatory infiltrates consisted of granulocytes and lymphocytes found in the wall of bile ducts/ductules and were also distributed in the fibrotic tissue between portal tracts. Bile plugs were also seen in every case and were accompanied by stromal oedema (Figure 3b). Immunohistochemical staining for cytokeratins CK7 (Figure 4a) and CK19 (Figure 4b) was performed in every case.

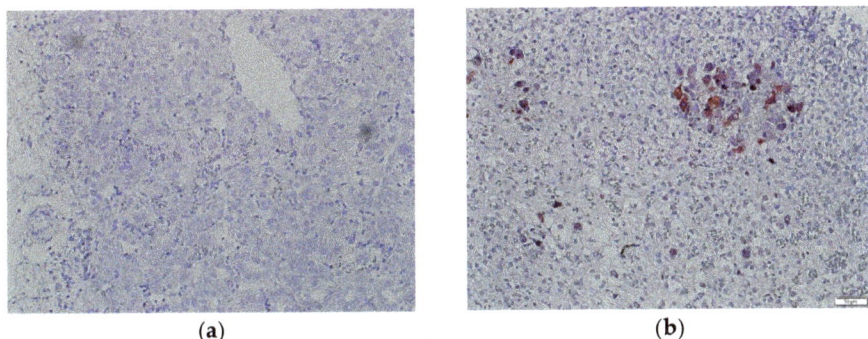

Figure 2. In situ hybridization for CMV in the liver tissue. The patient from Group I showing a negative reaction (**a**) and the positive control for CMV (**b**).

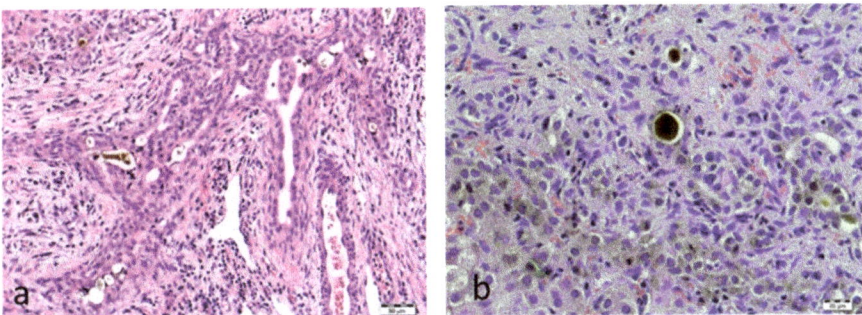

Figure 3. Bile duct and ductular proliferation in the portal tract (**a**). Lymphocytic and granulocytic infiltrates in the portal tract, bile clusters in the bile ducts, and fibrosis (Ishak fibrosis score 4) in the patient from Group I (**b**). Hematoxylin and eosin: 250× (**a**), 500× (**b**).

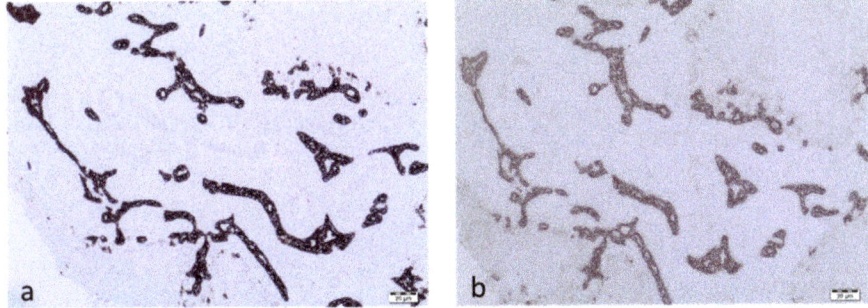

Figure 4. Immunohistochemical staining for CK7 (**a**) and CK19 (**b**) from the patient from group I.

3.3. CD8 Expression

Inflammatory cells were present in the portal tracts lying in the fibrotic tissue and infiltrating the bile ducts and ductules. The infiltration of lymphocytes CD8+ was more prominent in Group I with an active CMV infection compared to Group II without such infection (Figure 5). CD8+ cell infiltration dominated in portal areas in both groups. In the ductules, CD8+ lymphocytes were located between cholangiocytes. Morphometric analyses confirmed a statistically significant increase in the number of CD8+ lymphocytes both in the portal areas ($p = 0.002$) and in the bile ducts ($p = 0.002$) in patients with active CMV infection in comparison with the group of patients without infection (Group II). The number of lymphocytes expressing CD8 separately in the portal tracts and in the bile ducts is presented in Table 4.

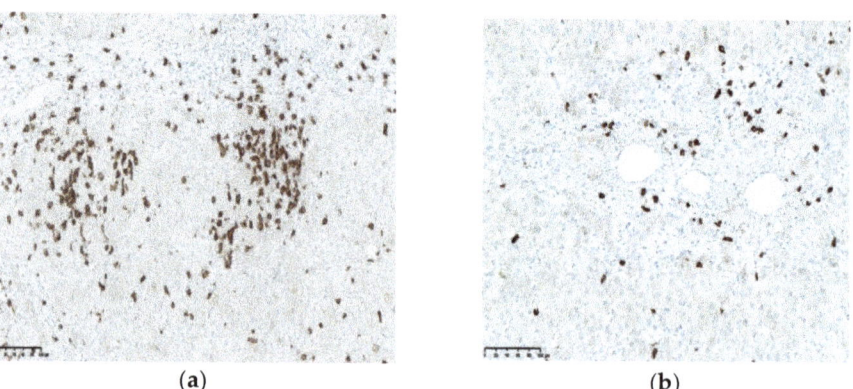

Figure 5. Presentation of the inflammatory infiltrates of CD8+ cells in the portal spaces, including bile ducts. IHC (Ventana, anti-CD8, clone SP57). Liver tissue from a patient with BA and with active CMV infection (**a**) and without active or past CMV/EBV infection (**b**).

Table 4. The number of CD8+ cells in the liver tissue of children with active CMV infection (Group I) and without CMV/EBV infection (Group II).

	The Surface of Slides (μm^2)	The Surface of Portal Areas (μm^2)	The Number of CD8+ Cells Per μm^2 of Portal Areas	The Surface of Bile Ducts in Portal Areas (μm^2)	The Number of CD8+ Cells Per μm^2 of Bile Ducts
Group I	17.67 ± 7.86	0.62 ± 0.35	206.92 ± 82.01 * $p = 0.0019$	2870.55 ± 3279.32	0.73 ± 1.23 # $p = 0.0019$
Group II	17.99 ± 5.06	0.41 ± 0.28	82.00 ± 38.98	2089.63 ± 1973.30	0.37 ± 0.62

The results are presented as arithmetical means ± SD. * Statistically significant difference in portal areas between the studied groups analyzed with the use of Student's t test, $p = 0.0019$ (d.f. = 18); # Statistically significant difference in bile ducts between studied groups analyzed with the use of the Mann–Whitney U test, $p = 0.0019$.

3.4. CD56 Expression

CD56 as a marker of immature bile ducts was expressed on the biliary epithelium of the bile ducts and bizarre forms of DPM in all cases, but was more prominent in Group I with CMV infection compared to Group II (Figure 6).

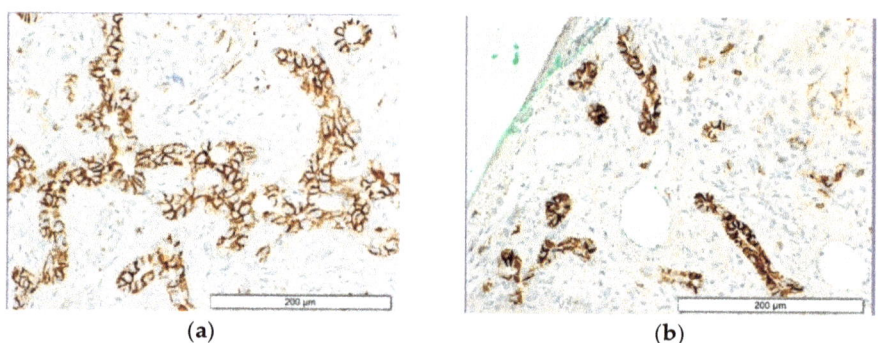

Figure 6. Expression of CD56 in the portal spaces. IHC (Cell Marque, anti-CD56, clone MRQ-42). Liver tissue from a patient with BA and with an active CMV infection (**a**) and without an active or past CMV/EBV infection (**b**).

The morphometric analysis confirmed statistical significance in CD56 expression between the groups ($p = 0.00003$) (Table 5).

Table 5. The CD56 expression in the livers of children with an active CMV infection (Group I) and without an active CMV/EBV infection (Group II).

Group I (n =4) (%)	Group II (n =4) (%)	p-Value
2.92 ± 1.43	1.43 ± 0.28	0.00003

The medium percentage (%) ± standard deviation of CD56 expression was measured as described in Material and Methods. Statistical differences were calculated with the use of the Mann–Whitney U test.

4. Discussion

Abnormal immune response in the pathogenesis of BA was reported before with the special role of CMV infection as an external trigger [1,10–12].

In our study, we presented a significant increase in CD8+ lymphocytes in both portal areas and bile ducts in patients with an active CMV infection vs. CMV-negative patients. This is in line with previous reports on the cytotoxicity of lymphocytes towards the biliary tract [11,13–15]. Mack et al. described the results of the transplantation of CD3+ cells (probably containing CD4+, CD8+, NK cells) into adult SCID mice. The transplanted cells lodged in the bile ducts, causing inflammation without losing the lumen of the ducts [11]. Shivakumar et al. showed that in response to a viral agent (Rotavirus Rhesus), CD8+ cells damage the bile ducts, leading to a BA-like phenotype in newborns. Interestingly, in CD8+-deficient mice, the disease did not progress and the bile duct lumen remained continuous [15].

Another study showed that the lymphocytic infiltration of the bile ducts in BA patients consists mainly of CD8+ T cells and NK cells. CD8+ cells can damage the bile duct epithelium as a result of NK cell activity [13]. The involvement of NK cells in biliary diseases has been repeatedly described [13,16–18]. CD56 glycoprotein is the differentiation antigen for these cells. One of the tasks of NK cells is to respond to infectious provocations in the liver. The proliferation and activation of these lymphocytes lead to the destruction of virus-infected cells [19]. In the study by Guo et al., abundant NK lymphocyte infiltration was found in the extrahepatic bile ducts of neonates with BA, including patients with CMV infection, compared to the controls [13]. We observed a similar relationship in our study. There was higher expression of CD56 in BA patients with a CMV infection than in those without infection.

On the other hand, CD56 is also a stem cell marker associated with biliary differentiation and ductal reaction [20], and it is considered an additional marker in the diagnosis of BA [21–25]. However, the increased expression of CD56 has also been observed in other cholestatic diseases, such as choledochal cyst and progressive familial intrahepatic cholestasis [25]. Zhang et al. observed in their study a positive correlation of CD56 expression with liver fibrosis [23]. Similar conclusions were presented by Ayyanara et al. [25]. We suggest that an increased expression of CD56 found in the portal space (including bile ducts in children with active CMV infection compared to children without infection) can be a sign of a newly formed bile structure often without lumen, suggesting the inhibition of the maturation process in BA. It is probable that CMV infection in patients with BA worsens the prognosis of the disease. In our study, patients with CMV infection required LTx at a much younger age than those in the group without CMV infection (32 vs. 83 weeks).

Study Limitations

Our study is limited by the small size of our group of patients. However, it is necessary to emphasize that three out of eight patients were extremely premature infants. Due to extreme prematurity and its complications, the diagnosis of BA in this group is difficult. For this reason, and due to the late referral of the patient to the reference center, KPE is performed in these patients at a later age compared to full-term newborns [26]. Other limitations include the lack of a control group and patients with other cholestatic diseases, non-BA and no confirmation of an increase in CD8+ number in peripheral blood, as well as no double immunohistochemical staining to visualize CD8+ lymphocytes in liver tissue co-stained with CD56, and cytokeratins such as CK7 or CK19. Immune profiles are different in the early and late stages of response [27], but in our study we focused on late-stage immune cells (CD8+ and CD56+), which is another limitation of our study. Further studies on a larger group of patients are needed to assess the role of individual effector cells in the pathogenesis of BA and the role of CMV infection in this process.

5. Conclusions

In conclusion, our observations indicate that active CMV infection induces an increased infiltration of cytotoxic CD8+ cells that could play role in BA immunopathogenesis. The expression of CD56 is not usually present in the mature biliary epithelium, but appears in the reactive and proliferative biliary epithelium. CD56+ can be a sign of a newly formed bile structure often without lumen, suggesting the inhibition of the maturation process in BA.

Author Contributions: Conceptualization, M.J., J.P. and J.C.-K.; methodology, M.J., J.C.-K., E.K., J.B.B., M.K. and A.W.-R.; formal analysis, J.P., B.C. and P.C.; investigation, M.J.; data curation, M.J., J.B.B., M.K. and E.K.; writing—original draft preparation, M.J. and J.C.-K.; writing—review and editing, M.J., J.B.B., J.P., P.C. and B.C.; visualization, J.C.-K. and M.K.; supervision, J.P., B.C. and J.C.-K. All authors have read and agreed to the published version of the manuscript.

Funding: This research was funded by the Children's Memorial Health Institute (Warsaw, Poland) internal grant number S154/2017.

Institutional Review Board Statement: This study was conducted in accordance with the Declaration of Helsinki and approved by the Ethics Committee of the Children's Memorial Health Institute in Warsaw, Poland (protocol code 17/KBE/2017 and date of approval 19 April 2017).

Informed Consent Statement: Informed consent was obtained from the parents or guardians of all subjects involved in the study.

Data Availability Statement: Not applicable.

Conflicts of Interest: The authors declare no conflict of interest.

References

1. Verkade, H.J.; Bezerra, J.A.; Davenport, M.; Schreiber, R.A.; Mieli-Vergani, G.; Hulscher, J.B.; Sokol, R.J.; Kelly, D.A.; Ure, B.; Whitington, P.F.; et al. Biliary atresia and other cholestatic childhood diseases: Advances and future challenges. *J. Hepatol.* **2016**, *65*, 631–642. [CrossRef] [PubMed]
2. Perlmutter, D.H.; Shepherd, R.W. Extrahepatic biliary atesia: A disease or a phenotype? *Hepatology* **2002**, *35*, 1297–1304. [CrossRef] [PubMed]
3. Petersen, C.; Davenport, M. Aetiology of biliary atresia: What is actually known? *Orphanet. J. Rare Dis.* **2013**, *8*, 128. [CrossRef] [PubMed]
4. Tarr, P.I.; Haas, J.E.; Christie, D.L. Biliary atresia, cytomegalovirus, and age at referral. *Pediatrics* **1996**, *97*, 828–831. [CrossRef] [PubMed]
5. Fischler, B.; Ehrnst, A.; Forsgren, M.; Örvell, C.; Nemeth, A. The viral association of neonatl cholestasis in Sweden: A possible link between cytomegalovirus infection and extrhepatic biliary atresia. *J. Pediatr. Gastroenterol. Nutr.* **1998**, *27*, 57–64. [CrossRef]
6. Xu, Y.; Yu, J.; Zhang, R.; Yin, Y.; Ye, J.; Tan, L.; Xia, H. The prenatal infection of cytomegalowirus is an important etiology for biliary atresia in China. *Clin. Pediatr.* **2012**, *51*, 109–113. [CrossRef]
7. Brindley, S.M.; Lanham, A.M.; Karrer, F.M.; Tucker, R.M.; Fontenot, A.P.; Mack, C.L. Cytomegalovirusspecific T-cell reactivity in biliary atresia at the time of diagnosis is associated with deficits in regulatory T cells. *Hepatology* **2012**, *55*, 1130–1138. [CrossRef]
8. Zani, A.; Quaglia, A.; Hadžić, N.; Zuckerman, M.; Davenport, M. Cytomegalovirus-associated biliary atresia: An aetiological and prognostic subgroup. *J. Pediatr. Surg.* **2015**, *50*, 1739–1745. [CrossRef]
9. Rauschenfels, S.; Krassmann, M.; Al-Masri, A.N.; Verhagen, W.; Leonhardt, J.; Kuebler, J.F.; Petersen, C. Incidence of hepatotropic viruses in biliary atresia. *Eur. J. Pediatr.* **2009**, *168*, 469–476. [CrossRef]
10. Bezerra, J.A.; Wells, R.G.; Mack, C.L.; Karpen, S.J.; Hoofnagle, J.H.; Doo, E.; Sokol, R.J. Biliary atresia: Clinical and research challenges for the twenty-first century. *Hepatology* **2018**, *68*, 1163–1173. [CrossRef]

11. Mack, C.L.; Tucker, R.M.; Lu, B.R.; Sokol, R.J.; Fontenot, A.P.; Ueno, Y.; Gill, R.G. Cellular and humoral autoimmunity directed at bile duct epithelia in murine biliary atresia. *Hepatology* **2006**, *44*, 1231–1239. [CrossRef] [PubMed]
12. Sokol, R.J.; Mack, C. Etiopathogenesis of biliary atresia. *Semin. Liver Dis.* **2001**, *21*, 517–524. [CrossRef]
13. Guo, C.; Zhu, J.; Pu, C.L.; Deng, Y.H.; Zhang, M.M. Combinatory effects of hepatic CD8+ and NK lymphocytes in bile duct injury from biliary atresia. *Pediatr. Res.* **2012**, *71*, 638–644. [CrossRef]
14. Mack, C.L.; Falta, M.T.; Sullivan, A.K.; Karrer, F.; Sokol, R.J.; Freed, B.M.; Fontenot, A.P. Oligoclonal Expansions of CD4+ and CD8+ T-Cells in the Target Organ of Patients With Biliary Atresia. *Gastroenterology* **2007**, *133*, 278–287. [CrossRef] [PubMed]
15. Shivakumar, P.; Sabla, G.; Mohanty, S.; McNeal, M.; Ward, R.; Stringer, K.; Caldwell, C.; Chougnet, C.; Bezerra, J.A. Effector role of neonatal hepatic CD8+ lymphocytes in epithelial injury and autoimmunity in experimental biliary atresia. *Gastroenterology* **2007**, *133*, 268–277. [CrossRef]
16. Miethke, A.G.; Saxena, V.; Shivakumar, P.; Sabla, G.E.; Simmons, J.; Chougnet, C.A. Post-natal paucity of regulatory T cells and control of NK cell activation in experimental biliary atresia. *J. Hepatol.* **2010**, *52*, 718–726. [CrossRef]
17. Davenport, M.; Gonde, C.; Redkar, R.; Koukoulis, G.; Tredger, M.; Mieli-Vergani, G.; Portmann, B.; Howard, E.R. Immunohistochemistry of the liver and biliary tree in extrahepatic biliary atresia. *J. Pediatr. Surg.* **2001**, *36*, 1017–1025. [CrossRef] [PubMed]
18. Shivakumar, P.; Sabla, G.E.; Whitington, P.; Chougnet, C.A.; Bezerra, J.A. Neonatal NK cells target the mouse duct epithelium via Nkg2d and drive tissue-specific injury in experimental biliary atresia. *J. Clin. Investig.* **2009**, *119*, 2281–2290. [CrossRef]
19. Vivier, E.; Tomasello, E.; Baratin, M.; Walzer, T.; Ugolini, S. Functions of natural killer cells. *Nat. Immunol.* **2008**, *9*, 503–510. [CrossRef] [PubMed]
20. Zhou, H.; Rogler, L.E.; Teperman, L.; Morgan, G.; Rogler, C.E. Identification of hepatocytic and bile ductular cell lineages and candidate stem cells in bipolar ductular reactions in cirrhotic human liver. *Hepatology* **2007**, *45*, 716–724. [CrossRef]
21. Torbenson, M.; Wang, J.; Abraham, S.; Maitra, A.; Boitnott, J. Bile ducts and ductules are positive for CD56 (N-CAM) in most cases of extrahepatic biliary atresia. *Am. J. Surg. Pathol.* **2003**, *27*, 1454–1457. [CrossRef] [PubMed]
22. Sira, M.M.; El-Guindi, M.A.; Saber, M.A.; Ehsan, N.A.; Rizk, M.S. Differential hepatic expression of CD56 can discriminate biliary atresia from other neonatal cholestatic disorders. *Eur. J. Gastroenterol. Hepatol.* **2012**, *24*, 1227–1233. [CrossRef] [PubMed]
23. Zhang, R.Z.; Yu, J.K.; Peng, J.; Wang, F.H.; Liu, H.Y.; Lui, V.C.; Nicholls, J.M.; Tam, P.K.; Lamb, J.R.; Chen, Y.; et al. Role of CD56-expressing immature biliary epithelial cells in biliary atresia. *World J. Gastroenterol.* **2016**, *22*, 2545–2557. [CrossRef] [PubMed]
24. Cielecka-Kuszyk, J.; Janowska, M.; Markiewicz, M.; Czubkowski, P.; Ostoja-Chyżyńska, A.; Bierła, J.; Cukrowska, B.; Pawłowska, J. The Usefulness of Immunohistochemical Staining of Bile Tracts in Biliary Atresia. *Clin. Exp. Hepatol.* **2021**, *7*, 41–46. [CrossRef]
25. Ayyanar, P.; Mahalik, S.K.; Haldar, S.; Purkait, S.; Patra, S.; Mitra, S. Expression of CD56 is Not Limited to Biliary Atresia and Correlates with the Degree of Fibrosis in Pediatric Cholestatic Diseases. *Fetal Pediatr. Pathol.* **2022**, *41*, 87–97. [CrossRef]
26. Van Wessel, D.B.; Boere, T.; Hulzebos, C.V.; de Kleine, R.H.; Verkade, H.J.; Hulscher, J.B. Preterm Infants With Biliary Atresia: A Nationwide Cohort Analysis From The Netherlands. *J. Pediatr. Gastroenterol. Nutr.* **2017**, *65*, 370–374. [CrossRef]
27. Yang, C.; Xing, H.; Tan, B.; Zhang, M. Immune Characteristics in Biliary Atresia Based on Immune Genes and Immune Cell Infiltration. *Front. Pediatr.* **2022**, *10*, 902571. [CrossRef]

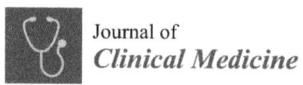

Article

Neonatal Hepatic Myeloid Progenitors Expand and Propagate Liver Injury in Mice

Anas Alkhani [1,2,†], Cathrine Korsholm [1,2,3,†], Claire S. Levy [1,2], Sarah Mohamedaly [1,2], Caroline C. Duwaerts [2,4,‡], Eric M. Pietras [5] and Amar Nijagal [1,2,6,7,*]

1. Department of Surgery, University of California, San Francisco, CA 94143, USA
2. The Liver Center, University of California, San Francisco, CA 94143, USA
3. Department of Comparative Pediatrics and Nutrition, University of Copenhagen, 1870 Frederiksberg C, Denmark
4. Department of Medicine, University of California, San Francisco, CA 94143, USA
5. Division of Hematology, University of Colorado Anschutz Medical Campus, Aurora, CO 80045, USA
6. The Pediatric Liver Center, UCSF Benioff Childrens' Hospital, San Francisco, CA 94143, USA
7. Eli and Edythe Broad Center of Regeneration Medicine, University of California, San Francisco, CA 94143, USA
* Correspondence: amar.nijagal@ucsf.edu; Tel.: +1-415-476-4086
† These authors contributed equally to this work.
‡ Current address: Gordian Biotechnology, South San Francisco, CA 94080, USA.

Abstract: Background: Biliary atresia (BA) is a progressive pediatric inflammatory disease of the liver that leads to cirrhosis and necessitates liver transplantation. The rapid progression from liver injury to liver failure in children with BA suggests that factors specific to the perinatal hepatic environment are important for disease propagation. Hematopoietic stem and progenitor cells (HSPCs) reside in the fetal liver and are known to serve as central hubs of inflammation. We hypothesized that HSPCs are critical for the propagation of perinatal liver injury (PLI). Methods: Newborn BALB/c mice were injected with rhesus rotavirus (RRV) to induce PLI or with PBS as control. Livers were compared using histology and flow cytometry. To determine the effects of HSPCs on PLI, RRV-infected neonatal mice were administered anti-CD47 and anti-CD117 to deplete HSPCs. Results: PLI significantly increased the number of common myeloid progenitors and the number of CD34[+] hematopoietic progenitors. Elimination of HSPCs through antibody-mediated myeloablation rescued animals from PLI and significantly increased survival (RRV+isotype control 36.4% vs. RRV+myeloablation 77.8%, Chi-test = 0.003). Conclusions: HSPCs expand as a result of RRV infection and propagate PLI. Targeting of HSPCs may be useful in preventing and treating neonatal inflammatory diseases of the liver such as BA.

Keywords: biliary atresia; perinatal liver injury; hematopoietic stem and progenitor cells; myeloid progenitor cells

Citation: Alkhani, A.; Korsholm, C.; Levy, C.S.; Mohamedaly, S.; Duwaerts, C.C.; Pietras, E.M.; Nijagal, A. Neonatal Hepatic Myeloid Progenitors Expand and Propagate Liver Injury in Mice. *J. Clin. Med.* **2023**, *12*, 337. https://doi.org/10.3390/jcm12010337

Academic Editor: Claus Petersen

Received: 2 December 2022
Revised: 24 December 2022
Accepted: 28 December 2022
Published: 1 January 2023

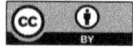

Copyright: © 2023 by the authors. Licensee MDPI, Basel, Switzerland. This article is an open access article distributed under the terms and conditions of the Creative Commons Attribution (CC BY) license (https://creativecommons.org/licenses/by/4.0/).

1. Introduction

Biliary atresia (BA) is the leading cause of pediatric liver transplants worldwide [1]. Though its exact etiology is unknown, the progressive perinatal liver injury (PLI) observed in patients with BA is caused by dysregulated immune responses to liver injury [2,3]. The rapid progression from liver injury to fulminant liver failure in children with BA suggests that factors specific to the perinatal hepatic environment are important for disease propagation. Therefore, understanding the perinatal hepatic immune environment in which inflammatory diseases such as BA develop and progress is important to identify promising treatment strategies for this devastating disease.

Our recent studies in mice indicate that the adaptive immune response plays a limited role in the pathogenesis of PLI [4], whereas the innate immune response, specifically myeloid populations, are critical for determining disease outcome as the relative proportions of pro-inflammatory and pro-reparative myeloid cells control disease severity [4].

Hematopoietic stem and progenitor cells (HSPCs) give rise to immune populations and reside in the liver of late-gestation human fetuses before emigrating to the bone marrow (BM) [5,6]; in mice, this transition occurs during the first weeks of postnatal life [7]. HSPCs react to inflammatory signals via Toll-like receptors, cytokines, and growth factors [8], and act as central hubs of inflammation by coordinating immune responses [9]. For example, IL-1ß binds to HSPCs and induces transcriptomic changes that skew HSPC differentiation towards myelopoiesis [8]. Through their rapid expansion and replenishment of mature myeloid populations, HSPCs are fundamental in facilitating the transition from inflammation to the resolution of liver disease [4,9–11]. Both human and murine models of liver injury show that monocytes derived from HSPCs transition from pro-inflammatory cells immediately after injury into pro-reparative monocytes once the injurious agent is no longer present [4,10–12]. Our group has previously elaborated on this observation by demonstrating that the abundance of pro-reparative Ly6C^{Lo} non-classical monocytes renders animals resistant to PLI and that reducing the number of Ly6C^{Lo} non-classical monocytes restores susceptibility to liver injury [4]. In addition to the rapid expansion of HSPCs and their differentiation into myeloid cells during inflammation, dysregulation of HSPCs can contribute to a feed-forward loop that leads to the pathologic expansion of inflammatory myeloid populations, resulting in chronic inflammation and tissue injury [9]. Taken together, these findings support the role of HSPCs and their mature myeloid progeny in propagating PLI.

In this study, we hypothesized that HSPCs propagate PLI in neonatal mice. To test this hypothesis, we used an infectious model of PLI to examine the role of HSPCs in neonatal liver injury. Using this model, we compared HSPCs and mature myeloid populations from the liver and BM in the setting of homeostasis and PLI. Our results demonstrate that HSPCs expand during PLI and that depletion of HSPCs prevents liver injury. These findings support our hypothesis that HSPCs play an important role in propagating PLI.

2. Materials and Methods

2.1. Mice

BALB/c mice were obtained from the National Cancer Institute (Wilmington, MA, USA), and received humane care according to the Guide for Care and Use of Laboratory Animals. Mouse experiments were approved by the University of California, San Francisco Institutional Animal Care and Use Committee, and all mice were euthanized according to humane end points.

2.2. Creation of Single-Cell Suspensions

P3 and P14 livers were isolated and mechanically dissociated in phosphate-buffered saline (PBS). Juvenile (P14) livers underwent additional enzymatic digestion using 2.5 mg/mL liberase (Roche Indianapolis, IN, USA, 05401119001) in 1 M CaCl2 HEPES buffer. BM was isolated from the tibia, fibula, hip, and lower spines of neonatal (P3) and juvenile (P14) animals, and mechanically dissociated in PBS. Both liver and BM single-cell suspensions were filtered through a 100 um strainer prior to further analysis.

2.3. Flow Cytometry

Single-cell suspensions from the liver and BM were divided into two fractions. One fraction was stained for surface markers on mature myeloid cells (Supplementary Table S1). To isolate HSPCs, the other fraction was depleted of lineage-positive (Lin$^+$) cells using a Direct Lineage Cell Depletion Kit (Miltenyi Biotec, Cambridge, MA, USA, 130-110-470) and stained for the following HSPCs: long-term hematopoietic stem cells (HSC^{LT}), common myeloid progenitors (CMP$^+$ and CMP$^-$), and terminal myeloid progenitors (TMPs: megakaryocytic-erythroid progenitors, MEP; monocytic-dendritic progenitors, MDP; granulocytic-monocytic progenitors, GMP; granulocytic progenitors, GP; monocytic and common monocytic progenitors, MP) using cell surface markers (Supplementary Table S2). Flow cytometry was performed on a LSR Fortessa X20 (BD Biosciences, San Jose, CA, USA) and data were analyzed in FlowJo (Ashland, OR, USA).

2.4. Colony-Forming Unit (CFU) Assays

Single-cell suspensions from P3 and P14 livers and BMs were cultured on Metho-Cult^{TM} media containing methylcellulose, recombinant mouse stem cell factor, IL-3, IL-6, and recombinant human EPO. 2×10^4 cells were plated and incubated at 37 °C in 5% CO_2 for 12 days. The proliferation and differentiation ability of HSPCs was assessed by a blinded observer who categorized CFU into granulocyte, macrophage (GM), granulocyte, erythrocyte, macrophage, megakaryocyte (GEMM), and macrophage (M) colonies.

2.5. Postnatal Model of Perinatal Liver Injury

Rotavirus (RRV) was grown and titered in *Cercopithecus aethiops* kidney epithelial (MA104) cells. PLI was induced by intraperitoneal injections (i.p.) of 1.5×10^6 focus forming units (ffU) RRV within 24 h of birth (P0). Controls were injected i.p. with PBS.

2.6. Histologic Analysis

Liver tissue was analyzed using immunohistochemistry (IHC) for $CD34^+$ cells or hematoxylin and eosin (H&E). H&E slides were examined for signs of inflammatory infiltrate and tissue injury (e.g., necrosis). IHC slides were imaged at 40× magnification and $CD34^+$ cells with large nuclei and little cytoplasm were counted as HSPCs by a blinded observer using QuPath [13]. Since CD34 is also present in vascular endothelial cells, all elongated cells with the morphologic appearance of endothelial cells were excluded [14]. The mean number of $CD34^+$ cells/cm^2 was calculated between all stained liver sections using QuPath [13].

2.7. Antibody-Mediated Myeloablation in Neonatal Mice

Myeloablation was induced by i.p. injections (20 µL) of anti-CD117 and anti-CD47. Anti-CD117 (0.20 µg/µL) was given only on day 0. Anti-CD47 was administered on day 0 (0.15 µg/µL), day 1 (0.20 µg/µL), day 2 (0.25 µg/µL), day 3 (0.30 µg/µL), and day 4 (0.35 µg/µL) post-RRV injection. Isotype controls were injected i.p. with isotype IgG2b (similar regimen as anti-CD117) and isotype IgG2a (similar regimen as anti-CD47). Escalating amounts of anti-CD47 and IgG2a were given to account for the natural increase in pup weight that occurs after birth. All antibodies for this experiment were purchased from BioXCell, West Lebanon, NH, USA.

2.8. Data Analysis

All graphs and statistics were generated using GraphPad Prism 9.3.1 (San Diego, CA, USA). Individual proportions of HSPCs were calculated based on absolute cell counts (ACC) as either a percentage (%) of the total lineage-negative progenitor compartment (Lin^{-ve} cells), or as a fraction of total HSC^{LT} and downstream myeloid progenitors (CMPs and TMPs). Mature myeloid cell proportions were calculated as a percentage of $CD45^+$ leukocytes based on ACC. p-values were calculated using unpaired, non-parametric tests (Mann–Whitney was used to compare the proportion and ACC of HSPCs) except for survival comparisons that were performed using chi-squared. A p-value of <0.05 was considered significant. Error bars represent mean ± standard deviation (SD). All authors had access to the study data and reviewed and approved the final manuscript.

3. Results

3.1. The Liver Is a Reservoir for Hematopoietic Progenitors in Neonatal Mice

To define the distribution of myeloid progenitors in neonatal animals under normal conditions, we quantified HSPCs (HSC^{LT}s, CMPs, TMPs) and their mature progeny in the liver and BM of neonatal (P3) and juvenile (P14) mice. All HSPC populations were identified using cell-surface markers: HSC^{LT} were defined as Sca-1$^+$. CMP and TMP populations were defined as Sca-1$^-$. Individual CMP and TMP populations were distinguished based on the expression of CD34, FcγR, Flt3, Ly6C, and CD115 (Figure 1a–c) [15]. Since our previous work demonstrated a limited role for T- and B-lymphocytes in the pathogenesis of PLI, lymphoid progenitors were not quantified in this study [4].

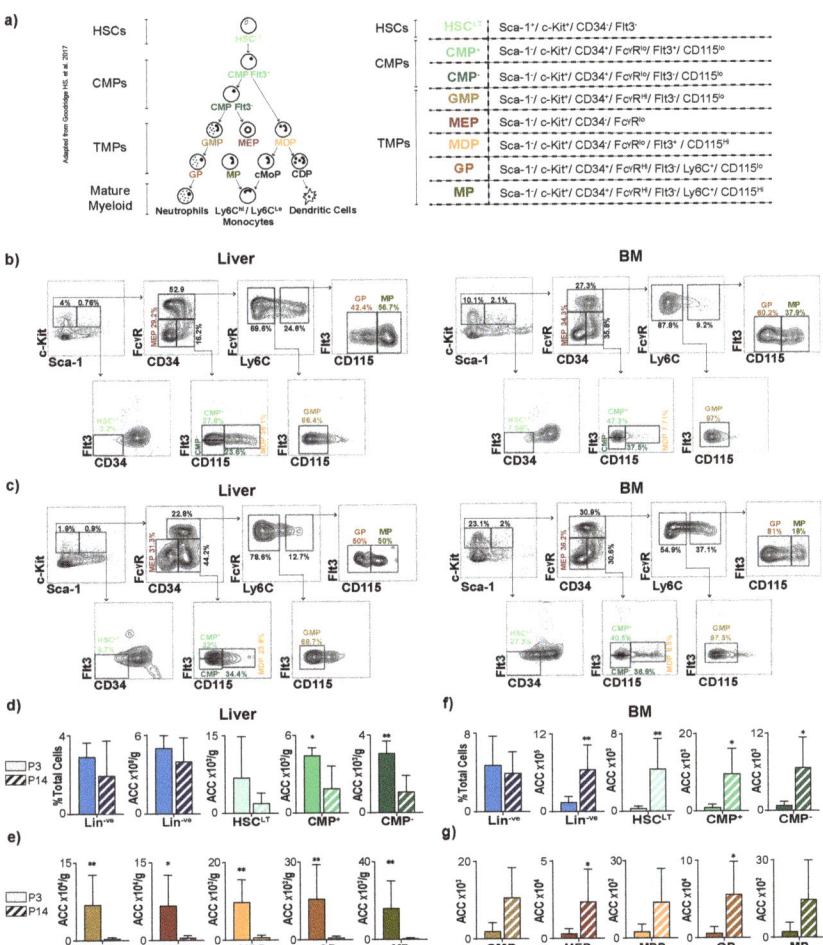

Figure 1. The liver is the main reservoir for myeloid progenitors in neonatal mice. (**a**) Schematic showing differentiation hierarchy and cell-surface markers of hematopoietic stem and progenitor cells (HSPCs): long-term hematopoietic stem cells (HSC^{LT}), common myeloid progenitors (CMP$^+$ and CMP$^-$), and terminal myeloid progenitors (TMP: megakaryocytic-erythroid progenitors, MEP; monocytic-dendritic progenitors, MDP; granulocytic-monocytic progenitors, GMP; granulocytic progenitors, GP; monocytic and common monocytic progenitors, MP), and mature myeloid populations [15]. Plots demonstrating flow cytometric gating strategy of HSC^{LT}s, CMPs, and TMPs in liver and bone marrow (BM) of PBS-injected mice on postnatal day 3 (P3) in (**b**) and postnatal day 14 (P14) in (**c**). Quantification of lineage negative (Lin^{-ve}) fraction and absolute cell counts (ACC) of Lin^{-ve}, HSC^{LT}, and CMP populations on P3 and P14 of life in (**d**) liver and (**f**) BM. Quantification of TMPs in P3 and P14 (**e**) liver and (**g**) BM. $n = 6$ for each group. p-value * < 0.05; ** < 0.01. Error bars represent mean ± SD.

We first quantified the Lin^{-ve} compartment in the liver and found that the percentage and number of Lin^{-ve} cells did not differ significantly between P3 and P14 livers (Figure 1d) and that the number of individual HSPC populations (CMPs and TMPs) were significantly lower at P14 compared to P3 (Figure 1d,e).

In contrast to these findings in the liver, both the number of Lin^{-ve} cells and downstream progenitor populations (specifically HSC^{LT}, CMP$^+$, CMP$^-$, MEP, and GP) in BM increased significantly between P3 and P14 (Figure 1f,g). In both the liver and BM, the mature myeloid populations mirrored the trends seen among progenitor populations as mature populations decreased in the liver and increased in the BM from P3 to P14; these differences, however, were not statistically significant (Supplementary Figure S1a,b).

Collectively, these findings quantify the extent to which the murine liver retains hematopoietic progenitors during early neonatal life. These findings are also consistent with the known migration of hematopoietic progenitors from the liver to the BM during the first 2–3 weeks of postnatal life in mice [16].

3.2. The Juvenile Liver Retains Common Myeloid Progenitors and Myeloid Differentiation Capacity

We next asked whether the relative proportions of individual HSPC populations in the liver and BM changed from P3 to P14. In the liver, both the percentage of CMPs out of all Lin^{-ve} cells (Figure 2a) and CMPs as a fraction of total HSC^{LT}s, CMPs, and TMPs (Figure 2b) significantly increased between P3 and P14. Meanwhile, all liver TMPs decreased, although this was only statistically significant for MDPs and MPs (Figure 2a,b). Unlike the liver, the BM exhibited a relative increase in the percentages of HSC^{LT}s, CMPs, and TMPs out of total Lin^{-ve} cells between P3 and P14 (Figure 2c). This increase was only significant for HSC^{LT}, MEPs, and GPs, and not for CMPs. The same trend was observed when we examined each population as a fraction of all HSC^{LT}s, CMPs, and TMPs (Figure 2d). These results indicate that CMPs in the liver increase relative to other Lin^{-ve} cells, at a time when the main site of hematopoiesis is transitioning to the BM.

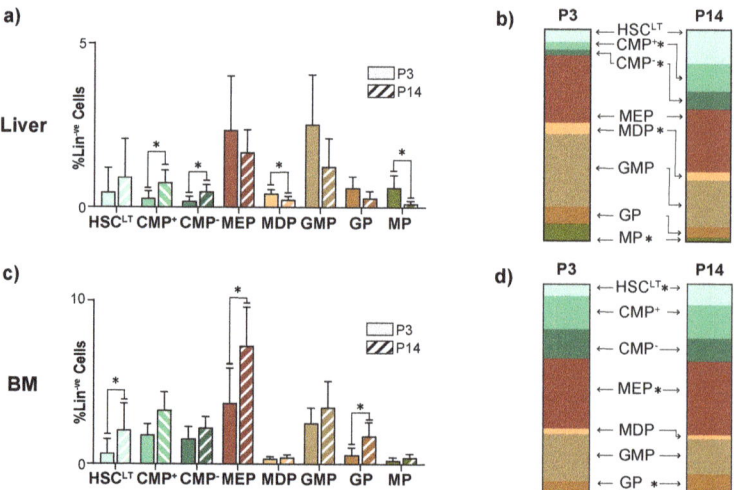

Figure 2. The juvenile mouse liver retains common myeloid progenitors. Percentage of hematopoietic stem cell (HSC^{LT}), common myeloid progenitor (CMP), and terminal myeloid progenitor (TMP) populations among lineage negative (Lin^{-ve}) cells in (**a**) liver and (**c**) bone marrow (BM) on postnatal day 3 (P3) and postnatal day 14 (P14). Relative proportions of HSC^{LT}, CMP, and TMP among HSC^{LT} and their downstream myeloid progenitors in the (**b**) liver and (**d**) BM (P3, P14, $n = 6$). p-value * < 0.05. Error bars represent the mean ± SD.

To test the differentiation potential of HSPCs from the liver and BM, we quantified colony-forming units of pro-myeloid colonies. The liver retained a similar pro-myeloid differentiation capacity at P14 compared to P3 as the number of granulocyte monocyte (GM) and granulocyte, erythrocyte, monocyte, megakaryocyte (GEMM) and megakaryocytes (M) colonies remain unchanged (Supplementary Figure S2a). In P14 BM, however, colonies from GM and GEMM increased, while the number of M colonies remained constant compared to P3 (Supplementary Figure S2b).

The increase in CMPs in the livers of juvenile mice and the maintenance of myeloid differentiation capacity led us to question whether HSPCs residing in the liver play a role in perinatal liver injury.

3.3. Perinatal Liver Injury Leads to Expansion of CMPs in the Neonatal Liver

Based on our observation that the liver is a reservoir for HSPCs in neonatal mice and the known role of HSPC populations as central hubs of inflammation, we hypothesized that HSPC populations in the liver would expand during PLI. We have previously used rhesus rotavirus infection (RRV) in neonatal mice to study the role of immune populations during PLI [4]. Neonatal pups injected with RRV within the first 24 h of life develop progressive liver injury and a periportal inflammatory infiltrate that resembles the histological findings observed in human BA [17].

To evaluate the effects of PLI, we analyzed the livers of RRV-injected pups using flow cytometry and histology three days after injury (P3). All HSPCs were identified from flow plots as shown in Figure 3a. PLI significantly increased the number of Lin^{-ve} cells in the liver (Figure 3b), which was reflected in downstream HSC^{LT}s and CMPs, though only CMPs reached statistical significance (Figure 3c). PLI had no effect on TMPs (Figure 3c). When we assessed each progenitor population as a fraction of total HSC^{LT}s, CMPs, and TMPs, we found that PLI led to increases in liver HSC^{LT} and CMP fractions, though these differences did not reach statistical significance (Figure 3d). Using immunohistochemistry to localize $CD34^+$ HSPCs in the P3 liver, we found that PLI significantly increased the number of $CD34^+$ HSPCs/cm^2 relative to controls and that these cells infiltrated all parts of the liver tissue with no identifiable pattern (Figure 3e,f). Notably, the expansion of CMPs did not lead to an increase in mature myeloid populations at P3 (Figure 3g–i).

We questioned whether RRV infection affected HSPC populations residing in the BM of neonatal mice, and observed no significant changes in the absolute cell counts or percentages of HSPC populations in the BM after RRV infection (Figure 4a–c). Similar to the liver, we also did not identify significant changes to mature myeloid populations in the BM after RRV injection (Figure 4e–g). Taken together, RRV infection led to an expansion of CMPs specifically in the livers of neonatal mice.

3.4. Perinatal Liver Injury Leads to Contraction of HSPCs and Expansion of Mature Myeloid Populations in the Juvenile Liver

We next determined whether the expansion of CMPs seen in the neonatal liver after RRV infection was persistent or temporary. We quantified HSPC populations in juvenile mice 14 days after RRV infection (P14, Figure 5a) and we observed an overall reduction in Lin^{-ve} cells (Figure 5b). The number of HSPCs, including CMP^+, MEPs, and MPs, decreased in RRV-infected P14 livers, compared to PBS-injected controls (Figure 5b). Despite the decrease in the number of these progenitor populations, MEP was the only progenitor population to decrease significantly as a percentage of Lin^{-ve} cells and as a fraction of total HSC^{LT}s, CMPs, and TMPs (Figure 5c,d). While the number of all mature myeloid populations remained constant (Figure 5e,f), the percentage of neutrophils, monocytes, and monocyte-derived macrophages out of $CD45^+$ leukocytes significantly increased in livers of RRV-infected juvenile mice, corresponding to the known peak of disease in RRV-infected animals (Figure 5e,g) [17]. These findings demonstrate that PLI causes a temporary expansion of CMPs in RRV-infected neonatal mice and that PLI results in a relative increase in mature myeloid populations 14 days after RRV infection.

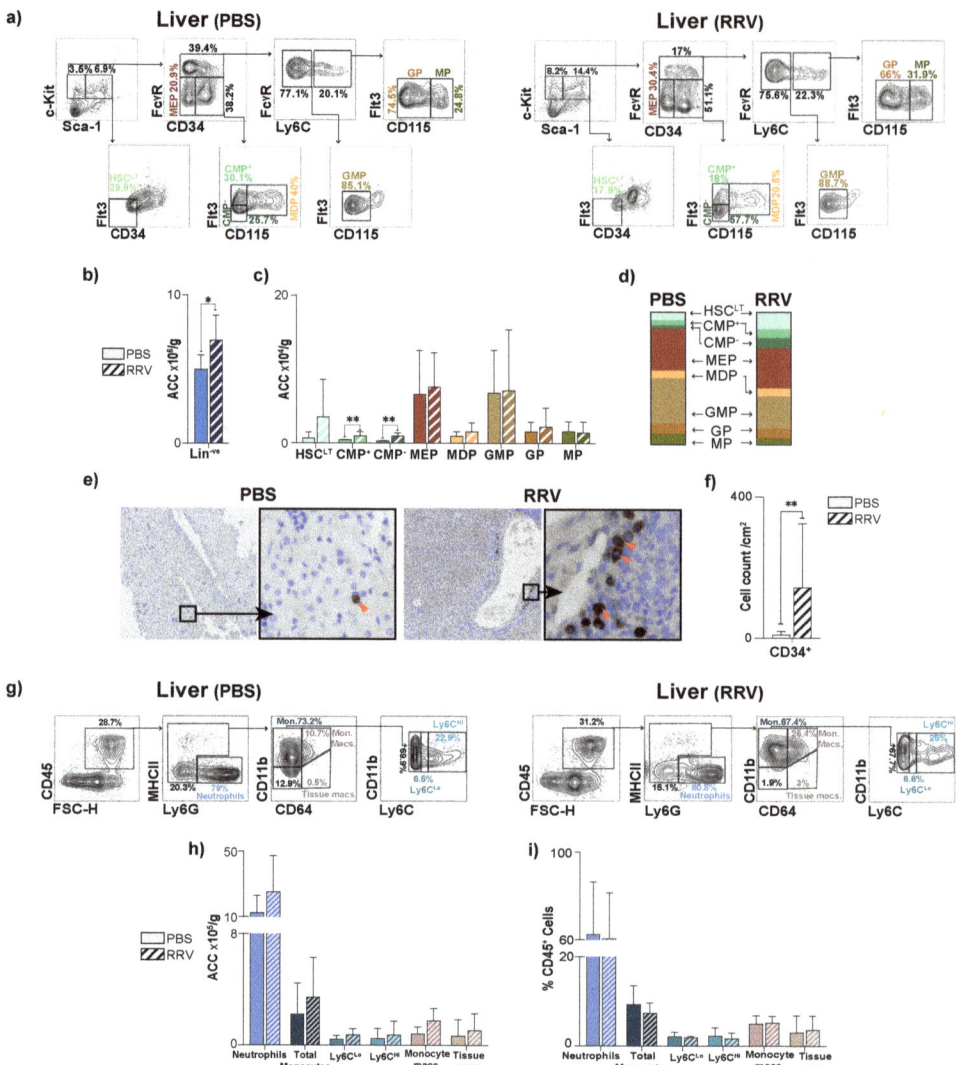

Figure 3. Perinatal liver injury results in the expansion of myeloid progenitors in the neonatal liver. (**a**) Representative flow plots demonstrating gating strategy of hematopoietic stem cells (HSC^{LT}), common myeloid progenitors (CMP), and terminal myeloid progenitors (TMP) in liver of PBS- and RRV-injected 3-day-old (P3) mice. Quantification of absolute cell counts (ACC) of (**b**) lineage negative (Lin^{-ve}) cells and (**c**) HSC^{LT}s, CMPs, TMPs in P3 livers from PBS- (n = 6) and RRV-injected (n = 7) mice. (**d**) Relative fractions of HSC^{LT}, CMP, and TMP populations in P3 livers from PBS- (n = 6) and RRV-injected (n = 7) mice. (**e**) Representative P3 livers in the setting of PBS and RRV with red arrows marking immunohistochemistry-stained CD34$^+$ cells. (**f**) Quantification of CD34$^+$ cells at P3 in PBS- (n = 6) and RRV-injected mice (n = 9). High-power images are at 40× magnification. (**g**) Representative flow plots demonstrating gating strategy of mature myeloid CD45$^+$ populations in liver of PBS- and RRV-injected 3-day-old (P3) mice. (**h**) Quantification of ACC of mature myeloid populations in the liver of PBS- (n = 3) and RRV-injected (n = 5) mice at P3. (**i**) Quantification of %CD45$^+$ leukocytes of mature myeloid populations in the liver of PBS- (n = 4) and RRV-injected (n = 8) mice at P3. p-value * < 0.05, ** <0.01. Error bars represent mean ± SD.

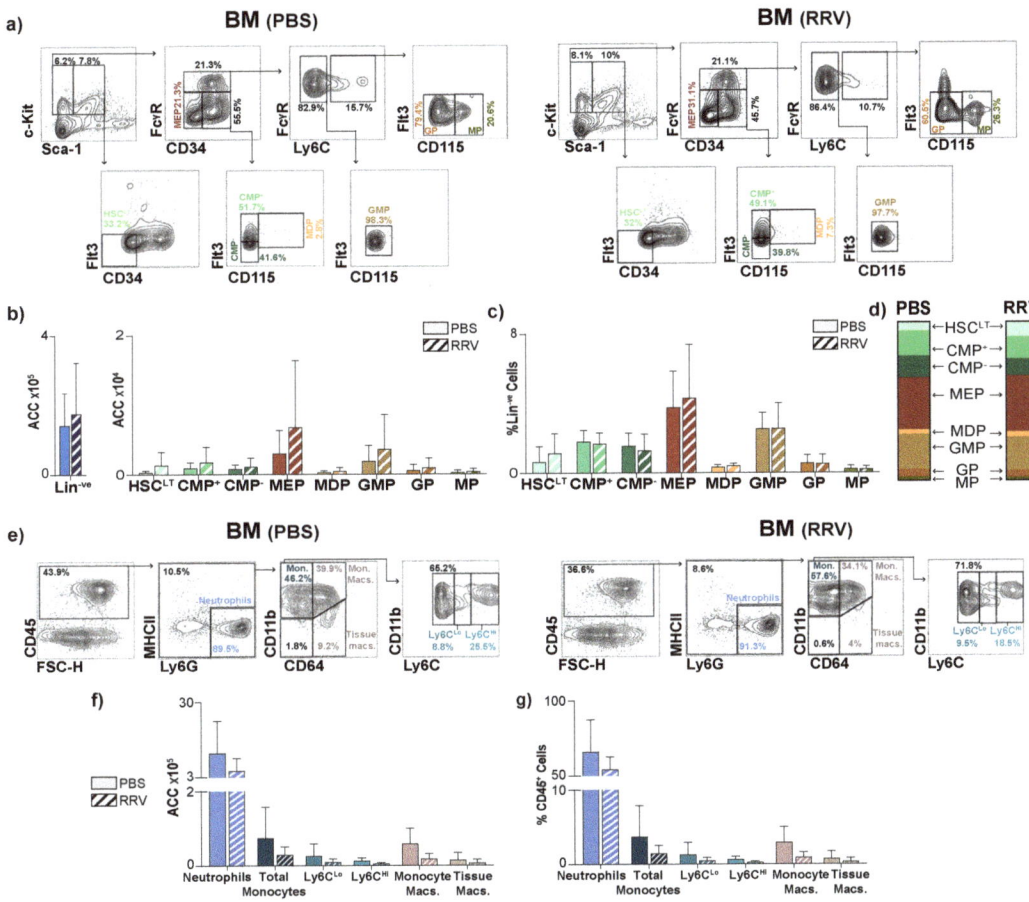

Figure 4. Perinatal liver injury causes no quantitative change to HSPCs in the BM of neonatal mice. (**a**) Representative flow plots demonstrating gating strategy of hematopoietic stem cells (HSC^{LT}), common myeloid progenitors (CMP), and terminal myeloid progenitors (TMP) in BM of PBS- and RRV-injected 3-day-old (P3) mice. (**b**) Absolute cell counts (ACC) of lineage negative (Lin^{-ve}) cells, hematopoietic stem cells (HSC^{LT}), common myeloid progenitors (CMPs), and terminal myeloid progenitors (TMPs) of the BM, (**c**) percentage of total Lin^{-ve} cells, (**d**) fraction of HSC^{LT}, CMPs, and TMPs. (**e**) Representative flow plots demonstrating gating strategy of mature myeloid CD45$^+$ populations in BM of PBS- and RRV-injected 3-day-old (P3) mice. (**f**) ACC of mature myeloid populations (PBS $n = 3$, RRV $n = 5$) of the BM and (**g**) percentage of individual mature myeloid populations out of all CD45$^+$ cells (PBS $n = 3$, RRV $n = 5$) at post-natal day 3 (P3). $n = 6$ for PBS and $n = 6$ for RRV unless otherwise stated. Error bars represent mean ± SD.

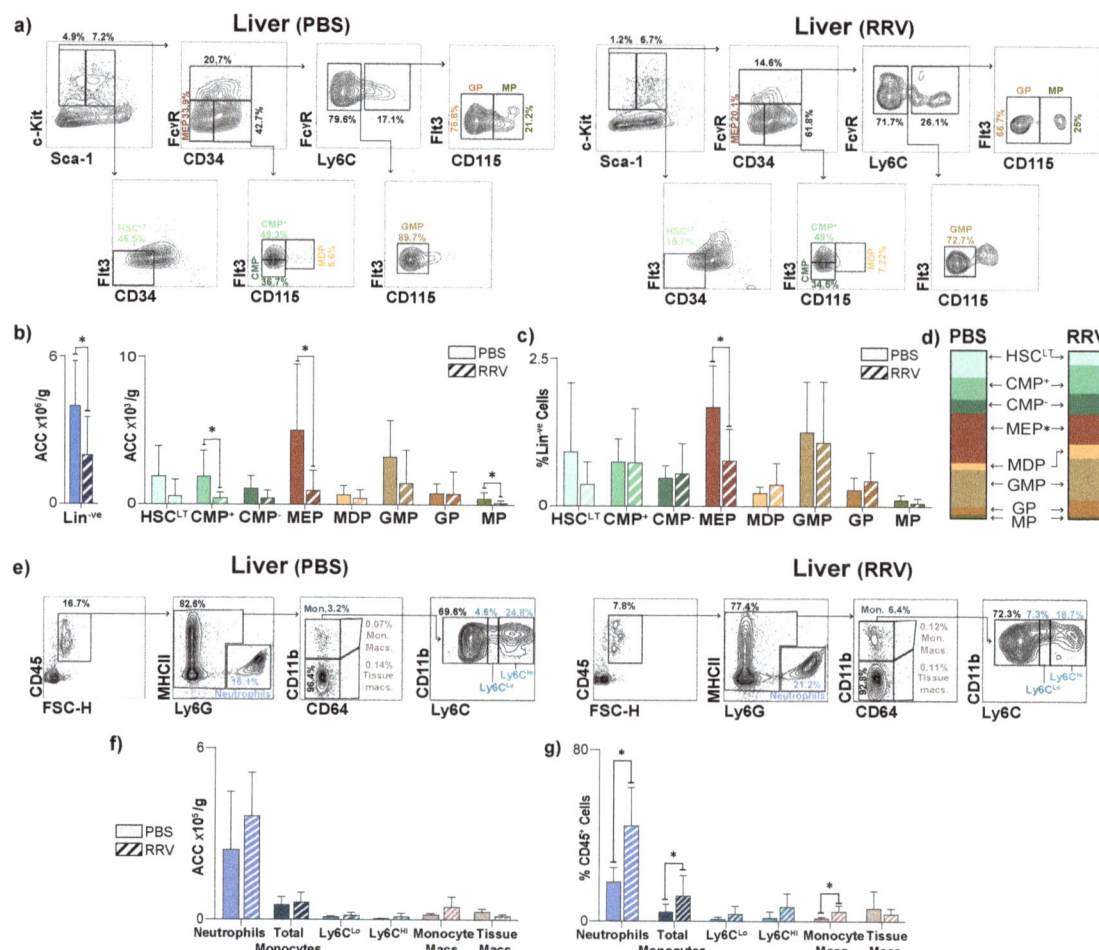

Figure 5. Perinatal liver injury leads to contraction of hematopoietic progenitors and expansion of mature myeloid cell proportions in the juvenile liver. (**a**) Representative flow plots demonstrating gating strategy of hematopoietic stem cells (HSC^{LT}), common myeloid progenitors (CMP), and terminal myeloid progenitors (TMP) in liver of PBS- and RRV-injected 14-day-old (P14) mice (**b**) Absolute cell count (ACC) of lineage negative (Lin^{-ve}) cells, hematopoietic stem cells (HSC^{LT}), common myeloid progenitors (CMPs), and terminal myeloid progenitors (TMPs) of the liver, (**c**) percentage of total Lin^{-ve} cells, and (**d**) fraction of whole for HSC^{LT}, CMPs, and TMPs. (**e**) Representative flow plots demonstrating gating strategy of mature myeloid CD45$^+$ populations in liver of PBS- and RRV-injected 14-day-old (P14) mice. (**f**) ACC of mature myeloid populations (PBS $n = 3$, RRV $n = 3$) of the liver and (**g**) percentage of individual mature myeloid populations out of all CD45$^+$ cells (PBS $n = 5$, RRV $n = 9$) at post-natal day 14 (P14). $n = 6$ for PBS and $n = 8$ for RRV unless otherwise stated. p-value * < 0.05. Error bars represent mean ± SD.

3.5. Myeloablation Protects Mice from RRV-Mediated Perinatal Liver Injury

The expansion of CMPs in the neonatal liver 3 days after RRV infection led us to question whether HSPCs play a role in propagating PLI. To test this, we evaluated the effect of depleting HSPCs on the progression of PLI, using synergistic, myeloablating anti-CD117 and anti-CD47 antibodies [18,19]. Myeloablation using anti-CD117 and anti-CD47 resulted in a reduction in all HSPC populations (Figure 6a,b). Though the reductions in HSC^{LT}

and CMPs did not reach statistical significance, four of the five downstream progenitors (GMP, MEP, GP, and MP) were significantly reduced after myeloablation (Figure 6a,b). We then tested the effects of myeloablation on RRV-infected mice. Neonatal pups were injected with RRV on day 0 to induce PLI. From day 0 to day 4, pups were also injected with anti-CD117 + anti-CD47 (MA) or IgG2b + Ig2a isotype controls (Iso) (Figure 6c). In the MA group, 78% of the pups survived RRV-mediated liver injury compared to only 36% in the isotype control group. (Figure 6d). MA pups also weighed more than isotype controls, but this difference was not statistically significant (Figure 6e). The improvement in survival and weight of the MA pups was corroborated by fewer moribund features, such as hair loss, dehydration, hunched appearance, and jaundice (Figure 6f). Finally, the extent of liver injury significantly decreased in the MA pups, as evidenced by lower levels of serum alanine transferase (Figure 6g), less periportal immune infiltrate, and fewer regions of hepatic necrosis (Figure 6h).

These results indicate that the propagation of PLI after RRV infection is dependent on HSPCs.

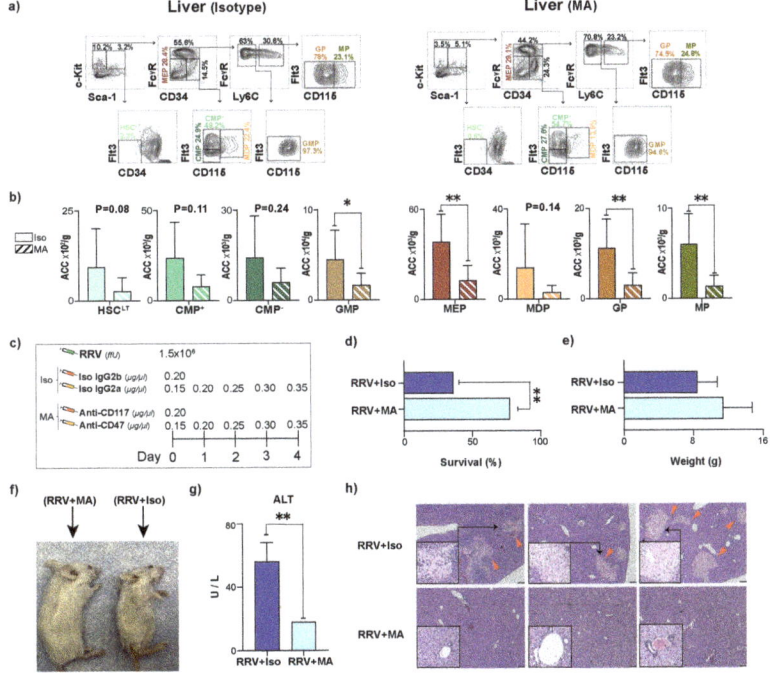

Figure 6. Antibody-mediated myeloablation depletes myeloid progenitor populations and protects mice from perinatal liver injury. (**a**) Representative flow plots demonstrating gating strategy of hematopoietic stem cells (HSC^{LT}), common myeloid progenitors (CMP), and terminal myeloid progenitors (TMP) in liver of isotype (Iso)- and myeloablative (MA)-injected 3-day-old (P3) mice. (**b**) Quantification of absolute cell counts (ACC) of HSC^{LT}s, CMPs, TMPs in P3 livers from Iso- ($n = 6$) and MA ($n = 8$) mice. (**c**) Dosage schedule illustrating rhesus rotavirus (RRV) injection, Iso, and MA. (**d**) Percent survival of RRV+MA ($n = 27$) vs. RRV+Iso ($n = 22$) injected controls at three weeks of life. (**e**) Pup weights of RRV+MA ($n = 15$) vs. RRV+Iso ($n = 5$) injected controls at three weeks of life. (**f**) Pictures illustrating phenotypic changes in mice after RRV+MA and RRV+Iso at three weeks of life. (**g**) Quantification of alanine transferase (ALT) in serum of RRV+MA ($n = 3$) treated mice vs. RRV+Iso ($n = 3$) injected controls at three weeks of life. (**h**) Histological H&E sections (5×) of livers from animals in both groups three weeks post-injection with either RRV + Iso or RRV + MA. Red arrows indicate necrotic foci. Black boxes indicate 20× magnified insets (necrotic foci are shown in RRV + Iso mice). *p*-value * < 0.05, ** < 0.01. Error bars represent mean ± SD.

4. Discussion

In this study, we defined the composition of HSPCs during homeostasis in neonatal and juvenile mouse livers, and we used an infectious mouse model of perinatal liver injury to define the changes that occur to HSPCs during liver injury. We found that (1) common myeloid progenitors reside in the livers of juvenile mice even after the main site of hematopoiesis has transitioned to the BM, (2) PLI leads to the expansion of common myeloid progenitors in neonatal mouse liver and causes an expansion of mature myeloid progenitors in juvenile mouse liver, and (3) targeted depletion of HSPCs using anti-CD117 and anti-CD47 prevents the development of RRV-induced PLI, as demonstrated by improved survival, increased jaundice clearance, and decreased liver injury.

Our results demonstrate the neonatal and juvenile mouse liver continues to act as a reservoir for common myeloid progenitors (CMPs) under homeostatic conditions. Furthermore, the differentiation capacity of HSPCs towards the myeloid lineage persists in the liver even after the main hematopoietic site has shifted to the BM. These findings corroborate the known role of the adult liver as a perpetual home for HSPCs [20]. The expansion of CMPs observed in P14 juvenile mouse livers also indicates that select HSPC populations may be important for the retention of myelopoiesis in the liver. Though the recruitment of myeloid cells (neutrophils, monocytes) during inflammation occurs from the bloodstream [12], our results also support the idea that remnant HSPCs in the liver may serve as central hubs of inflammation during PLI.

Our findings also support the idea that liver inflammation during perinatal life affects emigrating hepatic progenitor populations. In humans, the spatial and temporal overlap of liver development and hematopoiesis in the late-gestational fetus [21] may contribute to the devastating acute and chronic sequelae that affect liver- and immune function in progressive inflammatory diseases such as BA. In our study, perinatal liver injury led to an early increase in HSPCs and the depletion of these cells lessened clinical and histological signs of liver injury. Similar findings of HSPCs driving injury have previously been observed in the heart, where chronic inflammation directs HSPCs towards a pro-inflammatory phenotype that then enhances inflammation in a destructive feed-forward loop [9]. Our findings indicate that this detrimental feed-forward loop is similarly present in BA, where an injury to the fetal liver leads to dysregulation of HSPCs and propagation of tissue injury [22]. This theory is supported by the 'layered hygiene hypothesis' which suggests that fetal-derived HSPCs contribute to adult immune function and consequently, that impairment of fetal hematopoiesis can change the long-term trajectory of the immune system, potentially causing both autoimmunity and increasing disease susceptibility [23].

The current treatment of BA relies on early surgical treatment to restore bile flow after Kasai portoenterostomy, although most patients will continue to develop progressive liver injury requiring liver transplantation, highlighting the need for new and innovative treatments. Our results indicate that HSPCs propagate PLI in mice and suggest that HSPCs may also contribute to human BA. Intriguingly, the manipulation of HSPC populations has been found to influence disease outcome in human patients. In infants with BA who have undergone Kasai portoenterostomy, the effect of administering three consecutive days of granulocyte-colony-stimulating-factor (G-CSF) on liver inflammation was examined in a phase 1 trial demonstrating that peripheral neutrophils and HSPCs initially increased before decreasing to baseline levels after two weeks. Notably, G-CSF treatment was associated with reduced cholestasis one month after treatment but reverted to control levels after three months [24]. A phase 2 randomized controlled trial is currently underway to determine the efficacy of G-CSF in patients with BA (NCT04373941). Our findings combined with those from the phase I trial highlight that HSPC populations are dynamic during the course of an inflammatory insult and their functions change depending on the stage of disease and age of the patient. These findings also support the idea that manipulation of specific HSPC subsets may prove to be efficacious in resolving BA.

Our observed changes to HSPCs after RRV infection support the idea that early perinatal liver inflammatory insults have long-term consequences to immune function. Children with BA have an increased infection rate and decreased vaccine responses compared to healthy controls [25,26] and they are more likely than children with diseases other than BA who received liver transplants to reject donor livers [27]. In mice, a primary pathogenic stimulus has been found to cause changes in epigenetic and translational properties of HSPCs [28,29] resulting in a sustained myeloid lineage bias and an increased inflammatory response [8], which leads to a heightened response to similar secondary stimuli—a concept known as 'trained immunity' [28,29]. Maladaptive training of the myeloid compartment can result in increased susceptibility to other inflammatory conditions [8]. As myeloid cells account for the primary immune response during PLI [4], maladaptive trained immunity may similarly play a role in the long-term immune dysregulation observed in BA.

In our study, we eliminated HSCs and downstream hematopoietic progenitors using targeted antibodies directed against CD117 and CD47, thereby avoiding the devastating and non-specific tissue injury associated with traditional HSC-depleting strategies such as radiation and chemotherapy [18]. This approach does, however, have limitations that need to be addressed before considering its use in human patients. The intended removal of stem- and progenitor cells leads to a transient, secondary reduction in red blood cells [18]. Though previous studies have found anti-CD47 and anti-CD117 induced anemia to be mild and fully resolved within 2–3 weeks [30,31], further work will be needed to define the impact of neonatal anti-CD117 and anti-CD47 myeloablation on short and long-term anemia. Additional mild and temporary side effects of antibody-mediated myeloablation have also been reported, including hair color change and reduction in spermatogonia [18]. We expect that the short duration of myeloablation we used in neonatal mice would result in limited long-term toxicity; however, further studies would be needed to balance effective dosing and duration with side effects in human patients.

In conclusion, our study demonstrates that myeloid progenitors increase during PLI and that their depletion improves disease outcome. Future studies are necessary to investigate the specific effects of myeloablation on myeloid progenitor populations in neonates. Our study suggests that targeting hematopoietic progenitors may be useful in preventing and treating neonatal liver inflammatory diseases such as BA.

Supplementary Materials: The following supporting information can be downloaded at: https://www.mdpi.com/article/10.3390/jcm12010337/s1, Figure S1: Mature myeloid populations contract in the liver while expanding in the bone marrow of the juvenile mouse, Figure S2: HSPCs in the livers of juvenile mice maintain myeloid differentiation capacity, Table S1: Staining panel for mature myeloid cells, Table S2: Staining panel for hematopoietic stem- and progenitor cells (HSPCs): Long-term hematopoietic stem cells (HSC^{LT}), common myeloid progenitors (CMPs), and terminal myeloid progenitors (TMPs).

Author Contributions: Conceptualization, A.A., E.M.P. and A.N.; methodology, A.A., C.K., C.S.L., E.M.P. and A.N.; data analysis, A.A., C.K., S.M., C.S.L., C.C.D. and A.N.; manuscript preparation, A.A., C.K., C.C.D. and A.N.; supervision, C.C.D., E.M.P. and A.N. All authors have read and agreed to the published version of the manuscript.

Funding: C.K. was supported by a fellowship from the Lundbeck Foundation's Danish-American Research Exchange Program, administered by Innovation Center Denmark, Silicon Valley. Additional funding was provided by the FAVOR NIH T32 Training grant (5T32AI125222-05, SM), an American Pediatric Surgical Association Foundation Jay Grosfeld, MD Scholar Award (AN), an American College of Surgeons Faculty Research Fellowship (AN), a UCSF Liver Center Pilot Award (NIH P30 DK026743, AN), the UCSF Parnassus Flow Cytometry Core (DRC Center Grant NIH P30 DK063720), and core resources of the UCSF Liver Center (P30 DK026743).

Institutional Review Board Statement: The animal study protocol was approved by the Institutional Review Board of University of CA, San Francisco (protocol code AN183751-02E, approval date 17 March 2022).

Informed Consent Statement: Not applicable.

Data Availability Statement: The original contributions presented in the study are included in the article/supplementary material; further inquiries can be directed to the corresponding author.

Acknowledgments: The authors would like to thank Henry Greenberg (Stanford University, CA, USA) for providing MA104 cells and Rhesus rotavirus. The authors would also like to acknowledge Scott Kogan for assistance with CFU assay interpretation, Kyle Cromer, Vibeke Brix Christensen, and Pamela Derish for their critical review of the manuscript. C.K. was supported by a fellowship from the Lundbeck Foundation's Danish-American Research Exchange Program, administered by Innovation Center Denmark, Silicon Valley. Additional funding was provided by the American Pediatric Surgical Association Foundation Jay Grosfeld, MD Scholar Award (AN), an American College of Surgeons Faculty Research Fellowship (AN), a UCSF Liver Center Pilot Award (NIH P30 DK026743, AN), the UCSF Parnassus Flow Cytometry Core (DRC Center Grant NIH P30 DK063720), and core resources of the UCSF Liver Center (P30 DK026743).

Conflicts of Interest: The authors declare no conflict of interest.

Abbreviations

ACC	Absolute Cell Count
BA	Biliary Atresia
BM	Bone Marrow
CFU	Colony Forming Units
CMP	Common Myeloid Progenitors
ffU	Focus Forming Units
G-CSF	Granulocyte-colony-stimulating-factor
GEMM	Granulocyte, Erythrocyte, Macrophage, Megakaryocyte
GM	Granulocyte, Macrophage
GMP	Granulocytic-monocytic Progenitors
GP	Granulocytic Progenitors
H&E	Hematoxylin Eosin
HSC^{LT}	Long-term Hematopoietic Stem Cells
HSPC	Hematopoietic Stem and Progenitor cells
IHC	Immunohistochemistry
Iso	Isotype
Lin^{-ve}	Lineage negative hematopoietic compartment
Lin^{+}	Lineage positive hematopoietic compartment
$Ly6C^{Hi}$	$Ly6c^{Hi}$ classical monocytes
$Ly6C^{Lo}$	$Ly6C^{Lo}$ non-classical monocytes
M	Macrophage
MA	Myeloablation
MDP	Monocytic-dendritic Progenitors
MEP	Megakaryocytic-erythroid Progenitors
MP	Monocytic and common monocytic Progenitors
PLI	Perinatal Liver Injury
RRV	Rhesus Rotavirus
TMP	Terminal Myeloid Progenitors

References

1. D'Souza, R.; Grammatikopoulos, T.; Pradhan, A.; Sutton, H.; Douiri, A.; Davenport, M.; Verma, A.; Dhawan, A. Acute-on-chronic liver failure in children with biliary atresia awaiting liver transplantation. *Pediatr. Transplant.* **2019**, *23*, e13339. [CrossRef] [PubMed]
2. Bezerra, J.A. The Next Challenge in Pediatric Cholestasis: Deciphering the Pathogenesis of Biliary Atresia. *J. Pediatr. Gastroenterol. Nutr.* **2006**, *43*, S23–S29. [CrossRef] [PubMed]
3. Wehrman, A.; Waisbourd-Zinman, O.; Wells, R.G. Recent advances in understanding biliary atresia. *F1000Research* **2019**, *8*, 218. [CrossRef]
4. Alkhani, A.; Levy, C.S.; Tsui, M.; Rosenberg, K.A.; Polovina, K.; Mattis, A.N.; Mack, M.; Van Dyken, S.; Wang, B.M.; Maher, J.J.; et al. Ly6c(Lo) non-classical monocytes promote resolution of rhesus rotavirus-mediated perinatal hepatic inflammation. *Sci. Rep.* **2020**, *10*, 7165. [CrossRef]

5. Ciriza, J.; Thompson, H.; Petrosian, R.; Manilay, J.O.; García-Ojeda, M.E. The migration of hematopoietic progenitors from the fetal liver to the fetal bone marrow: Lessons learned and possible clinical applications. *Exp. Hematol.* **2013**, *41*, 411–423. [CrossRef]
6. Gao, S.; Liu, F. Fetal liver: An ideal niche for hematopoietic stem cell expansion. *Sci. China Life Sci.* **2018**, *61*, 885–892. [CrossRef] [PubMed]
7. Otsuka, K.S.; Nielson, C.; Firpo, M.A.; Park, A.H.; Beaudin, A.E. Early life inflammation and the developing hematopoietic and immune systems: The cochlea as a sensitive indicator of disruption. *Cells* **2021**, *10*, 3596. [CrossRef]
8. Li, X.; Wang, H.; Yu, X.; Saha, G.; Kalafati, L.; Ioannidis, C.; Mitroulis, I.; Netea, M.G.; Chavakis, T.; Hajishengallis, G. Maladaptive innate immune training of myelopoiesis links inflammatory comorbidities. *Cell* **2022**, *185*, 1709–1727.e18. [CrossRef]
9. Chavakis, T.; Mitroulis, I.; Hajishengallis, G. Hematopoietic progenitor cells as integrative hubs for adaptation to and fine-tuning of inflammation. *Nat. Immunol.* **2019**, *20*, 802–811. [CrossRef]
10. Eckert, C.; Klein, N.; Kornek, M.; Lukacs-Kornek, V. The complex myeloid network of the liver with diverse functional capacity at steady state and in inflammation. *Front. Immunol.* **2015**, *6*, 179. [CrossRef]
11. Weston, C.J.; Zimmermann, H.W.; Adams, D.H. The role of myeloid-derived cells in the progression of liver disease. *Front. Immunol.* **2019**, *10*, 893. [CrossRef] [PubMed]
12. Kubes, P.; Jenne, C.; Snyder, J. Immune Responses in the Liver. *Annu. Rev. Immunol.* **2018**, *44*, 247–277. [CrossRef] [PubMed]
13. Bankhead, P.; Loughrey, M.B.; Fernández, J.A.; Dombrowski, Y.; McArt, D.G.; Dunne, P.D.; McQuaid, S.; Gray, R.T.; Murray, L.J.; Coleman, H.G.; et al. QuPath: Open source software for digital pathology image analysis. *Sci. Rep.* **2017**, *7*, 16878. [CrossRef]
14. Sidney, L.E.; Branch, M.J.; Dunphy, S.E.; Dua, H.S.; Hopkinson, A. Concise review: Evidence for CD34 as a common marker for diverse progenitors. *Stem Cells* **2014**, *32*, 1380–1389. [CrossRef]
15. Yáñez, A.; Goodridge, H.S. Identification and isolation of oligopotent and lineage-committed myeloid progenitors from mouse bone marrow. *J. Vis. Exp.* **2018**, *2018*, e58061. [CrossRef]
16. Copley, M.R.; Eaves, C.J. Developmental changes in hematopoietic stem cell properties. *Exp. Mol. Med.* **2013**, *45*, e55. [CrossRef] [PubMed]
17. Oetzmann Von Sochaczewski, C.; Pintelon, I.; Brouns, I.; Dreier, A.; Klemann, C.; Timmermans, J.-P.; Petersen, C.; Kuebler, J.F. Rotavirus particles in the extrahepatic bile duct in experimental biliary atresia. *J. Pediatr. Surg.* **2014**, *49*, 520–524. [CrossRef] [PubMed]
18. Chhabra, A.; Ring, A.M.; Weiskopf, K.; Schnorr, P.J.; Gordon, S.; Le, A.C.; Kwon, H.-S.; Ring, N.G.; Volkmer, J.; Ho, P.Y.; et al. Hematopoietic stem cell transplantation in immunocompetent hosts without radiation or chemotherapy. *Sci. Transl. Med.* **2016**, *8*, 351ra105. [CrossRef] [PubMed]
19. Pang, W.W.; Czechowicz, A.; Logan, A.C.; Bhardwaj, R.; Poyser, J.; Park, C.Y.; Weissman, I.L.; Shizuru, J.A. Anti-CD117 antibody depletes normal and myelodysplastic syndrome human hematopoietic stem cells in xenografted mice. *Blood* **2019**, *133*, 2069–2078. [CrossRef]
20. Wang, X.Q.; Lo, C.M.; Chen, L.; Cheung, C.K.; Yang, Z.F.; Chen, Y.X.; Ng, M.N.; Yu, W.C.; Ming, X.; Zhang, W.; et al. Hematopoietic chimerism in liver transplantation patients and hematopoietic stem/progenitor cells in adult human liver. *Hepatology* **2012**, *56*, 1557–1566. [CrossRef] [PubMed]
21. Soares-da-Silva, F.; Peixoto, M.; Cumano, A.; Pinto-do-Ó, P. Crosstalk Between the Hepatic and Hematopoietic Systems During Embryonic Development. *Front. Cell Dev. Biol.* **2020**, *8*, 612. [CrossRef]
22. King, K.Y.; Goodell, M.A. Inflammatory modulation of HSCs: Viewing the HSC as a foundation for the immune response. *Nat. Rev. Immunol.* **2011**, *11*, 685–692. [CrossRef]
23. Apostol, A.C.; Jensen, K.D.C.; Beaudin, A.E. Training the Fetal Immune System Through Maternal Inflammation-A Layered Hygiene Hypothesis. *Front. Immunol.* **2020**, *11*, 123. [CrossRef]
24. Holterman, A.X.; Nguyen, H.P.A.; Nadler, E.; Vu, G.H.; Mohan, P.; Vu, M.; Trinh, T.T.; Bui, H.T.T.; Nguyen, B.T.; Quynh, A.T.; et al. Granulocyte-colony stimulating factor GCSF mobilizes hematopoietic stem cells in Kasai patients with biliary atresia in a phase 1 study and improves short term outcome. *J. Pediatr. Surg.* **2021**, *56*, 1179–1185. [CrossRef]
25. Liu, J.; Fei, Y.; Zhou, T.; Ji, H.; Wu, J.; Gu, X.; Luo, Y.; Zhu, J.; Feng, M.; Wan, P.; et al. Bile Acids Impair Vaccine Response in Children With Biliary Atresia. *Front. Immunol.* **2021**, *12*, 642546. [CrossRef]
26. Wu, J.F.; Ni, Y.H.; Chen, H.L.; Hsu, H.Y.; Lai, H.S.; Chang, M.H. Humoral immunogenicity to measles, rubella, and varicella-zoster vaccines in biliary atresia children. *Vaccine* **2009**, *27*, 2812–2815. [CrossRef]
27. Ruth, N.D.; Kelly, D.; Sharif, K.; Morland, B.; Lloyd, C.; McKiernan, P.J. Rejection is less common in children undergoing liver transplantation for hepatoblastoma. *Pediatr. Transplant.* **2014**, *18*, 52–57. [CrossRef]
28. Divangahi, M.; Aaby, P.; Khader, S.A.; Barreiro, L.B.; Bekkering, S.; Chavakis, T.; van Crevel, R.; Curtis, N.; DiNardo, A.R.; Dominguez-Andres, J.; et al. Trained immunity, tolerance, priming and differentiation: Distinct immunological processes. *Nat. Immunol.* **2021**, *22*, 2–6. [CrossRef]

29. Netea, M.G.; Domínguez-Andrés, J.; Barreiro, L.B.; Chavakis, T.; Divangahi, M.; Fuchs, E.; Joosten, L.A.B.; van der Meer, J.W.M.; Mhlanga, M.M.; Mulder, W.J.M.; et al. Defining trained immunity and its role in health and disease. *Nat. Rev. Immunol.* **2020**, *20*, 375–388. [CrossRef]
30. Derderian, S.C.; Togarrati, P.P.; King, C.; Moradi, P.W.; Reynaud, D.; Czechowicz, A.; Weissman, I.L.; MacKenzie, T.C. In utero depletion of fetal hematopoietic stem cells improves engraftment after neonatal transplantation in mice. *Blood* **2014**, *124*, 973–980. [CrossRef]
31. Liu, J.; Wang, L.; Zhao, F.; Tseng, S.; Narayanan, C.; Shura, L.; Willingham, S.; Howard, M.; Prohaska, S.; Volkmer, J.; et al. Pre-Clinical Development of a Humanized Anti-CD47 Antibody with Anti-Cancer Therapeutic Potential. *PLoS ONE* **2015**, *10*, e0137345. [CrossRef]

Disclaimer/Publisher's Note: The statements, opinions and data contained in all publications are solely those of the individual author(s) and contributor(s) and not of MDPI and/or the editor(s). MDPI and/or the editor(s) disclaim responsibility for any injury to people or property resulting from any ideas, methods, instructions or products referred to in the content.

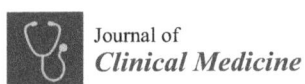 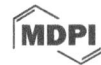

Review

Biliary Atresia in Adolescence and Adult Life: Medical, Surgical and Psychological Aspects

Deirdre Kelly [1,*], Marianne Samyn [2] and Kathleen B. Schwarz [3,4]

1. Liver Unit, Birmingham Women's & Children's NHS Hospital, University of Birmingham, Birmingham B15 2TT, UK
2. Paediatric Liver, Gastroenterology and Nutrition Unit, King's College Hospital NHS Foundation Trust, London WC2R 2LS, UK
3. Pediatric Liver Center, Johns Hopkins University School of Medicine, Baltimore, MD 21287, USA
4. Pediatric Liver Center, UCSD School of Medicine/Rady Children's Hospital, San Diego, CA 92123, USA
* Correspondence: deirdre@kellyda.co.uk

Abstract: Prior to 1955, when Morio Kasai first performed the hepatic portoenterostomy procedure which now bears his name, Biliary atresia (BA) was a uniformly fatal disease. Both the Kasai procedure and liver transplantation have markedly improved the outlook for infants with this condition. Although long-term survival with native liver occurs in the minority, survival rates post liver transplantation are high. Most young people born with BA will now survive into adulthood but their ongoing requirements for health care will necessitate their transition from a family-centred paediatric service to a patient-centred adult service. Despite a rapid growth in transition services over recent years and progress in transitional care, transition from paediatric to adult services is still a risk for poor clinical and psychosocial outcomes and increased health care costs. Adult hepatologists should be aware of the clinical management and complications of biliary atresia and the long-term consequences of liver transplantation in childhood. Survivors of childhood illness require a different approach to that for young adults presenting after 18 years of age with careful consideration of their emotional, social, and sexual health. They need to understand the risks of non-adherence, both for clinic appointments and medication, as well as the implications for graft loss. Developing adequate transitional care for these young people is based on effective collaboration at the paediatric–adult interface and is a major challenge for paediatric and adult providers alike in the 21st century. This entails education for patients and adult physicians in order to familiarise them with the long-term complications, in particular for those surviving with their native liver and the timing of consideration of liver transplantation if required. This article focusses on the outcome for children with biliary atresia who survive into adolescence and adult life with considerations on their current management and prognosis.

Keywords: liver; biliary atresia; transition; adolescence; adherence; readiness; professionals; parents

Citation: Kelly, D.; Samyn, M.; Schwarz, K.B. Biliary Atresia in Adolescence and Adult Life: Medical, Surgical and Psychological Aspects. *J. Clin. Med.* **2023**, *12*, 1594. https://doi.org/10.3390/jcm12041594

Academic Editor: Kenneth Siu Ho Chok

Received: 18 October 2022
Revised: 6 December 2022
Accepted: 23 December 2022
Published: 17 February 2023

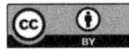

Copyright: © 2023 by the authors. Licensee MDPI, Basel, Switzerland. This article is an open access article distributed under the terms and conditions of the Creative Commons Attribution (CC BY) license (https://creativecommons.org/licenses/by/4.0/).

1. Introduction

The Kasai hepatic portoenterostomy, which was first performed in 1955 [1], markedly improved the outlook of children born with biliary atresia (BA). While there are a number of studies to determine short-term outcome following the Kasai, data have emerged more slowly regarding long-term outcomes. The purpose of this manuscript was to review overall actuarial survival data up to 30 years post-Kasai, the health status of survivors both with native liver and post-transplant, and predictors of outcome and strategies to improve it. To achieve this review, the first 100 papers listed in Pub Med under the search term "biliary atresia long term survival" were inspected and select ones were summarised, with emphasis on the most detailed papers published within the last five years.

2. Overall Survival Data up to 30 Years

One of the largest and most recent series published is that of Fanna et al. [2] who summarised results on the 1428 patients with BA managed in France from 1986 to 2015. In addition to their own series, the authors reported a comprehensive analysis of 11 BA registries in Europe, America and Asia. (Table 1). Survival with native liver after the Kasai operation at 10 years was 26 to 73% (average of means 44%); at 20 years after the Kasai in the 3 registries reporting was 24–28%, and at 30 years after the Kasai was 22% for France and 49% for Japan. Survival post liver transplant (LT) was 86% at 5 years to 79% at 30 years. In total, 10.2% died without LT.

Table 1. Reported outcomes of BA worldwide in main registries [2].

	Europe								America		Asia	
	France (this study)	France (last 3 cohorts)	UK (16)	Switzerland (19)	Netherlands (17)	Netherlands (18)	Nordic countries (20)	Canada (21,22)	USA: BARC (9 Expert centers) (23)	Taiwan (15)	Japan (13)
Years	1986–2015	1997–2015	1999–2009	1994–2004	1977–1988	1987–2008	2005–2016	1985–2002	1997–2000	2004–2009/2010 *	1989–2015
Max follow-up	30 y	20 y	10 y	10 y	31 y	22 y	12 y	18 y	2 y	7 y	28 y
N patients	1428	951	443	48	104	231	154	349	104 (All after KOp)	197 (170 *)	3160
N Kasai op	1340 (94%)	895 (94%)	424 (96%)	43 (90%)	104 (100%)	214 (93%)	148 (96%)	312 (89%)	104 (–)	193 (98%)	3090 (98%)
Age at KOp, days Median (range) or mean ± SD	59 (6–199)	57 (6–199)	54 (7–209)	68 (30–126)	59 (25–222)	59 (20–210)	60 (4–165)	65 (6–200)	61	Term: 53 +/− 19 Preterm: 72 +/− 28	68
Documented clearance of jaundice after Kasai op	38%	39%	55%	39.5%		34%	64%	NA	NA	Term: 62% Preterm 37% (bilirubin < 34 μmol/L)	58% †
SNL after K op At last follow-up	34%	41%	50%	40%		4 y: 46% (42–50)	55% ‡	27%	56%	18 months SNL: Term 73% Preterm: 50%	
10 y (CI 95%)	35% (34–36)	36% (34–38)	40% (34–46)	33% (26–40)	27% §		45% (35–55) ‡	26% (20–32)			
20 y (CI 95%)	26% (24–28)	26% (24–28)									49%
30 y (CI 95%)	22% (20–24)										
Death without LT	10%	7%	6%	8%	50%	8%	8%	12%	4% (all after KOp)		
N transplanted patients at last follow-up	793 (56%)	512 (54%)	194 (44%)	27 (56%)	26 (25%)	69 (32%) ‖	64 (42%)	210 (60%)	42 (40%)	41 (20%)	1236 (39%)
Survival after LT At last follow-up	84%	90%	93%	100%	73%	NA	86%	80%	88%	32 (78%)	1134 (92%)
5 y (CI 95%)	85% (84–86)	90% (89–91)	90% (88–93)	100%	‖	4 y: 79% ‖	84% (74–94)	4 y: 83% (77–88)			
10 y (CI 95%)	84% (83–85)	90% (89–91)	89% (86–93)	92% (87–96)	43%		84% (74–94)	80% (75–86)			
20 y (CI 95%)	80% (78–82)	89% (87–91)									
28 y	79 (77–81)										
Overall survival At last follow-up	81%	87%	91%	92%	43%	NA	87%	77%	91%		
5 y (CI 95%)	82% (81–83)	87% (86–88)	90% (88–93)	92% (87–96)		4 y: 73 (70–76) ‖	88% (83–94)	4 y: 77 (72–82)			
10 y (CI 95%)	80% (79–81)	86% (85–87)	89% (86–93)				87% (81–93)	75% (70–80)			89%
20 y (CI 95%)	78% (77–79)	85% (84–86)									
30 y (CI 95%)	76% (74–78)										
Population 2018 (million people)	68	66	8.6	17			27	36	326	24	127
Incidence of BA (CI 95%)	1/19,600 (1/18,200–1/21,100)	1/17,000	1/17,800 (1/13,900–1/24,800)		1/18,600			1/19,000 (1/17,800–1/20,300)		1/6600 (1/4200–1/7000)	1/13,500 (1/11,300–1/17,000)
% of BASM	8.2%	11% (37)	8%	5%	5%		12%	14%	11%		2%

BA = biliary atresia; BARC = Biliary Atresia Research Consortium; BASM = BA splenic malformation syndrome; KOp = Kasai operation; LT = liver transplantation; SNL = survival with native liver. * Value calculated from text and Figure 2 and Figure 4 of reference 13. ‡ Including 6 of 154 patients who did not undergo Kasai operation. § 20 y SNL: 1977–1982 20%; 1983–1988: 32%. ‖ Six patients who underwent LT abroad excluded from analysis.

3. Health Status of Survivors

3.1. Chronic Liver Disease

Kelay and Davenport [3] described the long-term health status of survivors with native liver. Only 11% had no signs of liver disease. Manifestations of chronic liver disease included cirrhosis in most after age 20 years, portal hypertension/varices, and recurrent cholangitis. Malignant transformation was rare but did occur: hepatocellular carcinoma developed in 0.8% and there were rare cases of hepatoblastoma and cholangiocarcinoma. Interestingly growth and development were usually normal.

3.2. Health Related Quality of Life (HRQOL)

Rodijk et al. [4] reviewed the literature on HRQOL in children with biliary atresia and noted that, in general scores in children with BA were lower than in healthy peers. They also performed their own study in Dutch BA patients ($n = 38$; age 10 ± 3 years), the parent-proxy physical score was significantly lower compared with healthy controls. It was also lower than in children with a variety of other medical conditions. Psychosocial HRQOL was lower than in healthy peers and largely comparable to children with other chronic conditions. Parent-proxy physical HRQOL was adversely related to adverse medical events in the past year, special education, and motor impairments; psychosocial HRQOL was adversely related to behavioural problems. Liang et al. [5] also observed that having other medical conditions impacted negatively on the HRQOL; an additional factor that impacted the HRQOL was the parents' knowledge of LT [5]. In general, HRQOL of parents of children with BA was adversely affected [6]; Wong et al. [7] performed similar analyses and noted that HRQOL scores did not differ in general between those with a native liver and those post LT.

3.3. Neurodevelopmental Outcome

The Childhood Liver Disease Research and Education Network (ChiLDREN) performed comprehensive neurodevelopmental testing on children with BA and their native liver, ages 3–12 [8]. As shown in Figure 1 [8], iIn general average IQ scores were above the expected. (as indicated by light gray). However, Ruuska et al. [9] found the opposite Rodiijk et al. [10] studied 46 Dutch children ages 6–12 years with BA in a group some of whom had had LT and some who were with native liver. Motor delays were particularly prominent [10]. No longer-term studies of neurodevelopmental testing in children with BA were identified.

3.4. Predictors of Outcome

One of the major determinants of long-term outcome is the age at Kasai (Figure 2). Survival up to 30 years was 38, 27, 22, and 19% in patients operated on at 1 month, 2, 3 and later [2]. The anatomic pattern of the biliary remnant and the presence or absence of Biliary Atresia Splenic Malformation (BASM) were also important determinants [2,3]. The data regarding the impact of these factors on long-term survival up to 30 years are shown in Table 2. As noted by Kelay [3], the etiology of BA also influenced outcome with worse outcome for cat eye syndrome (chromosome 22 aneuploidy), and better outcome for cystic BA. The type of anatomy influenced the type of operation and had an impact on 20-year survival: hepatic portocholecystostomy 35% cystojejunostomy 40%, Type IIIa 19%.

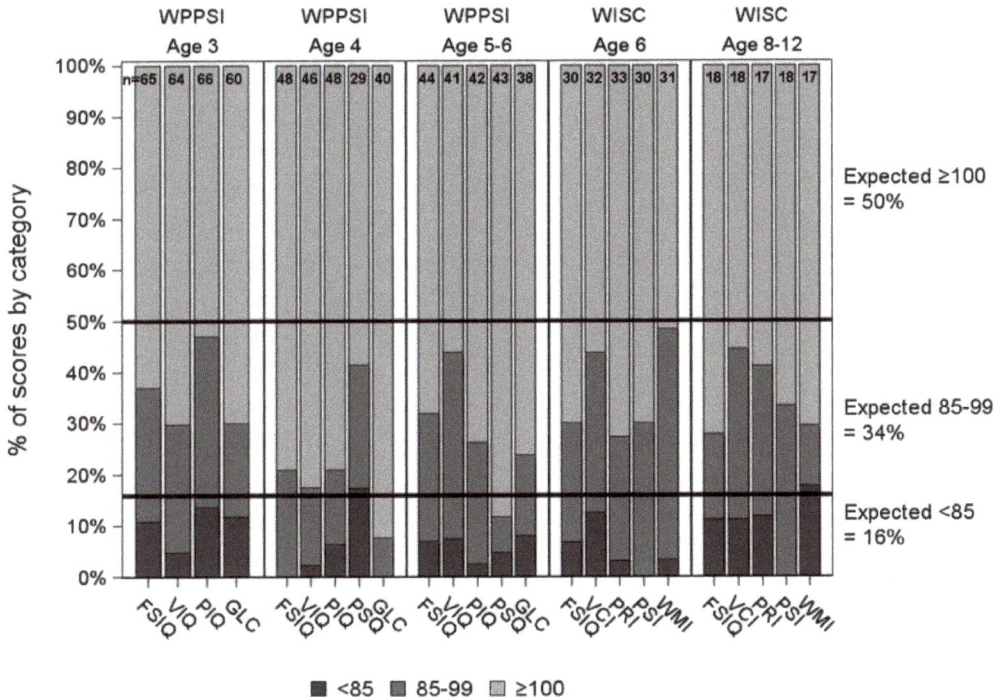

Figure 1. IQ scores in children with BA ages 3–12 years. Neurocognitive Score Distribution. Distribution of WPPSI-III and WISC-IV scores compared to population norms. FSIQ: Full Scale Intelligent Quotient; GLC: General Language Composite; PIQ: Performance Intelligent Quotient; VIQ: Verbal Intelligent Quotient; PSQ: Processing Speed Quotient; PRI: Perceptual Reasoning Index; PSI: Processing Speed Index; VCI: Verbal Comprehension Index; WMI: Working Memory Index [8].

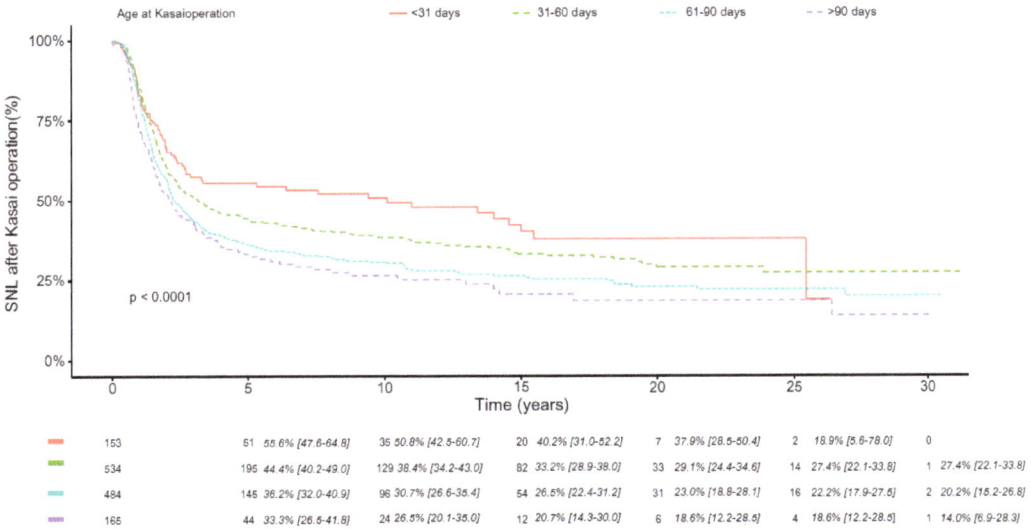

Figure 2. Survival with native liver according to age at Kasai operation [2]. At each point of follow-up: N patients alive with native liver, SNL after Kasai operation (CI 95%). SNL = survival with native liver [2].

Table 2. Predictors of long-term outcome of BA in survivors of the Kasai with a native liver up to 30 years post Kasai [2].

Univariate Analysis						
		SNL _ SE standard error (number of patients alive with native liver at follow-up)				
Prognostic factor	N patients	5-Y SNL	10-Y SNL	20-Y SNL	30-Y SNL	p
Anatomical pattern of the extra hepatic biliary remnant						<0.0001
Type 1	20	89.7% ± 6.9% (18)	84.1% ± 8.4% (16)	75.7% ± 11.2% (11)	75.7% ± 11.2% (11)	
Type 2	104	60.4% ± 5.1% (47)	51.6% ± 5.7% (26)	44.3% ± 6.3% (15)	36.9% ± 8.6% (6)	
Type 3	235	48.2% ± 3.4% (92)	42.9% ± 3.5% (68)	29.9% ± 3.8% (25)	29.9% ± 3.8% (25)	
Type 4	917	36.0% ± 1.7% (264)	30.7% ± 1.6% (184)	23.1% ± 1.8% (48)	18.1% ± 2.8% (11)	
Missing data	64					
BASM syndrome						<0.0001
No	1002	44.0% ± 1.6% (366)	38.5% ± 1.6% (258)	28.4% ± 1.8% (72)	24.7% ± 2.4% (19)	
Yes	118	20.8% ± 3.8% (20)	15.4% ± 3.7% (11)	15.4% ± 3.7% (11)	7.7% ± 5.7% (2)	
Missing data						
Age at Kasai operation						<0.0001
<31 days	153	55.6% ± 4.4% (60)	50.8% ± 4.6% (39)	37.9% ± 5.5% (17)	18.9% ± 13.7% (2)	
31–60 days	534	44.4% ± 2.2% (197)	38.4% ± 2.2% (134)	29.1% ± 2.6% (34)	27.4% ± 2.9% (17)	
61–90 days	484	36.2% ± 2.3% (146)	30.7% ± 2.2% (102)	23.0% ± 2.4% (35)	20.2% ± 2.9% (11)	
>90 days	165	33.3% ± 3.8% (45)	26.7% ± 3.7% (27)	18.6% ± 4.0% (10)	14.0% ± 5.0% (4)	
Missing data	4					
Multivariate analysis						
Prognostic factor		Hazard ratio		95% CI		p
Anatomical pattern of the extrahepatic biliary remnant						
Type 1		0.145		0.046–0.453		0.0009
Type 2		0.531		0.387–0.728		
Type 3		0.746		0.605–0.920		
Type 4		1				
BASM syndrome						
No		0.550		0.438–0.691		<0.0001
Yes		1				
Age at Kasai operation						
<31 days		0.538		0.388–0.745		0.0002
31–60 days		0.616		0.488–0.779		
61–90 days		0.766		0.604–0.971		
>90 days		1				

BASM = BA splenic malformation syndrome; CI = confidence interval; SE = standard error; SNL = survival with native liver.

A very recent report by van Wessel et al. [11] noted that the gut microbiota composition of BA patients pre-Kasai associated with outcome at 6 months. No data are yet available re the effect on long-term outcome. Interestingly enough, cytokines were not predictive of outcome Madadi-Sanjaniet al. [12]. Harumatsu et al. [13] recently reported that microvascular proliferation of the portal vein branches at the time of Kasai was associated with better outcome; Sasaki et al. [14] made similar observations. Finally, Johansson et al. [15] recently reported that reduction of hepatic FGF 19 at the time of Kasai predicted better outcome.

Wang et al. [16] noted a strong difference between the estimated 5-year native liver survival (NLS) rates of their successful Kasai group (defined as clearance of jaundice at 4 weeks post Kasai) and failed Kasai group: NLS rates at 5 years post Kasai were 90.1% vs. 10.7% for successful vs. failed Kasai ($p = 0.000$). Shneider et al. [17] noted similar findings for total serum bilirubin 3 months post-Kasai in the ChiLDReN BA cohort. Additionally, utilising data from the ChiLDReN study, Venkat et al. [18] found that long-term survival up to age 14 years could be modelled using platelet count, GGT, and predicted SE-free survival at age 7 years. (Figure 3).

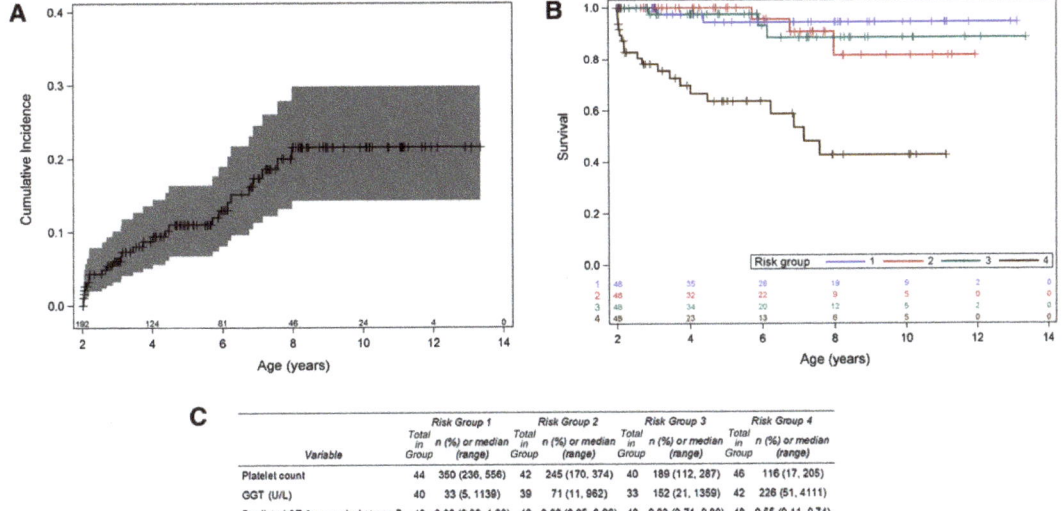

Figure 3. Incidence and risk for the SE-model (sentinel event) (**A**) Cumulative incidence of LTD among the 240 study participants. (**B**) Kaplan-Meier curves for LT-free survival stratified by quartile of risk score. Stratification of participants shows a high-risk group (group 4; brown) and a medium-risk group (group 3; green), with the remaining two quartiles showing a similar lower risk. (**C**) Risk factor distribution of participants in the analysis by quartiles of risk is provided. Venkat [18].

4. Adolescence and Transition

4.1. Adolescence

Adolescence is a challenging time for all young people and their families, as they progress through multiple physical, developmental and cultural changes in parallel [19]. It is a time of increasing independence and autonomy, with a belief in one's own immortality, struggles with peer pressure, a focus on body image, frequently undiagnosed mental health problems.

In contrast to biological and cognitive changes, the psychosocial changes of adolescence may be culturally determined and include the social "tasks" of adolescence such as establishing relationships, achieving independence from parents and establishing financial (i.e., vocational) independence [20,21]

Conversely, in the search for identity and independence, immature abstract thinking common in adolescence may make medical management difficult through poor adherence to medical regimens and "risky" health behaviours [22].

The additional burden of biliary atresia requiring regular hospital visits and medication can make this period even more difficult for young people to navigate, particularly when they move from family-centred paediatric care to adult services [23].

4.2. Transition

Transition is an active process that focusses on the medical, psychosocial and educational/vocational needs of adolescents as they move from child to adult-centred care [24,25].

The aims of transition are [26,27] to provide high quality, coordinated health care which is patient-centred, age and developmentally appropriate, flexible, and comprehensive; to encourage skills in communication, decision-making, self-care and self-advocacy; to develop a sense of control and independence in health care [28] and to maximise life-long physical and psychosocial health.

Transitional care acknowledges the reciprocal influences of adolescent development, the underlying chronic illness and/or the effects of transplantation. Patients may have been affected by their chronic liver disease with malnutrition or delayed puberty. Cognitive development may have been affected by their disease or by drug side effects (steroids and calcineurin inhibitors), pain, fatigue and repeated hospitalisation. The stage of cognitive development is important in planning health and disease education for such young people as well as their involvement in decision-making and self-care.

The combination of chronic liver disease/post-transplant and adolescent development (physical, cognitive and psychosocial) are important considerations for the multidisciplinary teams. Both paediatricians and adult physicians should monitor growth and pubertal development especially if there has been growth retardation due to the biliary atresia. Some of these patients may have a learning disability and health providers need to be skilled at both age and development appropriate management for this age-group.

Paediatric care focusses on the relationship with parent, professional and child, and needs to change to an adult relationship of patient and professional. As they mature, young people progress from using emotional strategies (such as wishful thinking or resignation) to problem-solving strategies which may be delayed by their chronic illness [24–27].

4.3. The Transitional Care Programme

Transitional care should start at around 12 years of age to promote resilience and self-determination in the young person and their families. There are no good measures of transition readiness and as transition is a process, there is no agreed age for the end of transition or the timing of transfer to adult care so it should be individualised for each patient. Discussion and preparation for transition needs should be at a time of good hepatic/graft function and transfer should not be implemented during an acute illness or rejection or graft failure [29].

Although the focus should be on the young person, family relationships and stability are important factors for resilience. Lack of parental support at this time has been associated with negative outcomes, e.g., greater non-adherence to medication.

As the adolescent negotiates the tasks and transitions detailed above, his/her parent are also managing the transition from being a parent of a dependent child to a parent of an independent young adult and need appropriate support [30,31].

Ideally, there should be an identified health professional for each young person, who can support the process in the paediatric and adult units and the primary health care team. Equally essential are other key players such as teachers, (including careers and vocational rehabilitation), social services and voluntary organizations who provide dedicated youth

Transition may take place in a variety of ways: via a transition clinic from paediatric to an adult care or a specific adolescent clinic or a young adult clinic before moving into adult care, but it is important that the Transition team, both adult and paediatric, work together.

Absolutely key to the success of the process is an interested and capable adult service, willing to continue the transitional process in adult care. Establishing a local network of interested and committed professionals is vital for the success of any transitional care programme [32,33].

4.4. Key Transitional Care Issues

4.4.1. Disease Education

Most young people with biliary atresia with or without a LT will have had their initial disease education directed to the parents and so need to be educated about their disease/post-transplant state. The use of age appropriate literature and a skilled play worker or teacher are invaluable to help young people to understand and accept difficult issues such as having a dead person's organ, or facing a life-time of medical monitoring and medication [34].

In addition, young people need to be aware of the signs and symptoms requiring urgent medical attention and how to access to medical care, which may be daunting for them in an adult unit. Information regarding drugs should include the importance of adherence and side effect profile and monitoring but also rationale and benefits [35].

4.4.2. Generic Health Education and Sexual Health

Generic health issues need consideration especially as many adult health-promoting behaviours become established during adolescence. Adolescents with chronic illness report more age- related concerns than their healthy peers: acne, alcohol and drug, periods, headaches, anxiety, contraception, insomnia, worry about height and weight and sexual health.

Greater levels of exercise are associated with well-being and long-term functioning in patients with chronic conditions [36] and are to be encouraged when feasible, particularly in view of the concerns of the metabolic syndrome post-transplant related to obesity and inactivity [37,38].

All young people should understand the implications of their disease/post-transplant state, e.g., immunosuppression and other treatments, on their sexual and reproductive health as they may be sexually active [35,39].

It is important to provide information about contraception. Although barrier methods are the safest, there is a high failure rate. It is safe for girls to take a low dose oestrogen/progesterone contraceptive pill or to take the 'morning after pill' [40]. Chronic liver disease may have delayed puberty but this will begin after a successful transplant. Most immunosuppressive drugs are not teratogenic or affect fertility apart from mycophenolate mofetil which should be avoided in adolescent girls. Many girls develop menorrhagia post-transplant and specific advice from a gynaecologist trained in managing contraception and pregnancy in patients with chronic liver disease or immunosuppression is useful.

4.4.3. Substance Misuse

Cigarette smoking should be discouraged as there may be an increased risk of lung cancer post-transplant. Substance misuse has been reported in young people who are non-adherent with medication and hence an important aspect of history taking. It is important to highlight the importance of sensible behaviour, e.g., LT recipients may drink alcohol with their peers in moderation [41].

4.4.4. Self-Advocacy and Psychosocial Issues

Self-advocacy skills are a key goal of transition, such as being independent from parents, having a full understanding of their illness, involvement in decision-making, self-medication, adherence, etc. The young person should begin to develop these skills within the transition clinic and become more confident in decision-making, managing their own health by developing communication skills, independent living skills, accessing the health and educational services to prepare them for adult life [42].

Seeing the young person independently from the parent helps provide the privacy for such discussions of generic health concerns such as sexual health, alcohol use.

Coping with teasing and/or bullying as well as disclosure issues are important issues to address with the young person during adolescence and transition. Transplant recipients may be particularly vulnerable because of their altered appearance from disease or medication, or because of time lost from school. Exploring and developing coping strategies for disclosure with a health professional can help the young person gain in confidence. Peer support may be a useful means of promoting well-being for such young people in addition to psychological support [43].

Despite the many potential problems, many long-term survivors with biliary atresia report satisfactory completion of education and high levels of employment [44].

4.4.5. Non-Adherence

Non-adherence is a key risk factor for maintaining good disease control and is a significant cause of post-transplant acute rejection, graft loss and death [45]. It remains one of the most challenging aspects of managing care in the adolescent and young adult population. It may be part of the spectrum of risk-taking behaviour or associated with other risk-taking behaviours such as alcohol and drug use. It may be intentional or non-intentional and include mean missing a dose, taking doses irregularly, changing the prescribed dose, taking a medication holiday or stopping medications altogether [46].

Management is complex but should not be judgmental as a lack of sensitivity or awareness of adolescent/young adult issues can be particularly damaging and may result in increased non-adherence and disengagement with health care services. Interventions should be tailored to the individual patient and use a combination of approaches such as wireless enabled pill-boxes, customised text reminders, provision of electronic feedback and individual behavioural sessions involving goal setting and motivational interviewing [47].

5. Medical and Surgical Management in Adolescence and Adult Life

Young adults with BA surviving with their native liver are likely to develop complications in adolescence and adult life. Reports vary from 60% of patients with BA surviving long term without LT [48] to nearly two-thirds of young adults with BA developing complications requiring LT [49]. The commonest complications were cholangitis (100%), portal hypertension (80%) and variceal bleeding (45%). In contrast to adults with cirrhosis, hepatocellular carcinoma was rare (1.3%). Synthetic liver failure, recurrent cholangitis and complications of portal hypertension were the main indications for Liver transplantation [50,51].

Cholangitis is a common complication post Kasai porto-enterostomy, seen in over 50% of children in first 2 years after surgery. Less information on its prevalence in adolescence or adulthood is available. In our series of 89 young people with BA surviving with their native liver after the age of 16 years, 10% developed at least one episode of cholangitis between the age of 12 and 16 years and this was found to be associated with a 4-fold risk of requiring liver transplantation during adulthood [51] The symptoms can be non-specific and liver function tests not helpful as 90% of BA patients will have some deranged liver function tests. Cholangitis should be suspected when presenting with right upper quadrant pain, general malaise and nausea. Imaging can demonstrate the presence of dilated biliary radicles or rarely intra-ductal debris or stones whereas bile lakes and bile duct dilation typically not seen. Roux-en-Y loop obstruction should be considered, and a nuclear medicine scan can help to assess hepatic excretion as well as function. Treatment with antibiotics, preferably via intravenous route, needs to be considered. Recurrent cholangitis is an indication for listing for liver transplantation.

The presence of portal hypertension and development of varices on endoscopy during adolescence has been shown to increase the risk of requiring liver transplantation in adulthood, 7 and 8.5 fold, respectively. Assessment of presence of oesophageal and gastric varices is particularly important in young women who are considering pregnancy as well as during pregnancy to assess the risk of GI bleeding and decide on further management. Westbrook et al. [52]. found that a platelet count of $<110 \times 10^9/L$ in women with cirrhosis predicted the presence of varices during pregnancy [53]. In addition, evidence of more advanced liver disease, defined as Model of end stage liver disease (MELD) score of >6 and United Kingdom end stage liver disease score (UKELD) >46, increased maternal and foetal risk during pregnancy [52]. In BA, 58 live births in 40 females have been reported to date and both cholangitis and variceal bleeding were risk factors for developing complications during pregnancy [53,54].

Less is known about pubertal development and menstruation in young people with biliary atresia. It is known that advanced liver disease alters the physiology of the hypothalamic–pituitary–gonadal axis and disturbs oestrogen metabolism, affecting sexual function. Prevalence of amenorrhoea in women with advanced liver disease has been estimated between 30 and 71%; however, case series are small [55,56]. After liver transplantation, the majority with have a normal menstrual cycle within the first year after transplantation.

More recently, fibroscan has been used to assess portal hypertension in children and young people with BA and liver stiffness > 24 kPa has been shown to be a good predictor of portal hypertension in older children with BA [57].

In addition to portal hypertension and cholangitis, serum bilirubin levels just above the upper limit of normal (>21 umol/L) at the age of 12 years have shown to predict the need for LT in adulthood. Interestingly, serum sodium and creatinine levels included in adult LT allocation models such as Model for End stage Liver Disease (MELD) and United Kingdom End stage Liver disease (UKELD) do not reflect the severity of liver disease in BA therefore these should be interpreted with caution in this setting [52]. A recent report from the Scientific Registry of Transplant Recipients (SRTR) found that out of 331 patients with biliary atresia listed for LT, including 114 adolescents (12–17 years) and 217 adults (>18 years), adults demonstrated increased risk of waiting list mortality compared with adolescents (10.9 higher risk on multivariate analysis) [58]. Additionally, in comparison to the adult cohort, adolescents had lower laboratory MELD/Paediatric End-stage Liver Disease (PELD) score at listing and at LT but demonstrated superior 5 year patient (98% vs. 84%) and graft (94% vs. 79.5%), respectively.

Jain et al. suggested that MELD > 8.5 and UKELD > 47 predicted LT > 16 years in 397 BA patients with 84% and 79% sensitivity and 73% and 73% specificity, respectively [59]. Other predictive scores were evaluated including Mayo Primary Sclerosing Cholangitis risk score (MayoPSC) which includes markers of portal hypertension and synthetic function. MayoPSC revealed predictive accuracy for LT (AUROC 0.859), with a score of >0.87 predicting LT with 85% sensitivity and 82% specificity. MELD and MayoPSC at the age of 12 years as well as change in MELD, PELD and MayoPSC between 12 and 16 years, was associated with the need for LT.

Adults with BA requiring LT also provide surgical challenges in particular related to the vascular system. In a review of 36 adults with BA undergoing LT, 57.6% was found to have significant enlargement of the splenic artery with 21% noted to have multiple splenic artery aneurysms [51]. Spontaneous visceral porto-systemic shunting (SPSS) was present in 72.7%. Survival was excellent with 10-year graft and patient survival exceeding 90%, highlighting the importance of careful donor selection and transplant surgical expertise in this condition.

What is not clear is whether the presence of SPSS is associated with the concept of covert or minimal hepatic encephalopathy, well described in adults with cirrhosis but less explored in children and adolescents. Considering that school functioning is lower compared to controls, with 2–48% of children requiring additional educational support further research initiatives should focus on cognitive function in patients with BA and its relation with disease severity in order to improve social outcomes [60].

6. Summary

Advances in both medicine and surgery have significantly improved the prognosis for infants born with biliary atresia. Although long-term survival with native liver occurs in the minority, survival rates post liver transplantation are high. Most young people born with BA are likely to survive into adulthood when they need to adapt to managing their own care within adult services. Key to this success is an integrated transition service between paediatric and adult care, supported by a multidisciplinary team to ensure good clinical and psychosocial outcomes. Adult hepatologists should be aware of the clinical management and complications of biliary atresia and the long-term consequences of liver transplantation in childhood and work closely with their paediatric colleagues to achieve a successful transition.

Author Contributions: D.K.: Sections 4 and 6 and general overview and submission, M.S.: Section 5, K.B.S.: Sections 1–3. All authors have read and agreed to the published version of the manuscript.

Funding: This review received no external funding.

Institutional Review Board Statement: Not applicable.

Conflicts of Interest: The authors declare no conflict of interest.

References

1. Kasai, M.; Suzuki, M. A new operation for non-correctable biliary atresia: Hepatic portoenterostomy. *Shujutsu* **1959**, *13*, 733–739.
2. Fanna, M.M.G.; Capito, C.; Girard, M.; Guerin, F.; Hermeziu, B.; Lachaux, A.; Roquelaure, B.; Gottrand, F.; Broue, P.; Dabadie, A.; et al. Management of Biliary Atresia in France 1986 to 2015: Long-Term Results. *J. Pediatr. Gastroenterol. Nutr.* **2019**, *69*, 416–424. [CrossRef]
3. Kelay, A.; Davenport, M. Long-term outlook in biliary atresia. *Semin. Pediatr. Surg.* **2017**, *26*, 295–300. [CrossRef]
4. Rodijk, L.H.; Schins, E.M.W.; Witvliet, M.J.; Verkade, H.J.; de Kleine, R.H.; Hulscher, J.B.F.; Bruggink, J.L.M. Health-Related Quality of Life in Biliary Atresia Patients with Native Liver or Transplantation. *Eur. J. Pediatr. Surg.* **2020**, *30*, 261–272. [CrossRef] [PubMed]
5. Liang, Y.; Yu, H.; Shu, F.; Huang, W.; Jiang, X.; Xu, Z.; Zhang, T.; Xiang, B.; Jin, S. Factors influencing the quality of life in children after biliary atresia treatment. *Transl. Pediatr.* **2021**, *10*, 2496–2505. [CrossRef] [PubMed]
6. Rodijk, L.H.; Schins, E.M.; Witvliet, M.J.; Alizadeh, B.Z.; Verkade, H.J.; de Kleine, R.H.; Hulscher, J.B.; Bruggink, J.L. Quality of Life in Parents of Children with Biliary Atresia. *J. Pediatr. Gastroenterol. Nutr.* **2020**, *71*, 641–646. [CrossRef]
7. Wong, C.W.Y.; Chung, P.H.Y.; Tam, P.K.H.; Wong, K.K.Y. Long-Term Results and Quality of Life Assessment in Biliary Atresia Patients: A 35-Year Experience in a Tertiary Hospital. *J. Pediatr. Gastroenterol. Nutr.* **2018**, *66*, 570–574. [CrossRef]
8. Squires, J.E.; Ng, V.L.; Hawthorne, K.; Henn, L.L.; Sorensen, L.G.; Fredericks, E.M.; Alonso, E.M.; Murray, K.F.; Loomes, K.M.; Karpen, S.J.; et al. Neurodevelopmental Outcomes in Preschool and School Aged Children With Biliary Atresia and Their Native Liver. *J. Pediatr. Gastroenterol. Nutr.* **2020**, *70*, 79–86. [CrossRef]
9. Ruuska, S.; Lähteenmäki, M.; Häyrinen, T.; Kanerva, K.; Jahnukainen, T.; Haataja, L.; Kolho, K.-L.; Pakarinen, M.P. Neurocognitive and Motor Functions in Biliary Atresia Patients: A Cross-Sectional, Prospective National Cohort Study. *J. Pediatr. Gastroenterol. Nutr.* **2021**, *73*, 491–498. [CrossRef]
10. Rodijk, L.H.; Heijer, A.E.D.; Hulscher, J.B.; Alizadeh, B.Z.; de Kleine, R.H.; Verkade, H.J.; Bruggink, J.L. Long-Term Neurodevelopmental Outcomes in Children with Biliary Atresia. *J. Pediatr.* **2020**, *217*, 118–124.e3. [CrossRef]
11. Van Wessel, D.; Nomden, M.; Bruggink, J.; de Kleine, R.; Kurilshikov, A.; Verkade, H.; Harmsen, H.; Hulscher, J. Gut Microbiota Composition of Biliary Atresia Patients Before Kasai Portoenterostomy Associates with Long-term Outcome. *J. Pediatr. Gastroenterol. Nutr.* **2021**, *73*, 485–490. [CrossRef] [PubMed]
12. Madadi-Sanjani, O.; Kuebler, J.F.; Dippel, S.; Gigina, A.; Falk, C.S.; Vieten, G.; Petersen, C.; Klemann, C. Long-term outcome and necessity of liver transplantation in infants with biliary atresia are independent of cytokine milieu in native liver and serum. *Cytokine* **2018**, *111*, 382–388. [CrossRef] [PubMed]
13. Harumatsu, T.; Muraji, T.; Masuya, R.; Ohtani, H.; Nagai, T.; Yano, K.; Onishi, S.; Yamada, K.; Yamada, W.; Matsukubo, M.; et al. Microvascular proliferation of the portal vein branches in the liver of biliary atresia patients at Kasai operation is associated with a better long-term clinical outcome. *Pediatr. Surg. Int.* **2019**, *35*, 1437–1441. [CrossRef] [PubMed]
14. Sasaki, H.; Nio, M.; Ando, H.; Kitagawa, M.; Kubota, M.; Suzuki, T.; Taguchi, T.; Hashimoto, T.; Society, T.J.B.A. Anatomical patterns of biliary atresia including hepatic radicles at the porta hepatis influence short- and long-term prognoses. *J. Hepato-Biliary-Pancreat. Sci.* **2021**, *28*, 931–941. [CrossRef]
15. Johansson, H.; Svensson, J.F.; Almström, M.; Van Hul, N.; Rudling, M.; Angelin, B.; Nowak, G.; Fischler, B.; Ellis, E. Regulation of bile acid metabolism in biliary atresia: Reduction of FGF19 by Kasai portoenterostomy and possible relation to early outcome. *J. Intern. Med.* **2020**, *287*, 534–545. [CrossRef]
16. Wang, Z.; Chen, Y.; Peng, C.; Pang, W.; Zhang, T.; Wu, D.; Shen, Q.; Li, M. Five-year native liver survival analysis in biliary atresia from a single large Chinese center: The death/liver transplantation hazard change and the importance of rapid early clearance of jaundice. *J. Pediatr. Surg.* **2019**, *54*, 1680–1685. [CrossRef]
17. Shneider, B.L.; Magee, J.C.; Karpen, S.J.; Rand, E.B.; Narkewicz, M.R.; Bass, L.M.; Schwarz, K.; Whitington, P.F.; Bezerra, J.A.; Kerkar, N.; et al. Total Serum Bilirubin within 3 Months of Hepatoportoenterostomy Predicts Short-Term Outcomes in Biliary Atresia. *J. Pediatr.* **2016**, *170*, 211–217.e2. [CrossRef]

18. Venkat, V.; Ng, V.L.; Magee, J.C.; Ye, W.; Hawthorne, K.; Harpavat, S.; Molleston, J.P.; Murray, K.F.; Wang, K.S.; Soufi, N.; et al. Modeling Outcomes in Children With Biliary Atresia With Native Liver After 2 Years of Age. *Hepatol Commun.* **2020**, *4*, 1824–1834. [CrossRef]
19. Steinberg, L. Cognitive and affective development in adolescence. *Trends Cogn. Sci.* **2005**, *9*, 69–74. [CrossRef]
20. Blum, R.W.; Garell, D.; Hodgman, C.H.; Jorissen, T.W.; Okinow, N.A.; Orr, D.P.; Slap, G.B. Transition from child-centered to adult health-care systems for adolescents with chronic conditions: A position paper of the Society for Adolescent Medicine. *J. Adolesc. Health* **1993**, *14*, 570–576. [CrossRef]
21. Radzik, M.S.S.; Neinstein, L. Psychosocial development in normal adolescents. In *Adolescent Health Care: A Practical Guide*; Neinstein, L.G.C., Katzman, D., Rosen, D., Woods, E., Eds.; Lippincott Williams & Wilkins: Philadelphia, PA, USA, 2007.
22. WHO. *Maternal, Newborn, Child and Adolescent Health*; WHO: Geneva, Switzerland, 2015.
23. Ruth, N.; Sharif, K.; Legarda, M.; Smith, M.; Lewis, P.; Lloyd, C.; Mirza, D.; Kelly, D. What is the long-term outlook for young people following liver transplant? A single-centre retrospective analysis of physical and psychosocial outcomes. *Pediatr. Transplant.* **2020**, *24*, e13782. [CrossRef] [PubMed]
24. American Academy of Pediatrics; American Academy of Family Physicians; American College of Physicians-American Society of Internal Medicine. A consensus statement on health care transitions for young adults with special health care needs. *Pediatrics* **2002**, *110 Pt 2*, 1304–1306. [CrossRef]
25. Kennedy, A.; Sawyer, S. Transition from pediatric to adult services: Are we getting it right? *Curr. Opin. Pediatr.* **2008**, *20*, 403–409. [CrossRef] [PubMed]
26. Crowley, R.; Wolfe, I.; Lock, K.; McKee, M. Improving the transition between paediatric and adult healthcare: A systematic review. *Arch. Dis. Child.* **2011**, *96*, 548–553. [CrossRef] [PubMed]
27. While, A.; Forbes, A.; Ullman, R.; Lewis, S.; Mathes, L.; Griffiths, P. Good practices that address continuity during transition from child to adult care: Synthesis of the evidence. *Child Care Health Dev.* **2004**, *30*, 439–452. [CrossRef]
28. Mayer, K.; Junge, N.; Goldschmidt, I.; Leiskau, C.; Becker, T.; Lehner, F.; Richter, N.; van Dick, R.; Baumann, U.; Pfister, E.-D. Psychosocial outcome and resilience after paediatric liver transplantation in young adults. *Clin. Res. Hepatol. Gastroenterol.* **2019**, *43*, 155–160. [CrossRef]
29. Fredericks, E.M.; Dore-Stites, D.; Well, A.; Magee, J.C.; Freed, G.L.; Shieck, V.; Lopez, M.J. Assessment of transition readiness skills and adherence in pediatric liver transplant recipients. *Pediatr. Transplant.* **2010**, *14*, 944–953. [CrossRef]
30. Fredericks, E.M.; Dore-Stites, D.; Lopez, M.J.; Well, A.; Shieck, V.; Freed, G.L.; Eder, S.J.; Magee, J.C. Transition of pediatric liver transplant recipients to adult care: Patient and parent perspectives. *Pediatr. Transplant.* **2011**, *15*, 414–424. [CrossRef]
31. Wright, J.; Elwell, L.; McDonagh, J.E.; Kelly, D.A.; Wray, J. Parents in transition: Experiences of parents of young people with a liver transplant transferring to adult services. *Pediatr. Transplant.* **2017**, *21*, e12760. [CrossRef]
32. Junge, N.; Migal, K.; Goldschmidt, I.; Baumann, U. Transition after pediatric liver transplantation—Perceptions of adults, adolescents and parents. *World J. Gastroenterol.* **2017**, *23*, 2365–2375. [CrossRef]
33. Wright, J.; Elwell, L.; McDonagh, J.; Kelly, D.; McClean, P.; Ferguson, J.; Wray, J. Healthcare transition in pediatric liver transplantation: The perspectives of pediatric and adult healthcare professionals. *Pediatr. Transplant.* **2019**, *23*, e13530. [CrossRef] [PubMed]
34. Toft, A.; Taylor, R.; Claridge, L.; Clowes, C.; Ferguson, J.; Hind, J.; Jones, R.; McClean, P.; McKiernan, P.; Samyn, M.; et al. The Experiences of Young Liver Patients Transferring from Children's to Adult Services and Their Support Needs for a Successful Transition. *Prog. Transplant.* **2018**, *28*, 244–249. [CrossRef] [PubMed]
35. Kelly, D.A.; Bucuvalas, J.C.; Alonso, E.M.; Karpen, S.J.; Allen, U.; Green, M.; Farmer, D.; Shemesh, E.; McDonald, R.A. Long-term medical management of the pediatric patient after liver transplantation: 2013 practice guideline by the American Association for the Study of Liver Diseases and the American Society of Transplantation. *Liver Transplant.* **2013**, *19*, 798–825. [CrossRef] [PubMed]
36. Stewart, A.L.; Hays, R.D.; Wells, K.B.; Rogers, W.H.; Spritzer, K.L.; Greenfield, S. Long-term functioning and well-being outcomes associated with physical activity and exercise in patients with chronic conditions in the medical outcomes study. *J. Clin. Epidemiol.* **1994**, *47*, 719–730. [CrossRef]
37. Choudhary, N.S.; Saigal, S. Preventive Strategies for Nonalcoholic Fatty Liver Disease After Liver Transplantation. *J. Clin. Exp. Hepatol.* **2019**, *9*, 619–624. [CrossRef]
38. Donnelly, J.E.; Hillman, C.; Castelli, D.; Etnier, J.L.; Lee, S.; Tomporowski, P.; Lambourne, K.; Szabo-Reed, A. Physical Activity, Fitness, Cognitive Function, and Academic Achievement in Children: A Systematic Review. *Med. Sci. Sports Exerc.* **2016**, *48*, 1223–1224. [CrossRef]
39. Naya, I.; Sanada, Y.; Katano, T.; Miyahara, G.; Hirata, Y.; Yamada, N.; Okada, N.; Onishi, Y.; Sakuma, Y.; Sata, N. Pregnancy Outcomes Following Pediatric Liver Transplantation: A Single-Center Experience in Japan. *Ann. Transplant.* **2020**, *25*, e921193. [CrossRef]
40. Le, H.L.; Francke, M.I.; Andrews, L.M.; de Winter, B.C.M.; van Gelder, T.; Hesselink, D.A. Usage of Tacrolimus and Mycophenolic Acid During Conception, Pregnancy, and Lactation, and Its Implications for Therapeutic Drug Monitoring: A Systematic Critical Review. *Ther. Drug Monit.* **2020**, *42*, 518–531. [CrossRef]
41. Lurie, S.; Shemesh, E.; Sheiner, P.A.; Emre, S.; Tindle, H.L.; Melchionna, L.; Shneider, B.L. Non-adherence in pediatric liver transplant recipients—An assessment of risk factors and natural history. *Pediatr. Transplant.* **2000**, *4*, 200–206. [CrossRef]

42. Croft, C.A.; Asmussen, L. A developmental approach to sexuality education: Implications for medical practice. *J. Adolesc. Health* **1993**, *14*, 109–114. [CrossRef]
43. Mellanby, A.R.; Phelps, F.A.; Crichton, N.J.; Tripp, J.H. School sex education: An experimental programme with educational and medical benefit. *BMJ* **1995**, *311*, 414–417. [CrossRef] [PubMed]
44. Sagar, N.; Leithead, J.A.; Lloyd, C.; Smith, M.; Gunson, B.K.; Adams, D.H.; Kelly, D.; Ferguson, J.W. Pediatric Liver Transplant Recipients Who Undergo Transfer to the Adult Healthcare Service Have Good Long-Term Outcomes. *Am. J. Transplant.* **2015**, *15*, 1864–1873. [CrossRef] [PubMed]
45. Hoegy, D.; Bleyzac, N.; Robinson, P.; Bertrand, Y.; Dussart, C.; Janoly-Dumenil, A. Medication adherence in pediatric transplantation and assessment methods: A systematic review. *Patient Prefer. Adherence* **2019**, *13*, 705–719. [CrossRef] [PubMed]
46. Meng, X.; Gao, W.; Wang, K.; Han, C.; Zhang, W.; Sun, C. Adherence to medical regimen after paediatric liver transplantation: A systematic review and meta-analysis. *Patient Prefer. Adherence* **2018**, *13*, 1–8. [CrossRef] [PubMed]
47. Annunziato, R.A.; Bucuvalas, J.C.; Yin, W.; Arnand, R.; Alonso, E.M.; Mazariegos, G.V.; Venick, R.S.; Stuber, M.L.; Shneider, B.L.; Shemesh, E. Self-Management Measurement and Prediction of Clinical Outcomes in Pediatric Transplant. *J. Pediatr.* **2018**, *193*, 128–133.e2. [CrossRef]
48. Chung, P.H.Y.; Chan, E.K.W.; Yeung, F.; Chan, A.C.Y.; Mou, J.W.C.; Lee, K.H.; Hung, J.W.S.; Leung, M.W.Y.; Tam, P.K.H.; Wong, K.K.Y. Life long follow up and management strategies of patients living with native livers after Kasai portoenterostomy. *Sci. Rep.* **2021**, *11*, 11207. [CrossRef]
49. Bijl, E.J.; Bharwani, K.D.; Houwen, R.H.J.; De Man, R.A. The long-term outcome of the Kasai operation in patients with biliary atresia: A systematic review. *Neth. J. Med.* **2013**, *71*, 170–173.
50. Samyn, M. Transitional care of biliary atresia. *Semin. Pediatr. Surg.* **2020**, *29*, 150948. [CrossRef]
51. Cortes-Cerisuelo, M.; Boumpoureka, N.; Cassar, N.; Joshi, D.; Samyn, M.; Heneghan, M.; Menon, K.; Prachalias, A.; Srinivasan, P.; Jassem, W.; et al. Liver Transplantation for Biliary Atresia in Adulthood: Single-Centre Surgical Experience. *J. Clin. Med.* **2021**, *10*, 4969. [CrossRef]
52. Westbrook, R.H.; Yeoman, A.D.; O'Grady, J.G.; Harrison, P.M.; Devlin, J.; Heneghan, M.A. Model for End-Stage Liver Disease Score Predicts Outcome in Cirrhotic Patients During Pregnancy. *Clin. Gastroenterol. Hepatol.* **2011**, *9*, 694–699. [CrossRef]
53. Matarazzo, L.; Assandro, P.; Martelossi, S.; Maggiore, G.; Ventura, A. Multiple successful pregnancies in a woman with biliary atresia and native liver. *Eur. J. Obstet. Gynecol. Reprod. Biol.* **2017**, *221*, 194–195. [CrossRef] [PubMed]
54. Sasaki, H.; Nio, M.; Hayashi, Y.; Ishii, T.; Sano, N.; Ohi, R. Problems during and after pregnancy in female patients with biliary atresia. *J. Pediatr. Surg.* **2007**, *42*, 1329–1332. [CrossRef] [PubMed]
55. Mass, K.; Quint, E.H.; Punch, M.R.; Merion, R.M. Gynecological and Reproductive Function after Liver Transplantation. *Transplantation* **1996**, *62*, 476–479. [CrossRef] [PubMed]
56. Jabiry-Zieniewicz, Z.; Kaminski, P.; Bobrowska, K.; Pietrzak, B.; Wielgos, M.; Smoter, P.; Zieniewicz, K.; Krawczyk, M. Menstrual Function in Female Liver Transplant Recipients of Reproductive Age. *Transplant. Proc.* **2009**, *41*, 1735–1739. [CrossRef]
57. Hukkinen, M.; Lohi, J.; Heikkilä, P.; Kivisaari, R.; Jahnukainen, T.; Jalanko, H.; Pakarinen, M.P. Noninvasive Evaluation of Liver Fibrosis and Portal Hypertension After Successful Portoenterostomy for Biliary Atresia. *Hepatol. Commun.* **2019**, *3*, 382–391. [CrossRef]
58. Moazzam, Z.; Ziogas, I.A.; Wu, W.K.; Rauf, M.A.; Pai, A.K.; Hafberg, E.T.; Gillis, L.A.; Izzy, M.; Matsuoka, L.K.; Alexopoulos, S.P. Delay in liver transplantation referral for adolescents with biliary atresia transitioning to adult care: A slippery slope. *Br. J. Surg.* **2021**, *108*, e324–e325. [CrossRef]
59. Jain, V.; Burford, C.; Alexander, E.C.; Dhawan, A.; Joshi, D.; Davenport, M.; Heaton, N.; Hadzic, N.; Samyn, M. Adult Liver Disease Prognostic Modelling for Long-term Outcomes in Biliary Atresia: An Observational Cohort Study. *J. Pediatr. Gastroenterol. Nutr.* **2021**, *73*, 93–98. [CrossRef]
60. Alexander, E.C.M.; Greaves, W.M.; Vaidya, H.J.M.; Burford, C.M.; Jain, V.M.; Samyn, M. Social and Educational Outcomes in Patients with Biliary Atresia: A Systematic Review. *J. Pediatr. Gastroenterol. Nutr.* **2021**, *74*, 104–109. [CrossRef]

Disclaimer/Publisher's Note: The statements, opinions and data contained in all publications are solely those of the individual author(s) and contributor(s) and not of MDPI and/or the editor(s). MDPI and/or the editor(s) disclaim responsibility for any injury to people or property resulting from any ideas, methods, instructions or products referred to in the content.

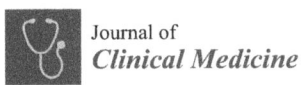

Article

Pediatric Liver and Transplant Surgery: Results of an International Survey and Expert Consensus Recommendations

Caroline P. Lemoine [1], Omid Madadi-Sanjani [2], Claus Petersen [2], Christophe Chardot [3], Jean de Ville de Goyet [4] and Riccardo Superina [1,*]

[1] Division of Transplant and Advanced Hepatobiliary Surgery, Ann & Robert H. Lurie Children's Hospital of Chicago, Northwestern University Feinberg School of Medicine, Chicago, IL 60611, USA
[2] Department of Pediatric Surgery, Hannover Medical School, 30625 Hannover, Germany
[3] Service de Chirurgie Pédiatrique Viscérale, Hôpital Necker—Enfants Malades, Université de Paris, 75015 Paris, France
[4] Department for the Treatment and Study of Pediatric Abdominal Diseases and Abdominal Transplantation, ISMETT, 90127 Palermo, Italy
* Correspondence: rsuperina@luriechildrens.org; Tel.: +1-312-227-4040; Fax: +1-312-227-9387

Abstract: Background: Pediatric liver surgery is a complex and challenging procedure and can be associated with major complications, including mortality. Best practices are not established. The aims of this study were to evaluate surgeons' individual and institutional practices in pediatric liver surgery and make recommendations applicable to the management of children who require liver surgery. Methods: A web-based survey was developed, focusing on the surgical management of children with liver conditions. It was distributed to 34 pediatric surgery faculty members of the Biliary Atresia and Related Disorders (BARD) consortium and 28 centers of the European Reference Network—Rare Liver. Using the Delphi method, a series of questions was then created to develop ideas about potential future developments in pediatric liver surgery. Results: The overall survey response rate was 70.6% (24/34), while the response rate for the Delphi questionnaire was 26.5% (9/34). In centers performing pediatric liver surgery, most pediatric subspecialties were present, although pediatric oncology was the least present (79.2%). Nearly all participants surveyed agreed that basic and advanced imaging modalities (including ERCP) should be available in those centers. Most pediatric liver surgeries were performed by pediatric surgeons (69.6%). A majority of participants agreed that centers treating pediatric liver tumors should include a pediatric transplant program (86%) able to perform technical variant grafts and living donor liver transplantation. Fifty-six percent of responders believe pediatric liver transplantation should be performed by specialized pediatric surgeons. Conclusion: Pediatric liver surgery should be performed by specialized pediatric surgeons and should be centralized in regional centers of excellence where all pediatric subspecialists are present. Pediatric hepatobiliary and transplant training needs to be better promoted amongst pediatric surgery fellows to increase this subspecialized workforce.

Keywords: pediatric liver surgery; pediatric liver transplantation; hepatoblastoma; hepatocellular carcinoma; pediatric surgery workforce; subspecialization

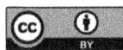

1. Introduction

Hepatoblastoma and hepatocellular carcinoma (HCC) are the two most common primary liver tumors affecting children and teenagers. However, despite this, those tumors constitute rare diseases. It is estimated that approximately 100 children are treated for hepatoblastoma at nearly 100 different institutions on an annual basis in the United States [1,2]. Therefore, the number of liver resections performed at each individual center and by individual pediatric surgeons is extremely low, and the management is not uniform. Pediatric liver surgery can also be performed for benign tumors or infectious conditions.

Over the last 33 years in the United States, the number of pediatric surgery training programs has increased by 278%, and the number of pediatric surgeons increased by 132% [3]. The consequence of this increase in the workforce has been a reduction in index cases per individual surgeon. On average, each U.S. surgeon performed less than one Kasai portoenterostomy or choledochal cyst excision per year. Liver resection was not evaluated in that study.

Studies from both the adult and pediatric surgery literature have shown improved outcomes with the increased surgeon and center volume for rare conditions [4,5]. In children, a relationship between volume and outcomes has been shown in Kasai portoenterostomy [6], congenital diaphragmatic hernia repair [7], and Wilms tumor resection [8]. The success of pediatric liver surgery is obviously not solely related to the surgeon performing the surgery but also to the presence of other pediatric specialists and appropriate resources at an institution to optimally diagnose, treat, and care for these children with complex conditions.

In this study, an international group of pediatric hepatobiliary and transplant surgeons aimed to evaluate and compare their individual and institutional practice in pediatric liver surgery and to elaborate expert recommendations in the management of children with liver tumors.

2. Methods

2.1. Development of the Questionnaire

A panel of experts consisting of pediatric hepatobiliary surgeons was created. Based on author consensus, a total of 31 questions were generated, focusing on different aspects of the management of pediatric liver conditions requiring either liver resection or transplantation: (1) institutional logistics related to the management of children with liver disease requiring surgical intervention; (2) surgical management, including indication for surgery, surgical technique, duration of surgical interventions and estimated blood loss, postoperative hospital stay; (3) oncology management for malignant conditions; (4) pediatric liver transplantation. The detailed content of the questionnaire is available in Supplementary Materials Document S1.

2.2. Study Design

The web-based questionnaire was developed in English. The questionnaire was a self-administered, web-based survey using the online tool SurveyMonkey (http://www.surveymonkey.com, accessed on 11 August 2020). Each participant could advance in the survey after skipping a question. There were no mandatory questions.

2.3. Study Population

The questionnaire was electronically distributed to 34 faculty members of the Biliary Atresia and Related Disorders (BARD) consortium and 28 centers of the European Reference Network—Rare Liver. The questionnaire did not differentiate between free-standing pediatric hospitals or pediatric departments part of an adult healthcare institution.

The survey was answered by a variety of surgeons: pediatric surgeons or transplant surgeons (either pediatric or adult surgeons performing pediatric liver transplant or pediatric hepatobiliary surgery) located in Europe, North America, Asia, and Australia.

2.4. Distribution of the Questionnaire

The survey was distributed by email. A cover letter clearly detailed the objectives of the survey. Survey administration followed the Dillman principles and recommendations of Burn et al. [9]. Participants were first contacted on 11 August 2020. A total of 2 reminder emails were sent 2 and 4 weeks later. The survey was closed on 9 December 2020. Only one participant was allowed to answer in each individual institution. Overall, 24 pediatric surgeons answered the survey.

2.5. Development of the Delphi Questionnaire

The variables assessed in the Delphi questionnaire were selected by consulting an international panel of experts in pediatric hepatobiliary surgery. The questionnaire was developed using a semi-structured interview with the aim of identifying redundant or poorly worded questions. Testing of the questionnaire was performed by running the questions to 10 other pediatric surgeons and hepatologists. Last, the reliability of the questionnaire was assessed by re-testing the same pediatric surgeons with the questionnaire at a 2-week interval. Participants were allowed to answer the Delphi questionnaire between 5 March 2021 and 29 April 2021. Nine surgeons answered the Delphi questionnaire (26.5% response rate, 9/34).

2.6. Pre-Meeting Working Group

A working group was created constituted of four surgeons (CL, OMS, RS, and CP). They analyzed the results of the Delphi questionnaire and organized a summary presentation of the survey and Delphi questionnaire results.

2.7. Expert Panel Meeting

The results of the survey and the Delphi questionnaire were presented and discussed within an expert panel meeting during the virtual BARD webinar held on 30 June 2021. Other participants in the webinar could also participate through online chat. Panelists were provided with a summary depicting the results of the survey and the Delphi questionnaire. RS served as moderator of the meeting session.

3. Results

3.1. Institutional Logistics Related to the Pediatric Liver Surgery

The survey was answered by 24 surgeons. The annual number of pediatric liver surgical interventions performed in each institution varied greatly from 2 to >100. Pediatric surgeons were present in 100% of institutions. The transplant surgery was present in 87.5% (21/24) of cases. Pediatric anesthesiology (95.8%), pediatric hepatology, and pediatric radiology (91.7%) were also often present. Pediatric oncology was the pediatric specialty that was the least present at those institutions (79.2%). A pediatric intensive care unit was present in all hospitals, while a pediatric ward was nearly always present (95.8%, 23/24). The number of beds dedicated to pediatric patients ranged from 10 to 500, while the number of beds for pediatric surgery patients ranged from 10 to 250.

General imaging modalities (computed tomography (CT) or magnetic resonance imaging (MRI)) were available in all centers. However, interventional radiology (IR) with the ability to perform advanced procedures (percutaneous transhepatic cholangiogram or portal vein embolization) was available in 91.7% (22/24) of institutions. Diagnostic endoscopic retrograde cholangiopancreatography (ERCP) was available in 87.5% of cases, but interventional gastroenterologists able to perform bile duct stenting in small infants were present in 66.7% of surveyed institutions (16/24).

When surveyed through the Delphi questionnaire, all participants agreed that centers performing pediatric liver surgery should provide ultrasound, CT, MRI, and diagnostic interventional radiology. Almost all agreed advanced IR interventions (98%) and ERCP (91%) should also be available.

3.2. Surgical Management

All surveyed participants reported that liver surgery for benign and malignant tumors was performed at their institution. Hepatoblastoma and HCC were the two most common indications. Trauma surgery (73.9%, 17/24) and surgery for infectious causes (abscess, hydatic cysts) (69.6%, 16/24) were performed less frequently.

Most pediatric liver surgeries were performed by a pediatric surgeon (69.6%). (Figure 1) Less frequently, a transplant surgeon (47.8%) or a pediatric surgeon assisted by a transplant surgeon (47.8%) performed the intervention. In no instance did an adult general surgeon perform liver surgery on children. Of note, the survey did not specifically evaluate pediatric surgeons with additional training in hepatobiliary and/or transplant surgery, nor did it identify dedicated transplant surgeons who perform only pediatric transplants.

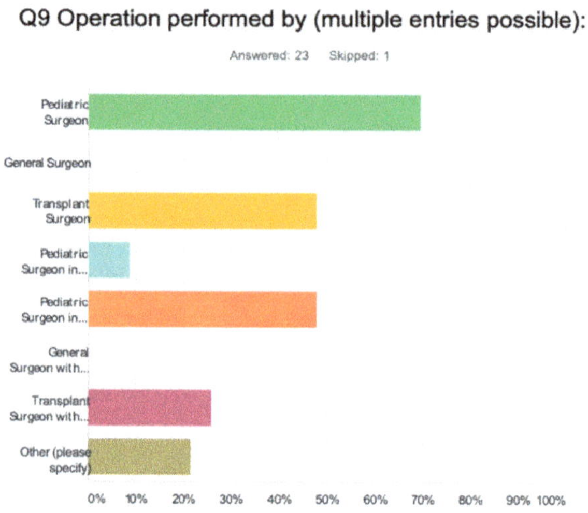

Q9 Operation performed by (multiple entries possible):

Answered: 23   Skipped: 1

ANSWER CHOICES	RESPONSES	
Pediatric Surgeon	69.57%	16
General Surgeon	0.00%	0
Transplant Surgeon	47.83%	11
Pediatric Surgeon in cooperation with General Surgeon	8.70%	2
Pediatric Surgeon in cooperation with Transplant Surgeon	47.83%	11
General Surgeon with assistance by Pediatric Surgeon	0.00%	0
Transplant Surgeon with assistance by Pediatric Surgeon	26.09%	6
Other (please specify)	21.74%	5
Total Respondents: 23		

Figure 1. Questionnaire asking which provider performs pediatric liver surgery at surveyed centers. (Each color represents a different answer).

Through the Delphi questionnaire, most surveyed participants (60%) answered that pediatric liver surgery should be performed by a pediatric surgeon rather than a transplant surgeon. (Figure 2) A majority of responders (64%) recommended that a pediatric liver tumor surgical team include a pediatric surgeon and a transplant surgeon.

All responders reported being able to perform pediatric liver surgery via laparotomy (most frequently through a transverse laparotomy with a midline extension; 40.9%), while only 47.8% reported also using a laparoscopic approach. The Delphi questionnaire revealed that the participants were evenly divided regarding which surgical approach should be used for pediatric liver surgery and if laparoscopic constitutes a valuable option for both minor and major pediatric liver surgical interventions (50%).

Standard left/right hepatectomy was performed at all institutions surveyed, while non-anatomical liver resection and extended left/right hepatectomy were performed in a majority of centers (22/24, 95.7%). The average operation duration ranged from 60 to 240 min for all liver resections except for the extended right (150–300 min) or left (150–360 min) hepatectomy. Estimated blood losses were lower for standard left/right hepatectomy or non-anatomical resection (20–500 mL) compared to extended hepatectomies (25–750 mL). The utilization of total vascular exclusion of the liver and inflow exclusion (Pringle maneuver) were utilized as needed. Five responders (22.7%) reported not utilizing any type of vascular exclusion for their liver resections, although the question did not specify in which instance vascular exclusion would or could be used. Most participants (72.7%, 16/24) reported using the Cavitron ultrasonic surgical aspirator (CUSA) for the parenchymal dissection. The non-stick bipolar diathermy (59.1%) and the "clamp crush" technique (50.0%) were other commonly used techniques. Most participants reported placing a surgical drain at the completion of liver resection (95.7%, 22/24). Overall hospital length of stay varied from 2 to 30 days, and intensive care unit stay ranged from 1 to 10 days.

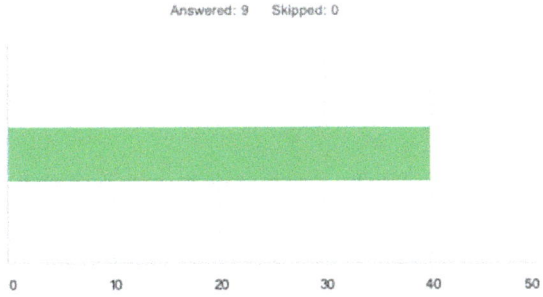

Figure 2. Questionnaire asking who should perform pediatric liver surgery: pediatric vs. transplant surgeons. (The color represents the proportion of answers provided).

The Delphi questionnaire showed that while most participants believe the knowledge of different vascular exclusion techniques is mandatory to perform pediatric liver surgery (83%), less than a third believe a Pringle maneuver is necessary during parenchymal dissection, and forty-two percent believe total vascular exclusion should be prepared for major liver resections. The majority (94%) thought the CUSA or other such equipment should be available in centers performing pediatric liver surgery.

3.3. Oncology Management

All surgeons answered that the oncological management of their pediatric patients with liver tumors is performed by a pediatric oncologist. However, the chemotherapy administration is performed at the same center in only two-thirds of cases. In the other third, patients are treated at another center. Most institutions (22/24, 95.7%) decide on postoperative oncological management at interdisciplinary oncology boards.

3.4. Pediatric Liver Transplantation

Pediatric liver transplantation was performed in most centers surveyed (20/24, 87.0%). In most instances, either a pediatric surgeon (57.1%) and/or a transplant surgeon (61.9%) performed the transplant. The post-transplant management was mostly performed by pediatric hepatologists (90.5%) and assisted by pediatric or transplant surgeons (52.4%). The survey did not specify if this question pertained to the short- or long-term management of transplant recipients.

All centers performed deceased donor liver transplants, while most also performed living donor liver transplants (95%, 19/20). Only 25% of centers accepted organs from donors after cardiac death. All participants responded that split liver transplantation was performed at their institution in addition to whole liver transplantation. (Figure 3) Most programs offered multi-organ transplants (simultaneous liver–kidney transplant: 17/18, 94.4%; less frequently intestinal or multivisceral transplant: 7/18, 38.9%).

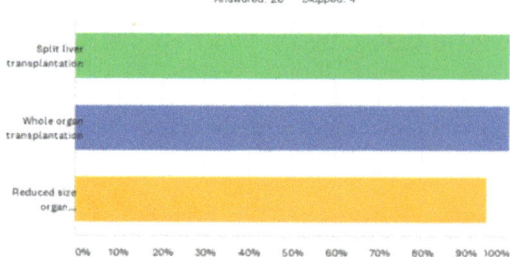

Figure 3. Different types of deceased donor liver transplantation graft types offered at surveyed centers. (Each color represents a different answer).

The Delphi questionnaire showed most responders believed centers treating pediatric liver tumors should include a pediatric transplant program (86%). (Figure 4) Although the distribution was almost equal, a slight majority of responders believed pediatric liver transplantation should be performed by specialized pediatric surgeons (56%). (Figure 5)

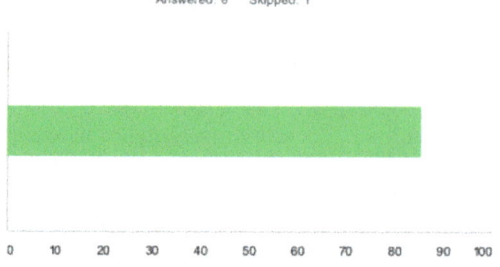

Figure 4. Questionnaire asking if centers treating pediatric liver tumors should include a pediatric transplant program. (The color represents the proportion of answers provided).

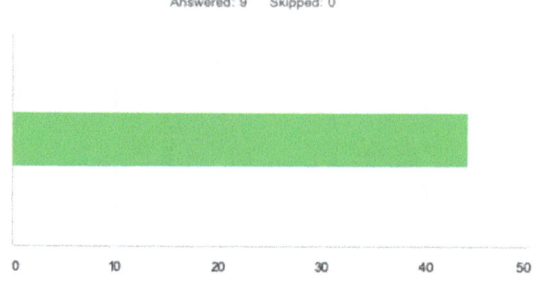

Figure 5. Questionnaire asking who should perform pediatric liver transplantation: pediatric vs. transplant surgeons. (The color represents the proportion of answers provided).

4. Discussion

Pediatric hepatobiliary surgery constitutes a challenging surgical intervention, with reported complication rates between 10–30% and a mortality rate of 5% [10–14]. In order to achieve the best outcomes for children with surgical liver conditions, a multidisciplinary team of pediatric specialists is needed. As presented by the World Federation of Associations of Pediatric Surgeons (WOFAPS) Declaration of Pediatric Surgery in 2001: "To provide the best surgical care for infants and children, complex pediatric surgical procedures should be carried out in specialized pediatric centers with appropriately equipped intensive care facilities staffed 24 h per day, 7 days per week. In addition to the trained pediatric surgeons, these facilities should be staffed with other pediatric specialists including radiologists, anesthesiologists, and pathologists" [15].

As previously presented, complex hepatobiliary surgeries are now less frequently performed by general pediatric surgeons. In the study by Abdullah et al., 60% of surveyed pediatric surgeons had not performed either a Kasai portoenterostomy or a choledochal cyst excision in the previous 12 months [3]. Liver resection is so rarely performed that it was not even compiled in the list of procedures evaluated in that study. A 2016 study focused on subspecialization in North American pediatric surgery groups showed that major liver resection (left/right hepatectomy or extended resection) was performed by any surgeon of a group in approximately 45% of cases and was performed by only certain dedicated surgeons in less than 10% [16]. Recently, a group from Texas reported an improvement in postoperative complications after major liver resection (52% to 20%) when they limited pediatric liver resections to be performed by only 2 surgeons rather than anyone in a group of 10 surgeons (previously creating an average of 3.3 cases/surgeon over a 10-year period) [2]. Limiting the number of surgeons performing liver resections in a group allows those hepatobiliary surgeons to increase their experience, becoming capable of performing all types of liver resections and offering the best outcomes to patients.

Subspecialization in hepatobiliary surgery is not yet recognized by most general pediatric surgeons. The most common specialties felt to be necessary are transplantation, fetal interventions, and bariatric surgery [17]. Most respondents of an American Pediatric Surgery Association (APSA) survey felt that specialists should not practice solely in their subspecialty but rather act as content experts and consult on relevant cases. Why pediatric surgeons are so reluctant to accept the benefits of subspecialization and concentrating cases on a subgroup of surgeons is multifactorial: it might not be easily applicable in rural settings or small groups/practices [16,18,19]. Additional years of formal training (hepatobiliary and/or transplant fellowship) can be difficult to achieve for personal or financial reasons. Nevertheless, in that same APSA survey, 50.8% of respondents responded that additional specialization training is necessary after completing a fellowship in general pediatric surgery.

Unlike adult general surgery, general pediatric surgery has been hanging on to the concept of the true general surgeon, even in academic centers. A 2010 survey of general surgery residency program directors reported that 71% of finishing general surgery residents entered a subspecialty residency [20]. Pediatric surgery subspecialty fellowships (fetal, colorectal, vascular anomalies, hepatobiliary, and trauma) are becoming more available, but the true translation of this concept into the reality of daily practice remains unfulfilled, particularly in the field of hepatobiliary surgery.

Hepatobiliary and pancreatic surgery deals with some of the most complicated and technically challenging operations. A survey of Canadian general surgeons showed that 91% of respondents would refer patients with the complicated hepatobiliary disease to a hepatobiliary expert [21]. Additionally, 95% of participants thought that some hepatobiliary procedures should be regionalized to high-volume, expert centers: pancreaticoduodenectomy, biliary reconstruction, and major hepatectomy (defined as two or more liver segments). In adult surgery, a relationship between outcomes and high-volume centers has been demonstrated.

Additionally, training in transplant surgery allows pediatric surgeons to offer all surgical treatment options to patients referred for the management of malignant liver tumors. Lautz et al. showed that of 18 patients, who were referred for liver transplantation by other pediatric surgeons and institutions because of what appeared to be unresectable tumors, all were resected, and their survival was equal or superior to that of patients treated with liver transplantation [22].

In the survey presented in this study, living donor liver transplantation was performed in 95% of centers and split liver transplantation in 100% of programs. This proportion is very different from most programs performing pediatric liver transplantation in the U.S. However, the authors believe that any pediatric liver transplant program should have the ability to offer all types of transplants, including technical variant grafts and living donor transplantation, in order to decrease the waitlist mortality as much as possible.

As reported in our international survey, some institutions rely on an adult transplant surgeon collaborating with a pediatric surgeon on liver resection in children and teenagers [19]. While the authors agree that the safety of the patient is the most important consideration in pediatric liver surgery and that a pediatric surgeon uncomfortable with performing a liver surgery should not attempt such an endeavor on their own, relying on an adult surgeon should not be the default solution. Again quoting Dr. Grosfeld in the WOFAPS Declaration of Pediatric Surgery, "Children are not just small adults and have medical and surgical problems and needs that often are quite different from those encountered by adult physicians. [15] Every infant and child who suffers from an illness or disease has the right to be treated [15] by a pediatric medical or surgical specialist" [15]. The American Academy of Pediatrics (AAP) also issued a policy statement regarding referral to pediatric surgical specialists [23]. The Surgical Advisory Panel recommended that "infants, children, and adolescents with solid malignancies should be cared for from the outset by a pediatric surgeon or a pediatric surgical specialist and a pediatric medical cancer specialist."

In conclusion, the authors and the participants of the BARD webinar propose the following recommendations for the management of pediatric patients with liver disorders requiring surgical treatment:

1. Pediatric liver surgery should be performed in institutions where all pediatric medical and surgical specialists are available on site to provide specialized pediatric care;
2. Pediatric liver surgery should be performed in centers where advanced interventional radiology and interventional gastroenterology are available to help provide all possible diagnostic and therapeutic adjuncts procedures to the management of children with liver conditions;
3. Pediatric liver surgery should be performed in centers where pediatric liver transplantation is performed (including technical variant grafts and living donor liver transplantation) and where surgical oncologists are present in order to offer the best oncological management;
4. Pediatric liver surgery should be performed by pediatric surgeons subspecialized in hepatobiliary and transplant surgery to allow knowledge and mastering of all surgical techniques, including vascular exclusion techniques;
5. Pediatric liver surgery should be centralized in regional centers of excellence in pediatric hepatobiliary surgery;
6. Subspecialization in hepatobiliary and transplant surgery should be promoted amongst pediatric surgery trainees; additionally, incentives or compensation strategies should be developed to help support pediatric surgeons through additional years of training and to avoid trainees being reluctant to complete subspecialty training.

Supplementary Materials: The following supporting information can be downloaded at: https://www.mdpi.com/article/10.3390/jcm12093229/s1, Figure S1: Liver Surgery Survey and Delphi questionnaire.

Author Contributions: Conceptualization, C.P.; Methodology, O.M.-S. and C.P.; Software, O.M.-S. and C.P.; Validation, C.P.L., O.M.-S., C.P., C.C., J.d.V.d.G. and R.S.; Formal Analysis, C.P.L., O.M.-S., C.P., C.C., J.d.V.d.G. and R.S.; Investigation, O.M.-S. and C.P.; Resources, O.M.-S. and C.P.; Data Curation, O.M.-S. and C.P.; Writing—Original Draft Preparation, C.P.L. and R.S.; Writing—Review and Editing, C.P.L., O.M.-S., C.P. and R.S.; Visualization, C.P.; Supervision, C.P. and R.S.; Project Administration, O.M.-S. and C.P.; Funding Acquisition, C.P. All authors have read and agreed to the published version of the manuscript.

Funding: This research received no external funding.

Institutional Review Board Statement: Not applicable for studies not involving humans or animals.

Informed Consent Statement: Not applicable for studies not involving humans.

Data Availability Statement: No new unavailable data were created, all datasets analyzed or generated during the study are included in this manuscript or in the supplemental material provided by the authors.

Conflicts of Interest: The authors declare no conflict of interest.

Abbreviations

CT	Computed tomography
CUSA	Cavitron ultrasonic surgical aspirator
ERCP	Endoscopic retrograde cholangiopancreatography
HCC	Hepatocellular carcinoma
IR	Interventional radiology
MRI	Magnetic resonance imaging
PTC	Percutaneous transhepatic cholangiogram

References

1. Spector, L.G.; Birch, J. The epidemiology of hepatoblastoma. *Pediatr. Blood Cancer* **2012**, *59*, 776–779. [CrossRef] [PubMed]
2. Whitlock, R.S.; Portuondo, J.I.; Commander, S.J.; Ha, T.A.; Zhu, H.; Goss, J.A.; Kukreja, K.U.; Leung, D.H.; Terrada, D.L.; Masand, P.M.; et al. Integration of a dedicated management protocol in the care of pediatric liver cancer: From specialized providers to complication reduction. *J. Pediatr. Surg.* **2022**, *57*, 1544–1553. [CrossRef] [PubMed]
3. Abdullah, F.; Salazar, J.H.; Gause, C.D.; Gadepalli, S.; Biester, T.W.; Azarow, K.S.; Brandt, M.L.; Chung, D.H.; Lund, D.P.; Rescorla, F.J.; et al. Understanding the Operative Experience of the Practicing Pediatric Surgeon: Implications for Training and Maintaining Competency. *JAMA Surg.* **2016**, *151*, 735–741. [CrossRef] [PubMed]
4. Pecorelli, N.; Balzano, G.; Capretti, G.; Zerbi, A.; Di Carlo, V.; Braga, M. Effect of surgeon volume on outcome following pancreaticoduodenectomy in a high-volume hospital. *J. Gastrointest. Surg.* **2012**, *16*, 518–523. [CrossRef] [PubMed]
5. Wang, H.H.; Tejwani, R.; Zhang, H.; Wiener, J.S.; Routh, J.C. Hospital Surgical Volume and Associated Postoperative Complications of Pediatric Urological Surgery in the United States. *J. Urol.* **2015**, *194*, 506–511. [CrossRef]
6. Davenport, M.; Ong, E.; Sharif, K.; Alizai, N.; McClean, P.; Hadzic, N.; Kelly, D.A. Biliary atresia in England and Wales: Results of centralization and new benchmark. *J. Pediatr. Surg.* **2011**, *46*, 1689–1694. [CrossRef] [PubMed]
7. Grushka, J.R.; Laberge, J.M.; Puligandla, P.; Skarsgard, E.D.; Canadian Pediatric Surgery, N. Effect of hospital case volume on outcome in congenital diaphragmatic hernia: The experience of the Canadian Pediatric Surgery Network. *J. Pediatr. Surg.* **2009**, *44*, 873–876. [CrossRef] [PubMed]
8. Gutierrez, J.C.; Cheung, M.C.; Zhuge, Y.; Koniaris, L.G.; Sola, J.E. Does Children's Oncology Group hospital membership improve survival for patients with neuroblastoma or Wilms tumor? *Pediatr. Blood Cancer* **2010**, *55*, 621–628. [CrossRef] [PubMed]
9. Burns, K.E.; Duffett, M.; Kho, M.E.; Meade, M.O.; Adhikari, N.K.; Sinuff, T.; Cook, D.J.; Group, A. A guide for the design and conduct of self-administered surveys of clinicians. *CMAJ* **2008**, *179*, 245–252. [CrossRef] [PubMed]
10. Towu, E.; Kiely, E.; Pierro, A.; Spitz, L. Outcome and complications after resection of hepatoblastoma. *J. Pediatr. Surg.* **2004**, *39*, 199–202. [CrossRef]
11. Zwintscher, N.P.; Azarow, K.S.; Horton, J.D. Morbidity and mortality associated with liver resections for primary malignancies in children. *Pediatr. Surg. Int.* **2014**, *30*, 493–497. [CrossRef] [PubMed]
12. Becker, K.; Furch, C.; Schmid, I.; von Schweinitz, D.; Haberle, B. Impact of postoperative complications on overall survival of patients with hepatoblastoma. *Pediatr. Blood Cancer* **2015**, *62*, 24–28. [CrossRef] [PubMed]
13. Grisotti, G.; Cowles, R.A. Complications in pediatric hepatobiliary surgery. *Semin. Pediatr. Surg.* **2016**, *25*, 388–394. [CrossRef] [PubMed]

14. Schnater, J.M.; Aronson, D.C.; Plaschkes, J.; Perilongo, G.; Brown, J.; Otte, J.B.; Brugieres, L.; Czauderna, P.; MacKinlay, G.; Vos, A. Surgical view of the treatment of patients with hepatoblastoma: Results from the first prospective trial of the International Society of Pediatric Oncology Liver Tumor Study Group. *Cancer* **2002**, *94*, 1111–1120. [CrossRef] [PubMed]
15. Grosfeld, J.L. World Federation of Associations of Pediatric Surgeons. Declaration of pediatric surgery. *J. Pediatr. Surg.* **2001**, *36*, 1743. [CrossRef] [PubMed]
16. Langer, J.C.; Gordon, J.S.; Chen, L.E. Subspecialization within pediatric surgical groups in North America. *J. Pediatr. Surg.* **2016**, *51*, 143–148. [CrossRef]
17. Rich, B.S.; Silverberg, J.T.; Fishbein, J.; Raval, M.V.; Gadepalli, S.K.; Moriarty, K.P.; Aspelund, G.; Rollins, M.D.; Besner, G.E.; Dasgupta, R.; et al. Subspecialization in pediatric surgery: Results of a survey to the American Pediatric Surgical Association. *J. Pediatr. Surg.* **2020**, *55*, 2058–2063. [CrossRef]
18. Alaish, S.M.; Powell, D.M.; Waldhausen, J.H.T.; Dunn, S.P. The Right Child/Right Surgeon initiative: A position statement on pediatric surgical training, sub-specialization, and continuous certification from the American Pediatric Surgical Association. *J. Pediatr. Surg.* **2020**, *55*, 2566–2574. [CrossRef] [PubMed]
19. Superina, R. The Shrinking Landscape of Pediatric Surgery: Is Less More? *J. Pediatr. Surg.* **2018**, *53*, 868–874. [CrossRef]
20. Bruns, S.D.; Davis, B.R.; Demirjian, A.N.; Ganai, S.; House, M.G.; Saidi, R.F.; Shah, B.C.; Tan, S.A.; Murayama, K.M.; Society for Surgery of the Alimentary Tract Resident Education Committee. The subspecialization of surgery: A paradigm shift. *J. Gastrointest. Surg.* **2014**, *18*, 1523–1531. [CrossRef]
21. Dixon, E.; Vollmer, C.M., Jr.; Bathe, O.; Sutherland, F. Training, practice, and referral patterns in hepatobiliary and pancreatic surgery: Survey of general surgeons. *J. Gastrointest. Surg.* **2005**, *9*, 109–114. [CrossRef] [PubMed]
22. Lautz, T.B.; Ben-Ami, T.; Tantemsapya, N.; Gosiengfiao, Y.; Superina, R.A. Successful nontransplant resection of POST-TEXT III and IV hepatoblastoma. *Cancer* **2011**, *117*, 1976–1983. [CrossRef] [PubMed]
23. Surgical Advisory Panel, A.A.o.P.; Klein, M.D. Referral to pediatric surgical specialists. *Pediatrics* **2014**, *133*, 350–356. [CrossRef] [PubMed]

Disclaimer/Publisher's Note: The statements, opinions and data contained in all publications are solely those of the individual author(s) and contributor(s) and not of MDPI and/or the editor(s). MDPI and/or the editor(s) disclaim responsibility for any injury to people or property resulting from any ideas, methods, instructions or products referred to in the content.

MDPI
St. Alban-Anlage 66
4052 Basel
Switzerland
www.mdpi.com

Journal of Clinical Medicine Editorial Office
E-mail: jcm@mdpi.com
www.mdpi.com/journal/jcm

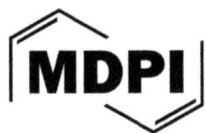

Disclaimer/Publisher's Note: The statements, opinions and data contained in all publications are solely those of the individual author(s) and contributor(s) and not of MDPI and/or the editor(s). MDPI and/or the editor(s) disclaim responsibility for any injury to people or property resulting from any ideas, methods, instructions or products referred to in the content.

www.ingramcontent.com/pod-product-compliance
Lightning Source LLC
LaVergne TN
LVHW070359100526
838202LV00014B/1347